Colon Cancer Diagnosis and Therapy

Ganji Purnachandra Nagaraju
Dhananjay Shukla • Naveen Kumar Vishvakarma
Editors

Colon Cancer Diagnosis and Therapy

Volume 1

Springer

Editors
Ganji Purnachandra Nagaraju
Department of Hematology
and Medical Oncology
Emory University
Atlanta, GA, USA

Naveen Kumar Vishvakarma
Department of Biotechnology
Guru Ghasidas Vishwavidyalaya
Bilaspur, India

Dhananjay Shukla
Department of Biotechnology
Guru Ghasidas Vishwavidyalaya
Bilaspur, India

ISBN 978-3-030-63368-4 ISBN 978-3-030-63369-1 (eBook)
https://doi.org/10.1007/978-3-030-63369-1

This Springer imprint is published by the registered company Springer Nature Switzerland AG
The registered company address is: Gewerbestrasse 11, 6330 Cham, Switzerland

This book is dedicated to our families, our teachers, and friends

Preface

Colorectal cancer (CRC) is the second most lethal cancer recorded for tumor-associated mortalities globally. The incidence and mortality are gradually increasing in the developing countries due to adaptation of western lifestyle. The increasing incidence of this heterogenous disease is due to various modifiable and unmodifiable risk factors that lead to the occurrence of CRC. In spite of advanced technologies in screening, surgery, and conventional therapies, the survival rate remains low due to asymptomatic conditions and delay in diagnosis. Additionally, development of resistance and tumor recurrence are major obstacles confronted by the present-day therapies. Therefore, a better surveillance of incidence, mortality, and survival of the population suffering from CRC would provide efficient preventive measures. A better understanding of the CRC progression at the molecular level would assist in developing effective therapeutic options. In this book, we will try to compile information thoroughly by exploring novel biomarkers, therapeutic options, and advanced nanomedicine for the treatment of CRC, which will benefit patients.

The volumes focus on elucidating a better understanding of the current epidemiological statistics of CRC. The incidence, mortality, and survival rate included define the population on varied disparities like race, sex, age, and geography. The data surveillance of the population suffering from CRC supports the clinicians as well the patients to be diagnosed at their early stage of disease to improve survival rate. The diagnosis of CRC performed by various screening techniques including sigmoidoscopy, colonoscopy, double contrast barium enema (DCBE), and fecal occult blood test (FOBT) is found to be efficient but exhibits limitations like minimal sensitivity and specificity. Therefore, discovery of non-metabolite signature patterns using NMR and MRI provides better understanding of imaging and progression of CRC. The chapters in this book focus on the novel advanced dynamic contrast enhanced-MRI and diffusion weighted imaging to study oncometabolites and angiogenesis. A better understanding of CRC growth and progression promotes the researchers and clinicians to develop efficient therapy strategies. Therefore, increased understanding of these processes and their related growth factors and transcription factors along with their dysregulated pathways reveal the complexity of the mechanism implicated. These also promote modifications in chief oncogenic and tumor suppressive miRNA that play a major role in regulating CRC. This knowledge will allow the development of novel biomarkers like exosome biomarkers that aid in early diagnosis of the diseases based on techniques like in-situ hybridization. It will also support ways to design more innovative therapeutic protein and compounds targeted against vital signaling cascades that play a crucial role in developing cancer angiogenesis and metastasis.

Conventional therapies including chemo and radiotherapies are found effective but the cytotoxicity developed by the chemodrugs is more disappointing. The main challenge for these conventional therapies is the resistance developed by the tumor cells due to the dysregulation of various transcription and growth factors. Therefore, improvements in techniques like targeted immunotherapy and nanotechnology are emerging to treat CRC patients for efficient results. Our authors will briefly compile information about these therapeutic options by systematically exploring the novel therapies for the betterment of patients. Finally, our book explores data pertaining to various advances integrated into a precision and personalized medicine treatment that can eventually enhance patient safety and efficacy.

We hope that our collection of novel therapeutic strategies reflects current research concept and we find immense pleasure in presenting our copy to the science community for the benefit of patients.

Atlanta, GA, USA — Ganji Purnachandra Nagaraju
Bilaspur, India — Dhananjay Shukla
Bilaspur, India — Naveen Kumar Vishvakarma

Contents

About the Editors

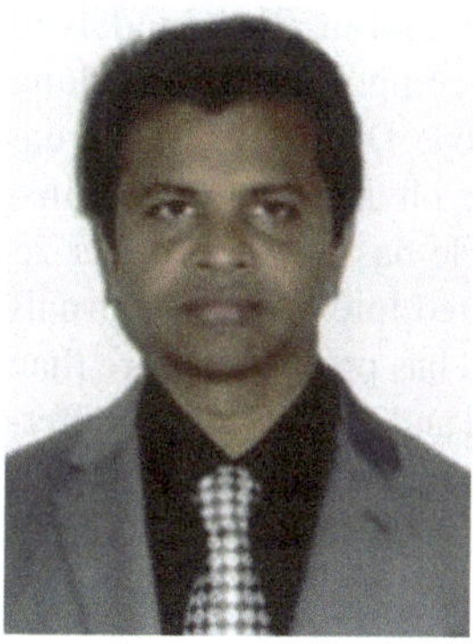

Ganji Purnachandra Nagaraju is a faculty member in the Department of Hematology and Medical Oncology at Emory University School of Medicine. He obtained his MSc and PhD, both in biotechnology, from Sri Venkateswara University in Tirupati, Andhra Pradesh, India. Dr. Nagaraju received his DSc from Berhampur University, Berhampur, Odisha, India. His research focuses on translational projects related to gastrointestinal malignancies. He has published over 100 research papers in highly reputed international journals and has presented more than 50 abstracts at various national and international conferences. Dr. Nagaraju is author and editor of several published books including (1) *Role of Tyrosine Kinases in Gastrointestinal Malignancies*, (2) *Role of Transcription Factors in Gastrointestinal Malignancies*, (3) *Breaking Tolerance to Pancreatic Cancer Unresponsiveness to Chemotherapy*, (4) *Theranostic Approach for Pancreatic Cancer*, and (5) *Exploring Pancreatic Metabolism and Malignancy*. He serves as an editorial board member of several internationally recognized academic journals. He is an associate member of the Discovery and Developmental Therapeutics research program at Winship Cancer Institute. Dr. Nagaraju has received several international awards including FAACC. He also holds memberships with the Association of Scientists of Indian Origin in America (ASIOA), the Society for Integrative and Comparative Biology (SICB), the Science Advisory Board, the RNA Society, the American Association for Clinical Chemistry (AACC), and the American Association of Cancer Research (AACR).

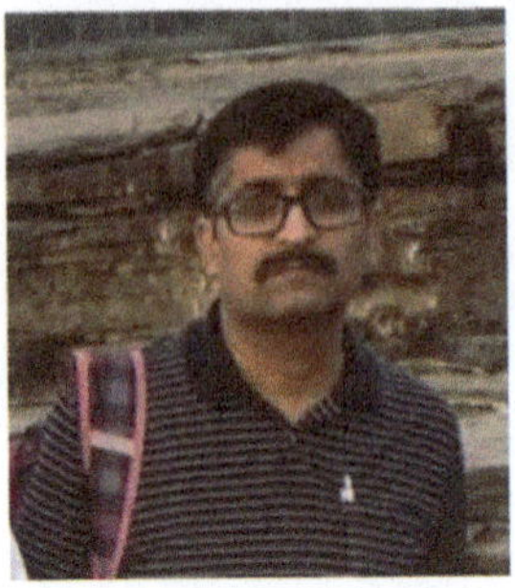

Dhananjay Shukla is an assistant professor in the Department of Biotechnology, Guru Ghasidas Vishwavidyalaya, Bilaspur, Chhattisgarh, India. He obtained his MSc in biotechnology from APS University Rewa, Madhya Pradesh. Dr. Shukla obtained his PhD in biotechnology from Defense Institute of Physiology and Allied Sciences, Defense Research and Development Organization, and Jamia Hamdard University, Delhi, India. Dr. Shukla did his postdoctoral research work at the Centre for DNA Fingerprinting and Diagnostics (CDFD), Hyderabad, Telangana, under DBT-Postdoctoral fellowship award. He received advanced research training from the Centre of Veterinary Health Sciences, Oklahoma State University, Stillwater, USA. He uses in vitro, in vivo, and in silico models to explore the role of bioactive compounds against lung diseases and cancer prevention. Dr. Shukla's current research interest is to evaluate phytomedicines against lung pathologies and cancer. He has published over 25 research papers in highly reputed International journals having high impact factors and has presented more than 15 abstracts at various national and international conferences. Dr. Shukla has been working as a faculty member since 2013 in the Department of Biotechnology, Guru Ghasidas Vishwavidyalaya.

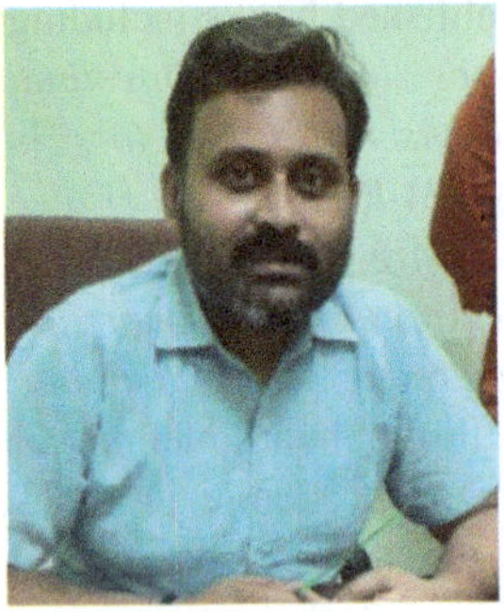

Naveen Kumar Vishvakarma is currently assistant professor of biotechnology at Guru Ghasidas Vishwavidyalaya. He earned his master's degree in microbiology and then did his doctoral research in tumor immunology. During his doctoral research, he worked in the area of tumor acidity–mediated immunosuppression. After completing doctoral research work, he worked as postdoctoral fellow/research associate at Banaras Hindu University, Manitoba Institute of Cell Biology (Canada), and Moffitt Cancer Center and Research institute (USA). During his work at Moffitt Cancer Center, he demonstrated the role of acidic tumor microenvironment in selection of aggressive phenotype with metabolic alterations. In 2013, he joined HNB Garhwal University as assistant professor and later moved to his current position at Guru Ghasidas Vishwavidyalaya in 2014. His current research interest includes modulation of tumor metabolism, evaluating derivative anticancer drugs, and chemosensitization.

Chapter 1
Epidemiology of Colorectal Cancer

Begum Dariya, Gayathri Chalikonda, and Ganji Purnachandra Nagaraju

Abstract Colorectal cancer (CRC) is a serious lethal disease and ranks third for cancer-related mortalities globally. As estimated for the year 2020 by the American Cancer Society, 147,950 new cases and 53,200 deaths are expected. The incidence of CRC has grown globally, especially in developing countries. The driving factors for CRC incidence are obesity, unhealthy food habits, smoking, and alcohol consumptions. Additionally, unmodifiable factors include personal history of inflammatory diseases and family history having cancer, diabetes, and inherited syndromes caused due to mutated genes. Age, sex, and geographical and race/ethnicity disparities play a crucial role in incidence and mortality. The novel advances regarding early diagnosis, screening, and therapy reduce incidence as well as mortality. Additionally, complete documentation of the family history, appropriate gene testing, and better predisposition of hereditary history aids for early diagnosis, preventive measures, and improved survival rate. In this chapter we have focused on current epidemiological trends of increasing incidence, mortality rates, and decreased survival rate. We have also focused on associated risk factors for CRC occurrence. Basing on the date surveillance, therapeutic plans can be scheduled for early screening and therapy at the benefit of patient survival.

Keywords Colorectal cancer · Epidemiology · Incidence · Mortality rate · Survival rate · Risk factors

B. Dariya
Department of Bioscience and Biotechnology, Banasthali University, Vanasthali, Rajasthan, India

G. Chalikonda
Internal Medicine, University of Nevada, Reno, NV, USA

G. P. Nagaraju (✉)
Department of Hematology and Medical Oncology, Winship Cancer Institute, Emory University, Atlanta, GA, USA
e-mail: pganji@emory.edu

G. P. Nagaraju et al. (eds.), *Colon Cancer Diagnosis and Therapy*, https://doi.org/10.1007/978-3-030-63369-1_1

Abbreviations

ACS	American Cancer Society
AI	American Indians
AN	Alaska Native
API	American Pacific Islanders
CRC	Colorectal cancer
FAP	Familial adenomatous polyposis
HDI	Human development index
HNPCC	Hereditary non-polyposis colorectal cancer
IBD	Inflammatory bowel disease
MAP	MUTYH-associated polyposis
NCHS	National Center for Health Statistics
NHBs	Non-Hispanic blacks
NHWs	Non-Hispanic white
PJS	Peutz-Jeghers syndrome

1.1 Introduction

Colorectal cancer (CRC) is a severe global health problem, ranking as the third leading cause for cancer-related mortalities [2]. It is the second most frequently diagnosed cancer in women and third in men; in 2019 over 140,000 cases were diagnosed in the United States [46]. Despite advances clinically and in research, the 5-year survival rate for localized CRC was 90% and 71% for regional-type CRC diagnosed at an early stage. However, in case of metastatic CRC, the 5-year survival rate is only about 14% [10]. CRC is a heterogenous disease with a varied array of mutations and mutagens. The incidence and mortality of CRC are steadily increasing in the developing nations due to varied risk factors, including environmental, epigenetic, and genetic factors. More or less the incidence and mortality of CRC are related to modifiable and unmodifiable risk factors. Therefore, a better understanding of CRC development and their associated genetic, epigenetic factors is essential, as the mortality and morbidity of CRC can be reduced through proper screening and surveillance. Epidemiology is the field of science that deals with the study of determinants and distribution of a disease in a specific population [49]. The main application of this study is to control the global health problems. In this chapter, we have included the determinants and distribution part of epidemiology related to CRC. This would suggest future efforts of public healthcare communities to bring out better screening methods basing on the epidemiological studies of CRC, in order to develop personalized therapeutic strategies.

1.2 Epidemiology

The incidence and mortality of CRC vary globally. The data of epidemiological studies establishes incidence of CRC based on the frequency data and risk factors of diseases in a specific population. The distribution of epidemiology includes the frequency that refers to the number of CRC cases in a population, allowing comparison across other population. On the other hand, the determinant includes risk factors that influence the occurrence of diseases.

1.2.1 Incidence

As per the data published by GLOBOCAN 2018, colon cancer is the fourth, and rectum cancer is the eighth most frequently diagnosed cancer in the world. As estimated from ACS for the year 2020, about 104,610 new cases for colon cancer and 43,340 new cases for rectal cancer were diagnosed [40]. Moreover, the number of individuals diagnosed with CRC per year has dropped since the mid-1980s, as many are opting for screening and lifestyle changes to reduce risk factors. While this trend is seen better in adults 55 years or older, with 3.6% drop, increased incidence of 2% was noted in those younger than 55 years [40]. Additionally, the incidence of CRC also varies by sex. CRC is most commonly diagnosed in males than in females. Thus, the incidence of CRC varies as per age, sex, race, and geographical disparities.

1.2.1.1 Age

The annual age-standardized incidence estimated for CRC from the year 2012–2016 was 38.7% among 100,000 individuals [40]. Similarly, the age-standardized incidence detected globally, per 100,000 CRC cases, was about 19.7; the incidence in 2018 was 23.6 for males and 16.3 for females [20]. As per the human development index (HDI) estimates, the age standardized incidence estimated for men is very high (30.1) when compared to female (8.4) for 100,000 cases of CRC [7]. Researchers estimated that the incidence of CRC increases with ages and approximately doubles for every 5 years until 50 years of age, while nearly 30% increase is detected among the individuals of age group of 55 years and older [39]. There is a drastic hike in the incidence of about 90.2 cases in 100,000 population aged between 60 and 64 years, 121.4 cases in those aged 65–69 years, and 258.8 in those 85 and older. However, only about 15% higher rate of incidence is detected in 55–59 years when compared to age group 50–54 years, as the age-associated risk factor is fluctuated in the age group of 50–54 years during their first-time screening for cancer. Moreover, if analyzed deeply, the age groups of 50–51 showed a higher incidence than age group of 52–55 years. The incidence also rose for the age group 20–49 years from 8.6 per 100,000 in the year 1992 in the United States to 13.2 per 100,000 in 2016 with a large increase in incidence among adults 40–49 years age [39]. Thus, this represents a decline in incidence in older aged group [39]. Additionally, the incidence for the age groups varies with the anatomical site. For instance, among CRC patients, half of the population aged 65 years and older had proximal colon cancer, while those 50 years and younger presented with distal colon cancer.

1.2.1.2 Sex

The risk for CRC occurrence is similar in men and women, with 4.4% and 4.1%, respectively. As women have longer life expectancy than men, a 31% higher incidence was noted in men. As with age, the anatomical site and incidence vary with sex. For instance, the incidence ratio for male/female (1.60:1.63) is large for rectal cancer, whereas for proximal colon cancer, the disparity is less 1.07:1.08. Moreover, for the year 2018, the incidence for colon cancer diagnosed was about 576,000 for men and 521,000 for women. Similarly, for rectal cancer about 274,000 and 430,000 were estimated for women and men, respectively [7]. Accordingly, the sex disparity also varies with the age. An age group of 74 years in both men and women showed a cumulative risk for colon cancer occurrence of about 1.51% and 1.12%, respectively, while for rectal cancer it is estimated as 1.2% and 0.65% for men and women, respectively [7]. The incidence estimated for men younger than 45 years age group showed 40–50% higher than in women of age group 55–74 years. The reason for higher incidence in males is not clearly understood; however sex hormones and the exposure to risk factors like smoking and alcohol may play a role [29, 31].

1.2.1.3 Race

Across all the racial/ethnic groups, the increase in incidence varies substantially. Researchers consider five racial groups of Asian Americans/Pacific Islanders (APIs), non-Hispanic blacks (NHBs), non-Hispanic whites (NHWs), American Indians/Alaska Native (AI/AN), and Hispanics. NHB showed higher incidence than AI/ANs; the lowest incidence detected in APIs. Whereas compared to NHB (45.7) and NHW (38.6), a higher incidence was seen in NHB during the period of 2012–2016. APIs were estimated to have 30.0 per 100,000 less incidence rate than both HNB and HNW race during the same period. The increased incidence in blacks is due to the risk factors and their low socioeconomic status. The socioeconomic status and annual income of the year 2018 for both NHBs and NHWs showed great variations having 21% and 8% respectively, leaving the later in poverty [37]. Another cause for these racial disparities is the prevalence of risk factors like smoking and obesity among different populations [17] and historical differences in relation to the delay in screening of diseases [26]. However, with risk factor control and timely screening of CRC, the NHBs are more likely than NHWs to develop CRC

[19, 25]. CRC incidence was found increased in NHW men significantly more than in API, who have 25% lower incidence. Moreover, for ANs the incidence is very high, estimated as 89 per 100,000 population number. The incidence in CRC for ANs was found significantly increased from the early 1970s due to increased risk factors, including low intake of fruits/vegetables, high intake of animal fats, diabetes, obesity, and smoking [23, 33]. Rural ANs are at higher risk for CRC occurrence due to the prevalence of *Helicobacter pylori* that is associated with inflammation in the stomach and are at risk for CRC occurrence [8, 44, 48]. Additionally, the incidence for CRC in AN is due to insufficient access to screening services [9, 14]. Furthermore, the screening test like stool testing that is considered the initial mode of diagnosing disease at Indian Health Service must be annually performed for effective diagnosis along with periodical endoscopy to reduce the mortality rate [28, 36].

1.2.1.4 Geographical Features

The incidence for CRC varies geographically due to the influence of lifestyle features [54]. Developed countries like Northern/Southern Europe, Australia, and New Zealand are at higher risk for colon cancer occurrence. Similarly, rectal cancer showed higher incidence in Eastern Asia, Australia/New Zealand, and Eastern Europe. The incidence was estimated to be higher in Appalachia, Mississippi Delta Region, and parts of the Midwest and South, while a lower incidence was detected in the west. This is due to higher poverty levels, poor access of healthcare, and unemployment in these regions. The geographic occurrence of CRC was similar for both NHW and NHB [38]. Within the United States, incidence and occurrence of CRC are due to variation in screening and healthcare as well the associated modifiable risk factors like obesity, smoking, and diet. As an example, data suggests that the incidence for Utah was 29.7 per 100,000 population and 49.2 in Kentucky per 100,000 population [4]. While the incidence in Hungarian males is 70.6 per 100,000 population, Norwegian females had an incidence of 29.3 per 100,000 population. An early onset of CRC was reported from the United Kingdom, Canada, Australia, and Asia. Men exceed women in CRC diagnosis in other countries like Qatar, UAE, Oman, Korea, Kuwait, South Korea, and Japan. In contrast, the incidence is highly diagnosed in both sexes in Africa and Southern Asia [7].

1.2.2 Mortality

The mortality and morbidity of CRC are altered through appropriate screening and surveillance analysis [52]. The CDC's National Center for Health Statistics (NCHS) maintains the US mortality data of CRC, collected since 1930 [15, 32, 53]. Additionally, SEER*Stat (version 8.3.6) maintains age-adjusted incidence and mortality on a geographical basis [15]. The NCI version 4.7.0.0 quantified the data for incidence and mortality using Joinpoint regression. Additionally, NCI's DevCan software version 6.7.7 maintains the data for lifetime probability of developing cancer [41].

CRC is considered as the second most lethal cancer globally. For the year 2018, mortality was an estimated 881,000. The annual CRC age standardized rate for mortality rate for the year 2013–2017 was 13.9 per 100,000 population. The mortality of CRC has decreased due to the advances in screening and therapies. A reduced mortality rate is detected in older adults (75+ years) but remained stable in younger adults at about 2.8 per 100,000 population [6–8]. Thus, the mortality trend varies by age group; young adults have increased mortality as compared to older adults. The analysis of data taken from 2008 to 2017 showed variations if estimated as per age. For instance, a 3% mortality decline is observed for individuals of age group 65 years and older, while an increase of 1.3% is observed for those 50 years and younger.

The mortality rate also varies significantly with race and ethnicity. The mortality rate for CRC is higher in blacks at 19.0 per 100,000 individuals, as compared to the NHWs (13.8) and APIs (9.5). The racial disparity for mortality is also due to risk factors, healthcare access, and socioeconomic status. Advanced screening tests, efficient colonoscopy, and risk factor control have led to reduced mortality rates. In addition to these, histology and anatomical site also contribute to racial disparities in mortality rate for CRC [12, 42, 43, 50]. The mortality for the year 2018 was evaluated for variations related to tumor anatomy, and significant differences were noted. For instance, colon cancer showed up with 551,000 mortalities comprising 5.8% making it fifth leading cause for cancer-related deaths. Similarly, rectal cancer stood as tenth leading cause for cancer-related mortalities with 310,000 deaths comprising of 3.2%. If we consider age and sex, 74 and younger age men have an estimated to have 0.66% mortality and women to have 0.44% mortality. Likewise, for rectal cancer, women had 0.26% and men has 0.46% death rate. Thus, a cumulative age standardized mortality rate for both the sexes estimated was 8.9 per 100,000 CRC population [7]. The mortality rate if analyzed, since 1947 a decline for women was observed, while a decline for men is seen only since 1980. As discussed, this difference in mortality rate as per the sex is due to the inconsistency of risk factors. However, there is decline in mortality of both the sexes since 2000 due to the advancements in technology of screening, therapies, and modifying patterns in CRC risk factors [54].

Furthermore, the mortality rate in both the sexes also varies as per the geographical disparity. For instance, in UAE, Saudi Arabia, and Oman, males showed higher mortality rate in CRC, whereas females in Spain, Algeria, Japan, Portugal, and Belarus showed higher mortality rates [7]. However, Hungary showed increased mortality rates comparatively for both men and women with 31.2 and 14.8, respectively. Considerably, the highest mortality rate is detected in Appalachia and some parts of South and Midwest while lowest in West. The mortality rate is 18.3 in Mississippi, 11.2 for Utah, and 11.0 for Connecticut for 100,000 people [47].

1.2.3 Trends in Incidence and Mortality

The association between incidence and mortality can be defined by HDI of nations characterized into three different global categories illustrated in Table 1.1 [4].

A high global burden is expected for the year 2030 with an increase of about 2.2 million new cases and 1.1 million mortalities annually. Growth is expected due to the transitions in economic developments and HDI nations from low-medium and environmental risk factors [4].

1.2.4 Survival Rate

Advancements in CRC therapies decrease the mortality rate of CRC, as determined for second and third categories of nations. The improvement of the survival rate is due to the advancement in screening techniques, including computer tomography, colonoscopy, fecal occult blood testing, and flexible sigmoidoscopies [18]. The incidence rate however found higher due to the diseased polyps that were undiagnosed initially, but are diagnosed later using the advancing screening techniques. However, the mortality is reduced due to the removal of these pre-cancerous polyps [4]. Thus, diagnosis at early stages plays a chief role in survival prediction. For instance, the 5-year survival rate was detected in 90% of CRC patients diagnosed with localized CRC while 14% for distant stage disease. Additionally, rectal cancer can be diagnosed easier than the colon cancer due to the symptoms detected in their early stages. Table 1.2 illustrates the survival rate data of the US patients diagnosed at different stages. Furthermore, in addition to diagnosis, age, race (black), low income status, and young age are also chief factors that determines the survival rate [3, 51]. Among the racial groups, black patient are most commonly diagnosed for distant or metastatic stages and showed minimum 5-year survival rate. This disparity is due to the inequalities in socioeconomic and lack of advanced therapies causing delay in diagnosis. Additionally, if analyzed among US population, the Native Americans, African Americans, and underprivileged minorities suffered with least survival rate for all the stages of CRC. This is due to poor access to

Table 1.1 Trends in CRC incidence and mortality

HDI category	Nations	Incidence	Mortality	Development
First category: Medium HDI	Philippines, Brazil, China, Baltics, Russia, and Latin America	Increased	Increased	Economic transition
Second category: High HDI	Singapore, United Kingdom, Canada, and Denmark	Increased	Decreased	Improved therapeutic options
Third category: Highest HDI	France, Iceland, Japan, and United State	Decreased	Decreased	Succeeded in prevention and advanced treatment options

Table 1.2 Colorectal cancer type, stage, and 5-year survival rate

Type of cancer	Stage	5-year survival rate (%)
Colon cancer	Stage I	92
	Stage IIA	87
	Stage IIB	65
	Stage IIIA	90
	Stage IIIB	72
	Stage IIIC	53
	Stage IV/metastatic	12
Rectal cancer	Stage I	88
	Stage IIA	81
	Stage IIB	50
	Stage IIIA	83
	Stage IIIB	72
	Stage IIIC	58
	Stage IV/metastatic	13

pre-emptive screening techniques, unhealthy food habits, and lack of availability for healthcare [34, 35].

The survival rate for 5 years is found higher for patients aged younger than 50 years. The overall survival rate was however found to be similar for both age groups: younger than 50 years having 68% and 69% for 50–64 years age group, as they are diagnosed in their later stages. If diagnosed in their distant or metastatic stages an approximate survival rate for age group 50 years and younger showed 26%, 23% for 50–64 years old group and 19% for 65 years and older. The survival rate for older patients (65 years and older) is very low even if they are diagnosed in their early stages, because age is a risk factor that plays a major role in determining survival rate. Additionally, older patients are unlikely to respond to surgeries or conventional therapies [1, 6].

1.3 Risk Factors

Race/ethnicity, sex, age, and geographical factors are consistently associated with incidence and survival in the epidemiological studies. In addition, there are several other factors including modifiable factors, smoking, alcohol, food habits, and obesity, and unmodifiable factors – being older, family history having cancer, personal history having inflammatory diseases, diabetes, mutations and inherited syndromes – that play a major role in CRC occurrence.

1.3.1 Modifiable Risk Factors

The lifestyle-associated factors like overweight BMI and physically inactive predispose patient to develop CRC [24, 40]. Unhealthy food habits include diet high in red and processed meat raise CRC risk [16]. Additionally, people using tobacco and using heavy alcohols are also associated with CRC occurrence. However, CRC can be prevented by lowering these risk factors, like having regular physical activities, healthy food patterns, and quitting smoking and alcohol [5, 13, 16].

1.3.2 Non-modifiable Risk Factors

These risk factors are those that cannot be changed or modified in causing CRC. The risk for CRC occurrence increases with the increase in individual's age. As discussed, 50 and older-aged people are at higher risk for CRC occurrence. Younger adults are also prone; however the exact reason for the occurrence is still unclear. People with non-insulin-dependent diabetes or type 2 diabetes are also at higher risk for CRC occurrence. Patients with personal history having diseases like inflammatory bowel disease (IBD) and adenoma/adenomatous polyps are at higher risk for CRC occurrence [11]. Furthermore, a family history particularly if his/her first-degree relative is diagnosed with CRC are also found at higher risk. As estimated about 5% of population who developed cancer were diagnosed with inherited gene mutations [27]. These mutations cause family cancer syndrome eventually developing into CRC. The inherited syndromes most commonly detected in CRC patients include familial adenomatous polyposis (FAP) and lynch syndrome/hereditary non-polyposis CRC/HNPCC. About 3% of CRC accounts for the presence of lynch syndrome in the patient [21, 22]. This is caused due to the aberrantly acting genes including MLH1 and MSH2/MSH6. Similarly, FAP accounts for 1% of CRC occurrence, which is caused due to the alterations or mutations in APC gene [30, 45]. Moreover, other rare inherited syndromes that are associated to the risk of CRC occurrence are Peutz-Jeghers syndrome (PJS) and MUTYH-associated polyposis (MAP).

1.4 Conclusion

CRC is the deadliest cancer among all other cancers, due to its increased incidence and mortality rate globally. For the year 2020, 147,950 diagnosed cases and 53,200 deaths were detected due to CRC. Even though CRC incidence and mortality rate declined with advanced techniques, they are found limited in older age groups.

Additionally, in case of race and geographical disparities, the mortality rate remains high for ANs when compared to NHWs. Although socioeconomic, sedentary lifestyles, and poor diet contribute to CRC occurrence in developed nations, the advanced diagnostic techniques and conventional therapies have allowed for reduced incidence and improved patient survival. Genetic testing done for the early-onset CRC patients supports the therapeutic guide and facilitates appropriate testing and screening. Additionally, a complete knowledge of birth cohort also indicates the lifestyle and environmental-related risk factors during patient's life that support for early-onset of CRC. Furthermore, future epidemiological studies evaluate a particular population to give better understanding about incidence, mortality, and survival rate. This promotes better screening approaches and therapeutic strategies to focus on low socioeconomic populations. Additionally, studies on molecular and genetic features will provide better understanding of CRC carcinogenesis and novel therapeutic approaches.

References

1. Abraham A, Habermann EB, Rothenberger DA, Kwaan M, Weinberg AD, Parsons HM, Gupta P, Al-Refaie WB. Adjuvant chemotherapy for stage III colon cancer in the oldest old: results beyond clinical guidelines. Cancer. 2013;119(2):395–403.
2. American Cancer Society. Global cancer facts and figures 4th edition. Am Cancer Soc. 2018;1:1–73.
3. Andrew AS, Parker S, Anderson JC, Rees JR, Robinson C, Riddle B, Butterly LF. Risk factors for diagnosis of colorectal cancer at a late stage: a population-based study. J Gen Intern Med. 2018;33(12):2100–5.
4. Arnold M, Sierra MS, Laversanne M, Soerjomataram I, Jemal A, Bray F. Global patterns and trends in colorectal cancer incidence and mortality. Gut. 2017;66(4):683–91.
5. Ballester V, Rashtak S, Boardman L. Clinical and molecular features of young-onset colorectal cancer. World J Gastroenterol. 2016;22(5):1736.
6. Boakye D, Walter V, Martens UM, Chang-Claude J, Hoffmeister M, Jansen L, Brenner H. Treatment selection bias for chemotherapy persists in colorectal cancer patient cohort studies even in comprehensive propensity score analyses. Clin Epidemiol. 2019;11:821.
7. Bray F, Ferlay J, Soerjomataram I, Siegel RL, Torre LA, Jemal A. Global cancer statistics 2018: GLOBOCAN estimates of incidence and mortality worldwide for 36 cancers in 185 countries. CA Cancer J Clin. 2018;68(6):394–424.
8. Butt J, Varga MG, Blot WJ, Teras L, Visvanathan K, Le Marchand L, Haiman C, Chen Y, Bao Y, Sesso HD. Serologic response to Helicobacter pylori proteins associated with risk of colorectal cancer among diverse populations in the United States. Gastroenterology. 2019;156(1):175–86. e172.
9. Carmichael H, Cowan M, McIntyre R, Velopulos C. Disparities in colorectal cancer mortality for rural populations in the United States: does screening matter? Am J Surg. 2020;219(6):988–92.
10. Carroll R, Zhao S. Trends in colorectal cancer incidence and survival in Iowa SEER data: the timing of it all. Clin Colorectal Cancer. 2019;18(2):e261–74.
11. Cohen M, Minsky B, Schilsky R. Cancer of the colon. In: DeVita VT, Hellman S, Rosenberg SA, editors. Cancer principals and practice of oncology. Philadelphia: Lippincott; 2001.
12. Coughlin SS, Blumenthal DS, Seay SJ, Smith SA. Toward the elimination of colorectal cancer disparities among African Americans. J Racial Ethn Health Disparities. 2016;3(4):555–64.

13. Dashti SG, Win AK, Hardikar SS, Glombicki SE, Mallenahalli S, Thirumurthi S, Peterson SK, You YN, Buchanan DD, Figueiredo JC. Physical activity and the risk of colorectal cancer in Lynch syndrome. Int J Cancer. 2018;143(9):2250–60.
14. Day LW, Espey DK, Madden E, Segal M, Terdiman JP. Screening prevalence and incidence of colorectal cancer among American Indian/Alaskan natives in the Indian Health Service. Dig Dis Sci. 2011;56(7):2104–13.
15. DeSantis CE, Miller KD, Goding Sauer A, Jemal A, Siegel RL. Cancer statistics for African Americans, 2019. CA Cancer J Clin. 2019;69(3):211–33.
16. DeVita VT, Rosenberg SA, Lawrence TS. DeVita, Hellman, and Rosenberg's cancer. Philadelphia: Lippincott Williams & Wilkins; 2018.
17. Doubeni CA, Major JM, Laiyemo AO, Schootman M, Zauber AG, Hollenbeck AR, Sinha R, Allison J. Contribution of behavioral risk factors and obesity to socioeconomic differences in colorectal cancer incidence. J Natl Cancer Inst. 2012;104(18):1353–62.
18. Edwards BK, Ward E, Kohler BA, Eheman C, Zauber AG, Anderson RN, Jemal A, Schymura MJ, Lansdorp-Vogelaar I, Seeff LC. Annual report to the nation on the status of cancer, 1975-2006, featuring colorectal cancer trends and impact of interventions (risk factors, screening, and treatment) to reduce future rates. Cancer. 2010;116(3):544–73.
19. Fedewa SA, Flanders WD, Jemal A, Doubeni CA, Goodman M. Racial and ethnic disparities in interval colorectal cancer incidence. Ann Intern Med. 2018;168(1):80.
20. Ferlay J, Ervik M, Lam F, Colombet M, Mery L, Piñeros M, Znaor A, Soerjomataram I, Bray F. Global cancer observatory: cancer today. Lyon: International Agency for Research on Cancer; 2018.
21. Hampel H, Frankel W, Panescu J, Lockman J, Sotamaa K, Fix D, Comeras I, La Jeunesse J, Nakagawa H, Westman JA. Screening for Lynch syndrome (hereditary nonpolyposis colorectal cancer) among endometrial cancer patients. Cancer Res. 2006;66(15):7810–7.
22. Haraldsdottir S, Rafnar T, Frankel WL, Einarsdottir S, Sigurdsson A, Hampel H, Snaebjornsson P, Masson G, Weng D, Arngrimsson R. Comprehensive population-wide analysis of Lynch syndrome in Iceland reveals founder mutations in MSH6 and PMS2. Nat Commun. 2017;8(1):1–11.
23. Kelly JJ, Alberts SR, Sacco F, Lanier AP. Colorectal cancer in Alaska native people, 2005–2009. Gastrointest Cancer Res. 2012;5(5):149.
24. Konishi M. Promotion of colorectal cancer screening completion through training of patient navigators. Honolulu: University of Hawai'i at Manoa; 2020.
25. Laiyemo AO, Doubeni C, Pinsky PF, Doria-Rose VP, Bresalier R, Lamerato LE, Crawford ED, Kvale P, Fouad M, Hickey T. Race and colorectal cancer disparities: health-care utilization vs different cancer susceptibilities. J Natl Cancer Inst. 2010;102(8):538–46.
26. Lansdorp-Vogelaar I, Kuntz KM, Knudsen AB, Van Ballegooijen M, Zauber AG, Jemal A. Contribution of screening and survival differences to racial disparities in colorectal cancer rates. Cancer EpidemiolBiomarkers Prev. 2012;21(5):728–36.
27. Lynch HT, De la Chapelle A. Hereditary colorectal cancer. N Engl J Med. 2003;348(10):919–32.
28. Martin J, Halm EA, Tiro JA, Merchant Z, Balasubramanian BA, McCallister K, Sanders JM, Ahn C, Bishop WP, Singal AG. Reasons for lack of diagnostic colonoscopy after positive result on fecal immunochemical test in a safety-net health system. Am J Med. 2017;130(1):93.e91–7.
29. Meissner HI, Breen N, Klabunde CN, Vernon SW. Patterns of colorectal cancer screening uptake among men and women in the United States. Cancer Epidemiol Biomarkers Prev. 2006;15(2):389–94.
30. Mork ME, You YN, Ying J, Bannon SA, Lynch PM, Rodriguez-Bigas MA, Vilar E. High prevalence of hereditary cancer syndromes in adolescents and young adults with colorectal cancer. J Clin Oncol. 2015;33(31):3544.
31. Murphy G, Devesa SS, Cross AJ, Inskip PD, McGlynn KA, Cook MB. Sex disparities in colorectal cancer incidence by anatomic subsite, race and age. Int J Cancer. 2011;128(7):1668–75.
32. National Institutes of Health. Surveillance, epidemiology, and end results (SEER) program SEER∗stat database: incidence-SEER 9 regs research data, Nov 2016 Sub (1973–2014). National Cancer Institute, D, Surveillance Research Program, 2017.

33. Perdue DG, Haverkamp D, Perkins C, Daley CM, Provost E. Geographic variation in colorectal cancer incidence and mortality, age of onset, and stage at diagnosis among American Indian and Alaska native people, 1990–2009. Am J Public Health. 2014;104(S3):S404–14.
34. Rawla P, Sunkara T, Muralidharan P, Raj JP. Update in global trends and aetiology of hepatocellular carcinoma. Contemp Oncol. 2018;22(3):141.
35. Rawla P, Sunkara T, Barsouk A. Epidemiology of colorectal cancer: incidence, mortality, survival, and risk factors. Prz Gastroenterol. 2019;14(2):89.
36. Redwood D, Provost E, Perdue D, Haverkamp D, Espey D. The last frontier: innovative efforts to reduce colorectal cancer disparities among the remote Alaska native population. Gastrointest Endosc. 2012;75(3):474–80.
37. Semega J, Kollar M, Creamer J, Mohanty A. US Census Bureau, Current population reports. Income and poverty in the United States: 2018. US Government Printing Office, 2019. https://www.census.gov/content/dam/Census ….
38. Siegel R, Ward E, Brawley O, Jemal A. Cancer statistics, 2011: the impact of eliminating socioeconomic and racial disparities on premature cancer deaths. CA Cancer J Clin. 2011;61(4):212–36.
39. Siegel RL, Fedewa SA, Anderson WF, Miller KD, Ma J, Rosenberg PS, Jemal A. Colorectal cancer incidence patterns in the United States, 1974–2013. J Natl Cancer Inst. 2017;109(8):djw322.
40. Siegel RL, Miller KD, Goding Sauer A, Fedewa SA, Butterly LF, Anderson JC, Cercek A, Smith RA, Jemal A. Colorectal cancer statistics, 2020. CA Cancer J Clin. 2020;70(3):145–64.
41. Simonson H. Statistical research and applications branch. National Cancer Institute. Headbang software. Version 3.0. 2015, 2016.
42. Sineshaw HM, Robbins AS, Jemal A. Disparities in survival improvement for metastatic colorectal cancer by race/ethnicity and age in the United States. Cancer Causes Control. 2014;25(4):419–23.
43. Sineshaw HM, Ng K, Flanders WD, Brawley OW, Jemal A. Factors that contribute to differences in survival of black vs white patients with colorectal cancer. Gastroenterology. 2018;154(4):906–15. e907.
44. Sonnenberg A, Genta RM. Helicobacter pylori is a risk factor for colonic neoplasms. Am J Gastroenterol. 2013;108(2):208–15.
45. Stoffel EM, Koeppe E, Everett J, Ulintz P, Kiel M, Osborne J, Williams L, Hanson K, Gruber SB, Rozek LS. Germline genetic features of young individuals with colorectal cancer. Gastroenterology. 2018;154(4):897–905. e891.
46. Street W. Cancer facts & figures 2019. Atlanta: American Cancer Society; 2019. p. 1–76.
47. Surveillance E, Program ER. SEER*stat database: North American Association of Central Cancer Registries (NAACCR) incidence data-CiNA analytic file, 1995–2015, for expanded races, custom file with county, ACS facts and figures projection project (which includes data from CDC's National Program of Cancer Registries [NPCR], CCCR's provincial and territorial registries, and the NCI's Surveillance, Epidemiology, and End Results [SEER] registries), 2018.
48. Tsukanov V, Mulvad G, Borresen M, Sacco F, Barrett D, Westby S, Parkinson A. The diagnosis and treatment of Helicobacter pylori infection in Arctic regions with a high prevalence of infection: expert. Epidemiol Infect. 2016;144:225–33.
49. U.S. Department of Health and Human Services. Principles of epidemiology in public health practice. Third edition. An introduction to applied epidemiology and biostatistics. Atlanta: U.S. Department of Health and Human Services; 2013. Available on the website: http://www.cdc.gov/ophss/csels/dsepd/SS1978.
50. Wallace K, Grau MV, Ahnen D, Snover DC, Robertson DJ, Mahnke D, Gui J, Barry EL, Summers RW, McKeown-Eyssen G. The association of lifestyle and dietary factors with the risk for serrated polyps of the colorectum. Cancer Epidemiol Biomarkers Prev. 2009;18(8):2310–7.
51. Ward E, Jemal A, Cokkinides V, Singh GK, Cardinez C, Ghafoor A, Thun M. Cancer disparities by race/ethnicity and socioeconomic status. CA Cancer J Clin. 2004;54(2):78–93.

52. Winawer SJ, Zauber AG. The advanced adenoma as the primary target of screening. Gastrointest Endosc Clin. 2002;12(1):1–9.
53. Wingo PA, Cardinez CJ, Landis SH, Greenlee RT, Ries LA, Anderson RN, Thun MJ. Long-term trends in cancer mortality in the United States, 1930–1998. Cancer. 2003;97(S12):3133–275.
54. Zauber AG, Lansdorp-Vogelaar I. Changes in risk factors and increases in screening contribute to the decline in colorectal cancer mortality, 1975 to 2000. Gastroenterology. 2010;139(2):698.

Chapter 2
Colorectal Cancer: A Model for the Study of Cancer Immunology

Pranav Kumar Prabhakar

Abstract Colorectal cancer is placed at the second place in terms of mortality by cancer. Even after the improvement and development in the colorectal cancer management, the prognosis of metastatic colorectal cancer is very poorly explored. And hence there is a requirement of very efficient, novel, and effective management strategies for the colorectal cancer, especially for metastatic colorectal cancer. Some of the recent studies has shown the efficacy of immunotherapy in some other types of tumors such as melanoma and the cancer of lungs and made this a practicable treatment strategy for the colorectal cancer and for clinical trials. The immunotherapy for the management of cancers is growing very rapidly due to advancement in the technological approaches. Here we are going to discuss the developmental status of immunotherapy for colorectal cancer. Some of the immunotherapy strategies which have shown success against the progression of colorectal cancer in some specific subsection of patients are different models for vaccine development, effector cell-based therapeutic strategies, and antibodies as checkpoint inhibition.

Keywords Colorectal cancer · Immunotherapy · Metastatic · Antibodies · Therapeutic · Checkpoint

2.1 Introduction

Colorectal cancer is the third most prevalent and diagnosed cancer. It is only the second most prevalent cancer in women and third in men [1]. According to the American Cancer Society, 1 out of 21 men and 1 out of 23 women of the USA have got colorectal cancer during their life time. As per one estimate out of 1.8 million colorectal cases detected, colorectal cancer caused more than 800,000 death in 2018 alone [2]. Even after the improvement and development in the management of

P. K. Prabhakar (✉)
Department of Medical Laboratory Sciences, Lovely Professional University, Phagwara, Punjab, India

G. P. Nagaraju et al. (eds.), *Colon Cancer Diagnosis and Therapy*, https://doi.org/10.1007/978-3-030-63369-1_2

colorectal cancer, the prognosis of metastatic colorectal cancer is very poorly explored, and it is the fifth leading cause of mortality among women and fourth in men [3]. It is expected that there is around 60% increases in global burden of colorectal cancer by 2030 [4]. Due to improvement and development of tools and techniques, the mortality rate due to colorectal cancer has been reduced over the time. The cancer might be of noncancerous type or benign and malignant (move from the original place). The major issue associated with the malignant cancer is that it can detach from their original site and move to other parts of the body and causes cancer and ultimately affects the organ physiologically.

The association of cancer genetics and the immunity has been very well elaborated with the distinction between the high and low mutation causing somatic mutations (Table 2.1). The category and magnitude of genetic variability seen in the case of colorectal cancer influence the immunity, immune components, and immune response in the cancer microenvironment and determine the clinical responses observed to cancer immunotherapy [4, 5].

More than ten mutations in every megabase lead to cancer with high burden and are responsible for more than 15–20% of total colorectal cancer prevalence. One of the main reasons for this is the defect in the DNA mismatch repair system (MMR) which can be genetically inherited, such as Lynch syndrome, or acquired. Hypermutated phenotype is also present in the small group of colorectal cancer (roughly 1%) and is due to somatic or germline mutations present in the gene responsible for the proofreading domain of DNA polymerase epsilon (POLE) or less commonly in the eukaryotic DNA polymerase delta-1 (POLD-1) enzyme [6, 7]. The defect in the MMR or POLE or POLD-1 enzymes results in the cumulative accumulations of a wide number of mutations which affect genomic region for protein coding. Insertion or deletion of a single nucleotide is very common in the case of defects of mismatch repair system, and if this happens in exon of the genes, it leads to frameshift mutation and results in a mutated protein with immunogenic potentials. The surplus of mutated proteins (neoantigens) in hypermutated cancers confers them an immunogenic character as demonstrated by their conspicuous infiltration with cytotoxic T cells [8, 9]. In any case, the vast dominant part of colorectal malignancies (up to 80% of cases) is MMR-capable and presents with low to direct

Table 2.1 Immunological spectrum of colorectal cancer with high and low somatic mutation burden

Immunological spectrum of colorectal cancer	
Colorectal cancers with high somatic mutation burden	Colorectal cancers with low somatic mutation burden
High rate of mutation (MOLE, MMR-d)	Low rate of mutation
High level of T cell infiltration	Low level of T cell infiltration
Response to checkpoint blockade	Refractory to checkpoint blockade
Good clinical prognosis	Poor clinical prognosis
Loss of HLA-I expression	Retention of HLA-I expression
Peritoneal metastasis	Hematogenous metastasis

MMR-d mismatch repair deficient, *HLA-1* human leukocyte antigen transformation trouble. This audit talks about how hereditary qualities and disease invulnerability are firmly entwined in colorectal malignancy and how this relationship impacts quiet anticipation and reaction to best in class immunotherapies.

2.2 Genetics of Colorectal Cancer

More than 90% of the case of colorectal cancer are sporadic and without any kinds of family history of genetic sensitivity, while only in less than 10% cases, the genetic predisposition has been identified. Roughly in the 25% of colorectal cases, an association of family history was found (known as familial CRC) [10]. Colorectal cancer involves a huge genetic heterogeneity which increases the complexity for the determination of clinical consequences for each single mutation [11]. The stability of genome of an organism is very essential for the maintenance of cellular integrity. The expiration of genetic stability resulted in the colorectal cancer advancement via the attainment of new mutations linked with the cancer phenotype. A number of attempts have been done to find the genetic features and molecular biology of the colorectal cancer, and there is more evidence available which shows the prognosis and also the response to therapeutic strategies. In the last 20 years, a large number of genetic mutation in the genes which regulates cell growth and its differentiation and maturation have been identified which reveals the association of genetic variation and mutation in the pathophysiology of different types of cancers including colorectal cancer [10, 12]. As we know, colorectal cancer is a heterogenous disorder which has three known major molecular groups, and these are (i) chromosomal instability, (ii) microsatellite instability, and (iii) aberrant DNA methylation.

(a) *Chromosomal instability*: The most common among these three are the chromosomal instability which is characterized by the cumulative accumulated mutations in the specific proto-oncogenes or tumor suppressor genes. It results in the variation and changes in the number of chromosome or structure of chromosomes. The mutation of proto-oncogenes converts them into oncogenes which lead to hyperactive protein product of these oncogenes, or overexpression of these oncogenes induces the cell cycle and results into cancer. The mutation in the case of wild tumor suppressor genes, whose normal function is to keep cell division under control, make them inactive and ultimately the regulation over the cell division doesn't work and results into cancerous growth. Some of the common tumor suppressor genes are adenomatous polyposis coli (APC), P53, SMAD4, etc. [13, 14]. Molecular process which comes after chromosomal instability includes the initiation of tumor formation, promotion, and tumor progression. These causative agents which cause chromosomal instability can be chemical agents, physical components, environmental factors, genetic factors, or acquired somatic mutations in colorectal epithelium.

(b) *Microsatellite instability*: Microsatellites are small parts of DNA where multiple repeated sequences of one to ten nucleotides are present. At the time of replication of DNA, these microsatellite sequences are highly susceptible for mutations such as single nucleotide insertion and deletion and results in frame-shift mutation. DNA mismatch repair system plays a very significant role in the recognition and rectification of these mutations in the microsatellite sequences, avoiding the alteration in genome [15]. The microsatellite instability is caused due to the abnormalities in the genes involved in the DNA mismatch repair system and causes genetic hypermutability. Studying mating errors in DNA bases in patients with colorectal cancer has observed that genes responsible for repairing were inactive. Those genes were called DNA mismatch repair genes (MMR). The occurrence of MSI is evaluated by the absence defective one MMR protein and is present in almost 15–20% of the colorectal cancer cases. The prevalence varies with the stage of cancers like highest in case of stage II (20%), in case of stage III (12%), and in the case of stage IV (4%). The inactivation can be inherited (hereditary non-polyposis cancer) or acquired. Loss of DNA mismatch repair function is associated with the so-called microsatellite instability phenomenon. Microsatellite instability refers to the change in the number of mono-, bi-, tri-, and tetraploid nucleotide which normally repeats in genomic DNA (microsatellites) or in the transcription of proteins [17]. Transformations of MLH 1, MSH 2, MSH 6, and PMS 2 qualities lead to the advancement of Lynch disorder, expanding malignant growth helplessness [18]. The greater part of these malignancies happens in the proximal colon and in older folks and is regularly connected with ladies. A much of the time accompanying inactivation of tumor silencer qualities is seen in these patients [16]. Consistently, more than 1 million patients will create colorectal malignancy, and 3% of them will have Lynch condition, inclining these patients to create HNPCC. Hereditary unsteadiness significantly underscores the musicality of malignant growth advancement in these patients, revealing instances of colorectal disease that was created in 3 years after a negative colonoscopy [19]. In 70–80%, the area is proximal to the splenic flexure, and the normal age at which malignancy creates is 45. Consequently, colonoscopy in these patients is yearly demonstrated or at like clockwork beginning from the age of 25 until 40 and every year beyond 40 years old. Given the high danger of simultaneous wounds and/or metachronous RCC in these patients, a subtotal colectomy might be required. Likewise, in light of the fact that 40–60% of female patients are in danger of creating endometrial malignancy, a prophylactic hysterectomy is suggested [17–19].

(c) *Aberrant DNA methylation*: The nucleotide island CpG is most vulnerable location for the methylation. The methylation at the fifth position of the pyrimidine ring of cytosine is a very common alteration in mammal at CpG Sequence Island. There is a progressive inversion of the methylation profile that results into the methylation of CpG islands and the loss of total methylation level during maturing; this change is also exceptionally pronounced, during the carcinogenesis process. Decrease in the methylation of cytosine and an aberrant considerable methylation at CpG islands is associated with the certain inducers found in the case of colorectal malignant growth. The physical epigenetic inactivation suppresses the MLH-1 expression in the case of sporadic colorectal malignancy with satellites shakiness. The exact molecular process behind this is not fully understood, but it has been found in almost 15% of the colorectal cancer patients, and it is also seen in the case of all tumor aberrant MLH-1 methylation [20, 21].

2.3 Classification of Colorectal Cancer

Colorectal cancer is a genetically heterogenous disorder that is associated with a number of different types of molecular pathways, such as the mechanism involves the initiation of tumor, growth, and development of tumor and its progression. On the basis of the molecular pathways involved in the pathophysiology of colorectal cancer, a consensus molecular subtype (CMS) classification scheme has been proclaimed on the basis of tumor, immune responses, and infiltrating gene expression [22]. On the basis of CMS classification scheme, there are four classes of colorectal cancers: (i) CMS-1 (14% of the colorectal cases; microsatellite instability immune) characterized by the hypermutation, defective mismatch repair system, mutated BRAF oncogene, activated Th1 and cytotoxic T cells (CTLs) signalling, and well-defined and activated immune evasion pathways; (ii) CMS-2 (37% of the colorectal cases; canonical) characterized by huge chromosomal instability and induction of Wnt and Myc cascade; (iii) CMS-3 (13% of the colorectal cases; metabolic) characterized by the not well-controlled metabolic pathways in cancer cells and KRAS mutations; and (iv) CMS-4 (23% of the colorectal cases; mesenchymal) characterized by the activation of TGF-β pathway, induced blood vessel formation (angiogenesis), and infiltration of inflammation (Fig. 2.1) [22]. Becht et al. have documented the composition of all the four CMSs and found a very significant difference between them [23]. CMS-1 and CMS-4 are hot tumors as immune system is activated significantly, whereas CMS-2 and CMS-3 are cold tumors as they lack immune activation. MCP-counter methodology has revealed the high rate of infiltrating CD8+ CTLs as well as CD68+ macrophage cells in the case of CMS-1 and CMS-4. CMS-4 has significantly high rate of infiltrating stromal cells when compared with other CMSs. The study and analysis of gene expression for cytokines and chemokines, inflammatory mediator molecules, product of immunoregulatory genes, MHC-1 expression and antigen presentation, complement system components, and the factors involving and affecting angiogenesis demonstrated the CMS-1 and CMS-4. CSM-1 have shown polarization of Th1 cells and chemokine for the attracting T cells, whereas CMS-4 have shown activated complement system, myeloid chemokine-chemokine ligand-2 motif, factors for angiogenesis, and some immunosuppressive regulator molecules [23]. The rise in expression level of checkpoint factors such as CTLS-4, PD-1, and PD-L1 explains the immune evasion strategy of the CMS-1 colorectal cancers cells [23]. The inhibitors of immune checkpoint can invert the blockade of immune system and induce an antitumor immunological response. CMS-4 has shown different types of immune infiltration process where

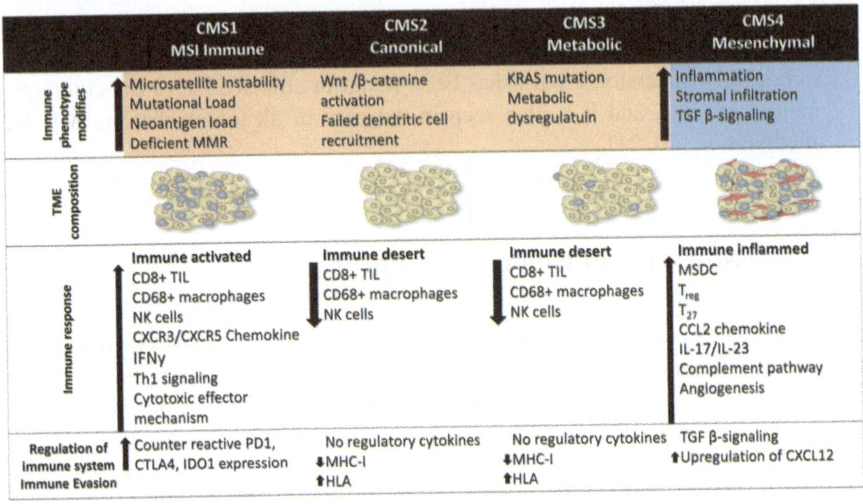

Fig. 2.1 Consensus molecular subtypes (CMS) of colorectal cancer. Immune modifiers can be either genetic origin (orange) or environmental (blue). "[MMR, mismatch repair; TGF-β, transforming growth factor beta; TILs, tumor-infiltrating lymphocytes; NK, natural killer; CXCR3/CCR5, chemokine (C-X-C motif) receptor 3/C-C chemokine receptor type 5; IFNy, interferon gamma; MSDCs, myeloid suppressor-derived cells; CCL2, chemokine (C-C motif) ligand 2; IL-17/IL-23, interleukin 17/interleukin 23; PD1, programmed death protein 1; CTLA4, cytotoxic T-lymphocyte-associated protein 4; IDO1, indoleamine-pyrrole 2,3-dioxygenase; MHC I, major histocompatibility complex 1; HLA, human leukocyte antigens; CXCL12, chemokine (C-X-C-motif) ligand 12]"

regulatory T cells (Treg), myeloid-derived suppressor cells (MDSCs), monocyte-derived cells, and T helper 17 (TH17) cells play a major role [24]. The CMS-4 which is an inflamed-type CMS is generally present in the tumor microenvironment of immune-resistant cancers and has a significantly high level of gene expression for the myeloid cell attracting chemokines along with the myeloid chemokine-chemokine ligand-2 motif, interleukins 17, and interleukin 23 [4]. Hence the possible immunological response in the case of CMS-4 can be blocked by the induction of various pathways in the stroma which supports the inflammatory microenvironment and ultimately decreases the immunological responses against the tumor cells. Here, TGF-β or other physiological activating molecules of the transition of epithelial to mesenchymal tissue and also angiogenesis might be a big player for the immune evasion strategy of tumor cells. Recently it has been experimentally proven in the mouse model that the growth, development, and progression of metastatic cancer in the colon is due to the key factor TGF-β activation in the tumor stroma which suppress the immunological responses [25]. Hence, a therapeutic strategy made of TGF-β and immunological checkpoint inhibitors combination can be able to reactivate immune response against colon cancer in this mouse model system [25]. Compared to CMS-1 and CMS-4, CMS-2 and CMS-3 tumor doesn't have sufficient immune activation and hence called immune desert tumors. A different mechanistic process might be responsible for this such as oncogenic induced cancer cell pathway, less expression or absence of MHC-1, and rise in the expression of HLA. These all together are responsible for immune evasion [25]. Hence there is a need of effective immunotherapeutic strategy to induce immune response especially against CMS-2 and CMS-3.

2.4 Additional Immunological Players in the Colorectal Cancer Microenvironment

Additional immunological subset such as regulatory T cells (Tregs) and macrophages are also associated with the clinical nature of colorectal cancers [26]. These regulatory T cells suppress the T-helper cell subtype-1-mediated immunological responses and also the function of cytotoxic T cell, but amazingly its presence has been associated with the ameliorated prognosis in the case of colorectal cancer, while poor prediction in case of other types to cancers [26–28]. Scientists have concluded that the presence of Tregs in the microenvironment of colorectal cancer is due to the result of immunological responses against cancer cells and tissue, where the TH1 inflammatory response is establishment is followed by the reduction and suppression mechanism to overcome inflammatory response. Saito and his team reported the arguable role of Tregs in the colorectal cancer due to the presence of two distinct but important FOXP3^{+} CD4^{+} T cell populations with opposite physiological functions: the immunosuppressive behavior of Tregs shows high expression of FOXP3 transcription factor and was counterbalanced by the inflammatory nature of FOXP3-low and CD4^{+} T cells in colorectal cancer tissues [29]. A normal semi-quantitative detection technique such as immunohistochemistry cannot differentiate these two subsets. More additional effort is required to analyze and address the individual role of Tregs in the case of colorectal cancers.

Just like the Tregs, the significance of macrophages and its strike in the prognosis of colorectal cancer patients need a clear explanation. On the basis of the phenotype and its physiology, macrophages have been classified into two classes: (i) M1 macrophage synthesizes and releases proinflammatory effector molecules such as TNF-α, nitric oxide (NO), and reactive oxygen species (ROS) which leads to the death of cancer cells [30], and (ii) M2 macrophage comes into the picture in response to the chronic inflammation and mainly responsible for the syntheses and releases of immunosuppressive, proangiogenic factors and the effector which induces cell growth, and these are responsible for pro-tumorigenic role [31]. Tumor associates predominant macrophages belonging to the M2 subset, and its occurrence has been linked with the weak prognosis in different types of cancer [31, 32].

In any case, some clashing reports have likewise exhibited that high macrophage invasion in tumors is related with improved patient endurance, especially in colorectal malignant growth [33, 34]. Such errors might be clarified by the work of particular markers across studies to characterize macrophage populaces or subsets. It is likewise now all around acknowledged that the dichotomization of macrophages into M1 and M2 subtypes is distorted and that these insusceptible cells display high phenotypic versatility [35]. Myeloid-derived suppressor cells (MDSC) are another populace of myeloid cells with phenotypical counterpart to macrophages and granulocytes however with youthful highlights. They are supposed a result from the expression of mature myeloid progenitor cell to ceaseless provocative signs like the ones gave by malignant growth tissues [36]. They have a strong suppressive activity due to the formation of components like arginase or prostaglandin E2 and of suppressing cytokines [36, 37]. Along these lines, their identification in disease patients has constantly been related with poor clinical results [38]. In colorectal malignancy, their quality in both fringe blood and tumor tissues has been related with cutting edge tumor stages [39, 40]. Besides, in metastatic colorectal malignancy patients, high measures of circulating MDSCs were prescient of helpless movement-free endurance following chemotherapy [41]. Like macrophages, the meaning of phenotypes which are discriminative of MDSC subsets has demonstrated testing and exceptionally factor between contemplates. Soon, it is normal that high-dimensional immunophenotyping innovations, for example, single-cell sequencing or multiplex imaging approaches, make significant commitments to propel our insight in this field [42, 43]. In spite of the fact that not part of the invulnerable framework, malignancy-related fibroblasts assume a vital job in the guideline of insusceptible reactions in the disease microenvironment. The investigation of worldwide quality articulation profiles in enormous associates of colorectal malignancy has uncovered four particular agreement sub-atomic subtypes (CMS) with natural and clinical importance [22]. The CMS1 subtype is generally made out of MMR-inadequate colorectal malignant growths with solid immunogenic highlights, while the CMS2 and CMS3 subtypes are related with WNT and MYC flagging initiation and articulated metabolic dysregulation, separately. The CMS4 subtype, thus, totals tumors with transcriptional marks suggestive of mesenchymal phenotypes that are driven by the TGF-β pathway. This subtype contains around one-fourth of every single colorectal malignancy and partners with more awful patient endurance. Critically, the mesenchymal marks that portray the CMS4 subtype are not solely reliant on the transcriptional program of malignancy cells and in any case, rather, are unequivocally determined by the stromal compartment of tumors and, especially, by disease related fibroblasts [44]. The reconstructing of fibroblasts through initiation of the TGF-β pathway brings about a positive-feedback where fibroblasts themselves become primary target of TGF-β, just as of other immunomodulatory particles, in this manner straightforwardly stifling the counter tumor action of natural and versatile impermeable cell compartments [45–47]. Appropriately, the restorative focusing of TGF-β can have a significant effect in the expanding of hostile to tumor insusceptible reactions in colorectal malignancy and other disease models [25, 48]. Besides, a desmoplastic stroma, made out of extracellular lattice proteins and malignancy-related fibroblasts, comprises a physical boundary that blocks the immediate contact among disease and invulnerable cells [49]. The proportion between malignant growth cells and stromal content has been appeared to convey prognostic importance in a few strong tumors, including colorectal disease [50, 51]. Going ahead, it would be critical that reviews planned for giving a complete outline of disease microenvironment represent the fibroblastic compartment. Further, when concentrating on colorectal malignant growth, it is fundamental to recognize the significant contrasts that recognize MMR-inadequate and MMR-capable tumors, especially when performing relationships with clinical boundaries.

2.5 Immunotherapy for Colorectal Cancer

Conventional therapies generally induce immune response against a specific antigen and contribute to the efficacy. Immunotherapy is particularly planned to induce anticancer immunological responses. Different types of strategies against various types of cancer have been evaluated for the active antitumor responses such as induction of immune response by cytokine treatment, immunological checkpoint inhibition, and vaccination. Some other approach for antitumor immunity development is through passive approach in which effector cell of immune system is developed and activated outside the patient's body including monoclonal antibody generation and adoptive T cell transfer against tumor-associated antigen. Till today immunocheckpoint approach is one of the very effective strategies against lung cancer, myeloma, renal carcinoma, melanoma, etc. [52].

In the case of colorectal cancer, infiltration of T cell into the microenvironment of tumor bed has been linked with the beneficial outcome; suggest the potential role for immunoediting in the regulating and managing the initiation, development and progression of tumor [53–55]. Our immune system is able to differentiate between self and non-self-tissues via the binding on the T cell receptor (TCR) present on the T cells surface to the MHC-1, which is present on the cell surface of all the eukaryotic cells including tumor cells. Binding and recognition of only TCR and MHC-1 is not sufficient for the activation of T cell responses. Along with TCR-MHC-1 recognition, it needs some additional association between T cell and MHC-1 containing cells, known as co-stimulatory signal or co-inhibitory signal. Tumor cells use these co-stimulatory signals to escape from the immune system [56, 57]. Immunocheckpoint inhibitors normally attack directly on the co-stimulatory receptors like cytotoxic T lymphocyte antigen 4 (CTLA4) and programmed cell death 1 (PD1) which is present on the surface of T cells and other immune cell subpopulations or its their substrate, like programmed cell death 1 ligand 1 (PDL1) which is present on the surface of tumor cells and various immune cells. Hence, immunological checkpoint inhibitors stop abnormal function of T cell and apoptosis and rather induce T cell activation, increasing the cytotoxic killing of tumor cells. On the basis of pattern of mutation and proportion of markers giving microsatellite instability, the colorectal cancer has been divided into two broad categories. Generally, cancers cells are deficient of MMR (dMMR) with high mutation rate (roughly 100–1000 times higher than normal cells) [58, 59]. Mostly these mutations occur in microsatellite region and hence known as dMMR-MSI-H [60]. Due to its high mutation rate, these dMMR-MSI-H cancers have neoantigens on MHC-1 and TCR along with co-stimulatory signal recognizes then as foreign. Simultaneously there are tumor cell with proficient MMR (pMMR) with very less mutation rates like 8.24 mutation per 106 base pairs [61, 62]. As there are less number of mutation present in the microsatellite region and hence known as pMMR-MSI-L, roughly 15% of colorectal cancer patients fall in the category of dMMR-MSI-H, and this rate decreases along with the cancer stages with approx. 5% of patients with mCRC demonstrating dMMR-MSI-H phenotype. Remaining 95% of the colorectal cases fall into pMMR-MSI-L category [63, 64].

At present a combination of cytotoxic along with the biological agents is the main therapeutic strategy for the management of colorectal cancers. There are a number of factors which influences and affect the treatment choice in colorectal cancer patients along with tumor and patients' characteristics.

The success of immunological checkpoint inhibitors in a high range of high mutated cancer like melanoma has been culminated in their exploration in various kinds of patients having colorectal cancers. Currently only a small group of patients with dMMR colorectal cancer responds positive for immunotherapy, and that is around 4–5% of the colorectal patients. Till today the currently approved immunological checkpoint inhibitors have shown a negative result in the pMMR-MSI-L phenotype which constitutes almost 95% of the colorectal cancer patients. This emphasizes the requirement of an effective and novel therapeutic strategy for such patients. Currently used immunotherapy is being evaluated which includes the combination of immunological checkpoint inhibitors with synthetic medicines, vascular endothelial growth factor inhibitors, cancer vaccines, adoptive cell transfer (ACT), biospecific T cells (BTC), etc. [64, 65]. Initially this cancer was treated as immunologically silent, and hence most of the immunotherapy against colorectal cancer is in early phage of its clinical trials. Now it has been clear that colorectal cancer can also be treated or managed by immunotherapy. Especially tumor caused due to microsatellite instability has shown a positive response for the treatment by anti-PD-1 or PD-L1 treatment. These tumors are targeted by immune system components mediated by immune checkpoint inhibitors as they have a tumor microenvironment which is characterized by the upregulation of immunologic constant of rejection (ICRs) genes and also by immune checkpoint molecules like PD-1, PD-L1, CTLA-4, and IDO [23]. Most of CMS-1 tumors display these characteristics, and hence these tumors are optimal candidate for the checkpoint inhibitions (Table 2.2). Recently the cancer management and treatment with anti-PD-1 has been approved by FDA for the cancers with microsatellite instability and defective MMR. Additionally, combination approach of checkpoint inhibitors with peptide vaccines against tumor-associated antigens (neoantigens) can increase the antitumor immunological responses.

A different scheme is required for the reengage the immune system for the CMS-4 cancer as the mechanism responsible for immunosuppression and already existing immunological cells components are different. A key component for the management of tumor microenvironment is TGF-β signaling and angiogenetic microenvironment, targeting these characteristics required for the conversion to

Table 2.2 Possible immunotherapy strategy for CMS of colorectal cancer

CMS1	CMS2	CMS3	CMS4
Immune checkpoint inhibition (anti-PD-1/PD-L1, anti-CTLA-4, anti-IDO)	Combined EGF pathway inhibition and immune checkpoint inhibition	Combined MEK-inhibitor and immune checkpoint inhibition	Combined TGF pathway inhibition and immune checkpoint inhibition
	Combined HDAC inhibitors and immune checkpoint inhibition	Combined HDAC inhibitors and immune checkpoint inhibition	Combined angiogenesis blockade and immune checkpoint inhibition
Combined neoantigen-based peptide vaccination and immune checkpoint inhibition	Immuno-chemotherapy	Immuno-chemotherapy	
	Passive immunotherapy (DCs vaccines, ACT)	Passive immunotherapy (DCs vaccines, ACT)	Anti-Treg and/or anti-MDSCs treatment

Proposed strategies to apply immunotherapeutic approaches across all types of CRC supported by preclinical or clinical evidence. PD-(L)1: programmed death (ligand) 1, CTLA-4, cytotoxic T-lymphocyte-associated antigen 4, IDO, indoleamine 2,3-dioxygenase, EGFR, epidermal growth factor receptor, HDAC, histone deacetylase, DC, dendritic cell; ACT, adoptive cell transfer; MEK, mitogen-activated protein kinase (MAPK) kinase; Treg, T-regulatory cells; MDSCs, myeloid-derived suppressor cells; TGF transforming growth factor

CMS-1-like immune tumor microenvironment. Experiments suggest that the inhibition of VEGF or TGF-β early in the tumor granuloma formation totally changes the suppressed immune contexture and restore the sensitivity toward immunological checkpoint inhibitors, suggesting that these are molecular drivers of immune responses [66]. Another study conducted in mouse model for mesenchymal CMS, TGF-β with PD-1 have shown synergistic effect [67]. At this moment multiple TGF-β targeted therapies are under various phases of clinical trials for colorectal cancer and the main mechanism of TGF-β taken under consideration is pro-metastatic effect [68]. The further step would be the evaluation of its combination along with the immune checkpoint inhibitors in the clinical trials. A number of clinical trials are being carried for the evaluation of safety and efficacy of combination of bevacizumab (anti-VEGF) along with atezolizumab (anti-PDL-1) in colorectal cancer cases. In case of renal cell carcinoma, a drug molecule sunitinib, which is tyrosine kinase inhibitor, has shown inhibitory effect and stopped myeloid-derived suppressor cells accumulation that leads to the restoration of TH1-type immune response and suppression of Treg cells [69]. The overall effect of Treg cells and suppression of myeloid-derived suppressor cells in the case of colorectal cancer patients and their synergistic combination effect need to be further evaluated.

CMS-2 and CMS-2 are immune desert cancer as they are very weak immunogenic and also devoid of immunological cell infiltrations. To manage and treat these tumors, first it needs to be converted from cold tumor to hot tumor so that it can be targeted by the immune system cells and effector components. One of the reasons for the less immunogenic nature of these cancers is the downregulation of MHC-1 and low presentation of tumor antigen on cell surface with MHC-1. This can be reversed with the help of some factors which can increase the expression of MHC-1, and so the tumor-associated antigen can also be presented [70]. Cobimetinib, an inhibitor for the mitogen-activated protein kinase (MAPK) kinase (MEK/MAP2K), has shown a positive response in the expression of MHC-1 and leads to the accruement of CD8+ cytotoxic T cells in the tumor microenvironment [71]. These MAPK signalling inhibition by cobimetinib is suggested for the KRAS-mutated colorectal cancers which belong to CMS-3. A clinical trial, conducted on 22 patients of metastasis colorectal cancer having mutated KRAS and one with wild type KRAS treated with the combination of cobimetinib and anti-PDL-1, resulted in the four partial responders [72]. Surprisingly, three out of four responders have intact MMR, supporting the combination treatment strategy can be applied in patients other than microsatellite instability colorectal cancer patients. Another property of the weekly infiltrated CMS-2 and CMS-3 cancers is decreased expression of chemokine which attracts cytotoxic T cells. In a preclinical study of various FDA-approved antitumor drugs, histone deacetylase (HDAC) inhibitors were found to induce the expression of T cell attracting multiple chemokines in case of tumor cells, macrophages and T cells that leads to the infiltration of T cell and increases PD-1 sensitivity. A combination approach for the treatment of advanced colorectal cancer with the HDAC inhibitor romidepsin and anti-PD-1 is under the clinical trial phase I and II.

2.6 Conclusion

Colorectal cancer is a wonderful model to analyze and study the genetics of cancer, cancer immunology, and immunotherapy for cancer. The etiological relationship between the gene mutation and anticancer immunological response deeply affects the clinical prognosis and the tumor response for immunotherapy. Since the time of the discovery of the role of immune checkpoint inhibitors in the activation of out immune response, immunotherapy for the cancer management is one of the very novel therapeutic strategies. Fast-moving advancement in the technologies considerably sharpen and deepen our knowledge and understanding for this cancer by favoring whole genome as a source of immunogenic antigens. The checkpoint-based anticancer therapy has reached to a plateau, and hence it can be felt that the anticancer therapy based on immune system and immunological response is novel and effective for the management of colorectal cancers. The use of anti-PD-1, anti-PD-L1 alone, or in combination with the anti-CTLA4 monoclonal antibodies has been a revolution in the field management and treatment of several types of cancers with a maximum efficacy seen in case of melanoma and alveoli cancer. Even in the case of these cancers, immunotherapy does not work evenly in all the patients, and hence the biomarker selection is very important step for the treatment optimization. The immunotherapy has not shown very effective results in the case of colorectal cancer treatment and management. A better understanding of the molecular process of immune competence of colorectal cancer is required for the development of predictive biomarker and better therapeutic combination approach with a better efficacy.

References

1. Ferlay J, Colombet M, Soerjomataram I, Mathers C, Parkin DM, Piñeros M, Znaor A, Bray F. Estimating the global cancer incidence and mortality in 2018: GLOBOCAN sources and methods. Int J Cancer. 2019;144(8):1941–53.
2. Bray F, Ferlay J, Soerjomataram I, Siegel RL, Torre LA, Jemal A. Global cancer statistics 2018: GLOBOCAN estimates of incidence and mortality worldwide for 36 cancers in 185 countries. CA Cancer J Clin. 2018;68(6):394–424.
3. Arnold M, Sierra MS, Laversanne M, Soerjomataram I, Jemal A, Bray F. Global patterns and trends in colorectal cancer incidence and mortality. Gut. 2017;66(4):683–91.
4. Angelova M, Charoentong P, Hackl H, Fischer ML, Snajder R, Krogsdam AM, Waldner MJ, Bindea G, Mlecnik B, Galon J, Trajanoski Z. Characterization of the immunophenotypes and antigenomes of colorectal cancers reveals distinct tumor escape mechanisms and novel targets for immunotherapy. Genome Biol. 2015;16(1):64.
5. Le DT, Durham JN, Smith KN, Wang H, Bartlett BR, Aulakh LK, Lu S, Kemberling H, Wilt C, Luber BS, Wong F. Mismatch repair deficiency predicts response of solid tumors to PD-1 blockade. Science. 2017;357(6349):409–13.
6. Cancer Genome Atlas Network. Comprehensive molecular characterization of human colon and rectal cancer. Nature. 2012;487(7407):330.
7. Rayner E, van Gool IC, Palles C, Kearsey SE, Bosse T, Tomlinson I, Church DN. A panoply of errors: polymerase proofreading domain mutations in cancer. Nat Rev Cancer. 2016;16(2):71.
8. de Miranda NF, Goudkade D, Jordanova ES, Tops CM, Hes FJ, Vasen HF, van Wezel T, Morreau H. Infiltration of Lynch colorectal cancers by activated immune cells associates with early staging of the primary tumor and absence of lymph node metastases. Clin Cancer Res. 2012;18(5):1237–45.
9. Dolcetti R, Viel A, Doglioni C, Russo A, Guidoboni M, Capozzi E, Vecchiato N, Macrì E, Fornasarig M, Boiocchi M. High prevalence of activated intraepithelial cytotoxic T lymphocytes and increased neoplastic cell apoptosis in colorectal carcinomas with microsatellite instability. Am J Pathol. 1999;154(6):1805–13.
10. Munteanu I, Mastalier B. Genetics of colorectal cancer. J Med Life. 2014;7(4):507.
11. Markowitz SD, Bertagnolli MM. Molecular basis of colorectal cancer. N Engl J Med. 2009;361(25):2449–60.
12. Mastalier B, Simion S, Brătucu E. Surgical treatment results in rectal cancer-experience of last 10 years. J Med Life. 2011;4(special issue):68–78.
13. Yan H, Yuan W, Velculescu VE, Vogelstein B, Kinzler KW. Allelic variation in human gene expression. Science. 2002;297(5584):1143.
14. Kinzler KW, Vogelstein B. Colorectal tumors. In: Vogelstein B, Kinzler KW, editors. The genetic basis of human cancer. 2nd ed. New York: McGraw-Hill; 2002. p. 583–612.
15. Vilar E, Gruber SB. Microsatellite instability in colorectal cancer—the stable evidence. Nat Rev Clin Oncol. 2010;7(3):153.
16. Hampel H, Frankel WL, Martin E, Arnold M, Khanduja K, Kuebler P, Nakagawa H, Sotamaa K, Prior TW, Westman J, Panescu J. Screening for the Lynch syndrome (hereditary nonpolyposis colorectal cancer). N Engl J Med. 2005;352(18):1851–60.
17. Boland CR, Goel A. Microsatellite instability in colorectal cancer. Gastroenterology. 2010;138(6):2073–87.

18. Chen WS, Chen JY, Liu JM, King KL, Whang-Peng J, Yang WK. Microsatellite instability in sporadic colon cancer patients with and without liver metastases. Int J Cancer. 1997;74(4):470–4.
19. Lynch HT, Lynch JF, Lynch PM, Attard T. Hereditary colorectal cancer syndromes: molecular genetics, genetic counseling, diagnosis and management. Familial Cancer. 2008;7(1):27–39.
20. Järvinen HJ, Aarnio M, Mustonen H, Aktan-Collan K, Aaltonen LA, Peltomäki P, et al. Controlled 15-year trial on screening for colorectal cancer in families with hereditary nonpolyposis colorectal cancer. Gastroenterology. 2000;118(5):829–34.
21. Weisenberger DJ, Siegmund KD, Campan M, Young J, Long TI, Faasse MA, et al. CpG island methylator phenotype underlies sporadic microsatellite instability and is tightly associated with BRAF mutation in colorectal cancer. Nat Genet. 2006;38(7):787–93.
22. Guinney J, Dienstmann R, Wang X, De Reyniès A, Schlicker A, Soneson C, Marisa L, Roepman P, Nyamundanda G, Angelino P, Bot BM. The consensus molecular subtypes of colorectal cancer. Nat Med. 2015;21(11):1350–6.
23. Becht E, de Reyniès A, Giraldo NA, Pilati C, Buttard B, Lacroix L, et al. Immune and stromal classification of colorectal cancer is associated with molecular subtypes and relevant for precision immunotherapy. Clin Cancer Res. 2016;22(16):4057–66.
24. Dienstmann R, Vermeulen L, Guinney J, Kopetz S, Tejpar S, Tabernero J. Consensus molecular subtypes and the evolution of precision medicine in colorectal cancer. Nat Rev Cancer. 2017;17(2):79–92.
25. Tauriello DV, Palomo-Ponce S, Stork D, Berenguer-Llergo A, Badia-Ramentol J, Iglesias M, Sevillano M, et al. TGFβ drives immune evasion in genetically reconstituted colon cancer metastasis. Nature. 2018;554(7693):538–43.
26. Fridman WH, Zitvogel L, Sautes-Fridman C, Kroemer G. The immune contexture in cancer prognosis and treatment. Nat Rev Clin Oncol. 2017;14(12):717–34.
27. Frey DM, Droeser RA, Viehl CT, Zlobec I, Lugli A, Zingg U, Oertli D, et al. High frequency of tumor-infiltrating FOXP3+ regulatory T cells predicts improved survival in mismatch repair-proficient colorectal cancer patients. Int J Cancer. 2010;126(11):2635–43.
28. Salama P, Phillips M, Grieu F, Morris M, Zeps N, Joseph D, et al. Tumor-infiltrating FOXP3+ T regulatory cells show strong prognostic significance in colorectal cancer. J Clin Oncol. 2009;27(2):186–92.
29. Saito T, Nishikawa H, Wada H, Nagano Y, Sugiyama D, Atarashi K, et al. Two FOXP3+ CD4+ T cell subpopulations distinctly control the prognosis of colorectal cancers. Nat Med. 2016;22(6):679–84.
30. Mantovani A, Sica A, Sozzani S, Allavena P, Vecchi A, Locati M. The chemokine system in diverse forms of macrophage activation and polarization. Trends Immunol. 2004; 25(12):677–86.
31. Qian BZ, Pollard JW. Macrophage diversity enhances tumor progression and metastasis. Cell. 2010;141(1):39–51.
32. Bingle L, Brown NJ, Lewis CE. The role of tumour-associated macrophages in tumour progression: implications for new anticancer therapies. J Pathol. 2002;196(3):254–65.
33. Edin S, Wikberg ML, Dahlin AM, Rutegård J, Öberg Å, Oldenborg PA, et al. The distribution of macrophages with a M1 or M2 phenotype in relation to prognosis and the molecular characteristics of colorectal cancer. PLoS One. 2012;7(10):e47045.
34. Forssell J, Öberg Å, Henriksson ML, Stenling R, Jung A, Palmqvist R. High macrophage infiltration along the tumor front correlates with improved survival in colon cancer. Clin Cancer Res. 2007;13(5):1472–9.
35. Aras S, Zaidi MR. TAMeless traitors: macrophages in cancer progression and metastasis. Br J Cancer. 2017;117(11):1583–91.
36. Veglia F, Perego M, Gabrilovich D. Myeloid-derived suppressor cells coming of age. Nat Immunol. 2018;19(2):108–19.
37. Huang B, Pan PY, Li Q, Sato AI, Levy DE, Bromberg J, et al. Gr-1+ CD115+ immature myeloid suppressor cells mediate the development of tumor-induced T regulatory cells and T-cell anergy in tumor-bearing host. Cancer Res. 2006;66(2):1123–31.

38. Zhang S, Ma X, Zhu C, Liu L, Wang G, Yuan X. The role of myeloid-derived suppressor cells in patients with solid tumors: a meta-analysis. PLoS One. 2016;11(10):e0164514.
39. Sun HL, Zhou X, Xue YF, Wang K, Shen YF, Mao JJ, Guo HF, Miao ZN. Increased frequency and clinical significance of myeloid-derived suppressor cells in human colorectal carcinoma. World J Gastroenterol: WJG. 2012;18(25):3303.
40. Zhang B, Wang Z, Wu L, Zhang M, Li W, Ding J, Zhu J, Wei H, Zhao K. Circulating and tumor-infiltrating myeloid-derived suppressor cells in patients with colorectal carcinoma. PLoS One. 2013;8(2):e57114.
41. Tada K, Kitano S, Shoji H, Nishimura T, Shimada Y, Nagashima K, Aoki K, Hiraoka N, Honma Y, Iwasa S, Okita N. Pretreatment immune status correlates with progression-free survival in chemotherapy-treated metastatic colorectal cancer patients. Cancer Immunol Res. 2016;4(7):592–9.
42. Finotello F, Eduati F. Multi-omics profiling of the tumor microenvironment: paving the way to precision immuno-oncology. Front Oncol. 2018;8:430.
43. Ijsselsteijn ME, Brouwer TP, Abdulrahman Z, Reidy E, Ramalheiro A, Heeren AM, Vahrmeijer A, Jordanova ES, de Miranda NF. Cancer immunophenotyping by seven-colour multispectral imaging without tyramide signal amplification. J Pathol Clin Res. 2019;5(1):3–11.
44. Calon A, Lonardo E, Berenguer-Llergo A, Espinet E, Hernando-Momblona X, Iglesias M, et al. Stromal gene expression defines poor-prognosis subtypes in colorectal cancer. Nat Genet. 2015;47(4):320–9.
45. Hawinkels LJ, Paauwe M, Verspaget HW, Wiercinska E, Van Der Zon JM, Van Der Ploeg K, et al. Interaction with colon cancer cells hyperactivates TGF-β signaling in cancer-associated fibroblasts. Oncogene. 2014;33(1):97–107.
46. Herrera M, Herrera A, Domínguez G, Silva J, García V, García JM, Gómez I, Soldevilla B, Muñoz C, Provencio M, Campos-Martin Y. Cancer-associated fibroblast and M2 macrophage markers together predict outcome in colorectal cancer patients. Cancer Sci. 2013;104(4):437–44.
47. Thomas DA, Massagué J. TGF-β directly targets cytotoxic T cell functions during tumor evasion of immune surveillance. Cancer Cell. 2005;8(5):369–80.
48. Mariathasan S, Turley SJ, Nickles D, Castiglioni A, Yuen K, Wang Y, Kadel EE III, Koeppen H, Astarita JL, Cubas R, Jhunjhunwala S. TGFβ attenuates tumour response to PD-L1 blockade by contributing to exclusion of T cells. Nature. 2018;554(7693):544–8.
49. Elahi-Gedwillo KY, Carlson M, Zettervall J, Provenzano PP. Antifibrotic therapy disrupts stromal barriers and modulates the immune landscape in pancreatic ductal adenocarcinoma. Cancer Res. 2019;79(2):372–86.
50. Huijbers A, Tollenaar RA, Van Pelt GW, Zeestraten EC, Dutton S, McConkey CC, et al. The proportion of tumor-stroma as a strong prognosticator for stage II and III colon cancer patients: validation in the VICTOR trial. Ann Oncol. 2013;24(1):179–85.
51. Vangangelt KM, Van Pelt GW, Engels CC, Putter H, Liefers GJ, Smit VT, Tollenaar RA, Kuppen PJ, Mesker WE. Prognostic value of tumor–stroma ratio combined with the immune status of tumors in invasive breast carcinoma. Breast Cancer Res Treat. 2018;168(3):601–12.
52. Roelands J, Kuppen PJ, Vermeulen L, Maccalli C, Decock J, Wang E, et al. Immunogenomic classification of colorectal cancer and therapeutic implications. Int J Mol Sci. 2017;18(10):2229.
53. Galon J, Costes A, Sanchez-Cabo F, Kirilovsky A, Mlecnik B, Lagorce-Pagès C, et al. Type, density, and location of immune cells within human colorectal tumors predict clinical outcome. Science. 2006;313(5795):1960–4.
54. Pagès F, Berger A, Camus M, Sanchez-Cabo F, Costes A, Molidor R, et al. Effector memory T cells, early metastasis, and survival in colorectal cancer. N Engl J Med. 2005;353(25):2654–66.
55. Galon J, Fridman WH, Pagès F. The adaptive immunologic microenvironment in colorectal cancer: a novel perspective. Cancer Res. 2007;67(5):1883–6.
56. Sharma P, Allison JP. The future of immune checkpoint therapy. Science. 2015;348(6230):56–61.
57. Wei SC, Duffy CR, Allison JP. Fundamental mechanisms of immune checkpoint blockade therapy. Cancer Discov. 2018;8(9):1069–86.

58. Le DT, Uram JN, Wang H, Bartlett BR, Kemberling H, Eyring AD, Skora AD, Luber BS, Azad NS, Laheru D, Biedrzycki B. PD-1 blockade in tumors with mismatch-repair deficiency. N Engl J Med. 2015;372(26):2509–20.
59. Eshleman JR, Lang EZ, Bowerfind GK, Parsons R, Vogelstein B, Willson JK, Veigl ML, Sedwick WD, Markowitz SD. Increased mutation rate at the hprt locus accompanies microsatellite instability in colon cancer. Oncogene. 1995;10(1):33.
60. Overman MJ, Ernstoff MS, Morse MA. Where we stand with immunotherapy in colorectal cancer: deficient mismatch repair, proficient mismatch repair, and toxicity management. Am Soc Clin Oncol Educ Book. 2018;38:239–47.
61. Pawlik TM, Raut CP, Rodriguez-Bigas MA. Colorectal carcinogenesis: MSI-H versus MSI-L. Dis Markers. 2004;20(4, 5):199–206.
62. Salipante SJ, Scroggins SM, Hampel HL, Turner EH, Pritchard CC. Microsatellite instability detection by next generation sequencing. Clin Chem. 2014;60:1192–9.
63. Venderbosch S, Nagtegaal ID, Maughan TS, Smith CG, Cheadle JP, Fisher D, et al. Mismatch repair status and BRAF mutation status in metastatic colorectal cancer patients: a pooled analysis of the CAIRO, CAIRO2, COIN, and FOCUS studies. Clin Cancer Res. 2014;20(20):5322–30.
64. Tabernero J, Melero I, Ros W, Argiles G, Marabelle A, Rodriguez-Ruiz ME, et al. Phase Ia and Ib studies of the novel carcinoembryonic antigen (CEA) T-cell bispecific (CEA CD3 TCB) antibody as a single agent and in combination with atezolizumab: preliminary efficacy and safety in patients with metastatic colorectal cancer (mCRC). J Clin Oncol. 2017;35:3002.
65. Kaufman HL, Lenz HJ, Marshall J, Singh D, Garett C, Cripps C, et al. Combination chemotherapy and ALVAC-CEA/B7. 1 vaccine in patients with metastatic colorectal cancer. Clin Cancer Res. 2008;14(15):4843–9.
66. Courau T, Nehar-Belaid D, Florez L, Levacher B, Vazquez T, Brimaud F, Bellier B, Klatzmann D. TGF-β and VEGF cooperatively control the immunotolerant tumor environment and the efficacy of cancer immunotherapies. JCI Insight. 2016;1(9):e85974.
67. Schaer D, Li Y, Castaneda S, Inigo I, Surguladze D, Xu X, Nugent D, Murphy M, Hall G, Benhadji K, Guba S. Targeting the TGFβ pathway with galunisertib, a TGFβRI SMI, promotes anti-tumor immunity leading to durable, complete responses, as monotherapy and in combination with checkpoint inhibition. J Immunother Cancer. 2015;3(S2):P402.
68. Tauriello DV, Batlle E. Targeting the microenvironment in advanced colorectal cancer. Trends Cancer. 2016;2(9):495–504.
69. Ko JS, Zea AH, Rini BI, Ireland JL, Elson P, Cohen P, et al. Sunitinib mediates reversal of myeloid-derived suppressor cell accumulation in renal cell carcinoma patients. Clin Cancer Res. 2009;15(6):2148–57.
70. Watson NF, Ramage JM, Madjd Z, Spendlove I, Ellis IO, Scholefield JH, Durrant LG. Immunosurveillance is active in colorectal cancer as downregulation but not complete loss of MHC class I expression correlates with a poor prognosis. Int J Cancer. 2006;118(1):6–10.
71. Ebert PJ, Cheung J, Yang Y, McNamara E, Hong R, Moskalenko M, Gould SE, Maecker H, Irving BA, Kim JM, Belvin M. MAP kinase inhibition promotes T cell and anti-tumor activity in combination with PD-L1 checkpoint blockade. Immunity. 2016;44(3):609–21.
72. Bendell JC, Kim TW, Goh BC, Wallin J, Oh DY, Han SW, Lee CB, Hellmann MD, Desai J, Lewin JH, Solomon BJ. Clinical activity and safety of cobimetinib (cobi) and atezolizumab in colorectal cancer (CRC). J Clin Oncol. 2016;34:3502.

Chapter 3
Impact of Covid-19 Pandemic on Gastrointestinal Cancer Patients: An Emphasis on Colorectal Cancer

Krishna Patel, Nuri Hamby, Sohail Siraj, Ananya Kurri, and Riyaz Basha

Abstract Gastrointestinal (GI) cancers originate in the GI track, ranging from the esophagus to rectum. Together, these cancers account for a quarter of cancer incidences and more than a third of cancer-related deaths. Of GI cancers, colorectal cancer (CRC) comprises the largest of GI cancer incidence and death burden. Due to the vast array of GI cancers, the survival rate and risk factors vary. The COVID-19 pandemic began in early December 2019 in Wuhan, China. Originally the virus was reported to the World Health Organization as multiple cases of pneumonia. It was later found to be a novel strain of the coronavirus. Since December, there have been more than 28.3 million cases worldwide spread over 214 countries, and this number is consistently increasing. The main method of transmission of COVID-19 is through respiratory droplets, which has made it very difficult to contain. The incidence of COVID-19 is highest among the adult population with the median age of patients between 34 and 59. However, COVID is more likely to affect those with chronic comorbidities and immunosuppression, such as cancer. Due to the novelty of coronavirus and the vagueness of symptoms (cough, congestion, fever, nausea, vomiting), many clinics have stopped doing unnecessary procedures such as endoscopies and colonoscopies. This has led to a decrease in CRC detection and screening. Delayed screenings can be detrimental to the survival of patients with CRC. It has been shown that surgical delays greater than 7–8 weeks have resulted in lower

K. Patel · S. Siraj
Texas College of Osteopathic Medicine, The University of North Texas Health Sciences Center at Fort Worth, Fort Worth, TX, USA

N. Hamby · A. Kurri
Texas College of Osteopathic Medicine, The University of North Texas Health Sciences Center at Fort Worth, Fort Worth, TX, USA

Department of Pediatrics and Women's Health, Texas College of Osteopathic Medicine, The University of North Texas Health Sciences Center at Fort Worth, Fort Worth, TX, USA

R. Basha (✉)
Department of Pediatrics and Women's Health, Texas College of Osteopathic Medicine, The University of North Texas Health Sciences Center at Fort Worth, Fort Worth, TX, USA
e-mail: Riyaz.Basha@unthsc.edu

G. P. Nagaraju et al. (eds.), *Colon Cancer Diagnosis and Therapy*,
https://doi.org/10.1007/978-3-030-63369-1_3

survival rates. It is vital that medical professionals implement safety protocols and provide safe ways for patients to receive routine checkups.

Keywords Colorectal cancer · COVID-19 · Colonoscopy · Diagnosis

3.1 Introduction

Gastrointestinal (GI) cancers are an abnormal proliferation of cells anywhere along the gastrointestinal tract. The location of GI cancers ranges from the esophagus to the rectum, and as a result, they are the most common type of cancer and the second highest leading cause of cancer-related deaths in the United States (https://www.gicancersalliance.org/resources/gastrointestinal-cancers-an-urgent-need/). Early screenings and surgical intervention are extremely important to the survival of patients diagnosed with GI cancer. The SARS-CoV-2 (COVID-19) pandemic has put a hindrance on screenings and treatment due to hospitals being overloaded with COVID-19 patients. Additionally, newly implemented social distancing and safety guidelines have caused clinics to limit their patient load. This has caused the timeline of diagnosis and treatment to be delayed, which could result in deadly outcomes for some individuals. In the time of COVID-19, it is important to adapt quickly; otherwise it may be the patients who suffer.

GI cancers refer to cancers affecting the following organs: esophagus, stomach, pancreas, biliary system, liver, small intestine, large intestine, rectum, and anus. Cumulatively, the cancers derived from these structures account for a quarter of cancer incidence and more than a third of cancer-related deaths [1].

3.2 Types of GI Cancers

Esophageal cancer (EC): cancer arising from the cells of the esophagus. Two dominant sub-types of EC are esophageal squamous-cell carcinoma (ESCC) and esophageal adenocarcinoma (EAC).

Gastric cancer: cancer affecting the stomach lining. Gastric adenocarcinoma is the most common gastric cancer sub-type [2].

Pancreatic cancer: digestive enzyme producing cells of the pancreas differentiate into ductal cells and develop into ductal adenocarcinoma [3].

Liver cancer: cancer formed from hepatic cells. The two dominant sub-types of liver cancer are hepatocellular carcinoma (HCC) and cholangiocarcinoma [4].

Colorectal cancer (CRC): cancers that develop in the parts of the large intestine, colon, and rectum. Colorectal adenocarcinoma develops from epithelium from the large intestine that has differentiated and become hyperproliferative [5].

3.3 Incidences and Survival Rates

Globally, GI cancers make up 26% of total cancer incidence and 35% of cancer-related deaths in 2018. Teasing out the statistics, colorectal cancers comprise the largest of the GI cancer incident and death burden with 1.8 million new cases (10.2%) and almost three hundred thousand deaths (9.2%) in 2018. Respectively, the incidence and mortality rate for the remaining four major GI cancers: gastric (5.7%, 8.2%), liver (4.7%, 8.2%), esophagus (3.2%, 5.3%), and pancreatic (2.5%, 4.5%) cancers [1].

The five-year relative survival is an estimate of the percentage of patients expected to survive the effects of cancer greater than 5 years after their diagnosis. GI cancers have broad five-year relative survival in the United States. Surveillance, Epidemiology, and End Results and Centers for Disease Control and Prevention US mortality data revealed that from 2010 through 2016 CRC patients showing 64.6% relative survival rate while only 10% of pancreatic cancer patient survival rate during the same period. Relative survival rates for gastric, liver, and esophageal cancer are, respectively, 32.0%, 19.6%, and 19.9%.

3.4 Risk Factors

GI cancer risk factors can be categorized under two big tents: environmental and host-related factors. Environmental factors include soil, air, water, chemical exposures from the home and workplace, lifestyle, and behavioral aspects. Host-related factors are innate traits that increase a host's susceptibility to carcinogenesis [6]. Types of GI cancers, common risk factors for each type of GI cancers, and expected incidence/deaths in 2020 are listed in Table 3.1.

Table 3.1 Information on GI cancer types, risk factors, and incidences/deaths in 2020

Type of gastrointestinal cancer	Esophageal	Gastric	Colorectal	Pancreatic	Liver
Risk factors	Tobacco use Smoked or pickled foods GERD Obesity	*H. pylori* infection Tobacco use Smoked/salted foods Type A blood	Obesity Heavy red meat consumption High BMI High alcohol intake	Heavy alcohol consumption Tobacco use Chronic Pancreatitis Type II diabetes	Hepatitis B Hepatitis Alcoholic liver disease Aflatoxin exposure
Expected incidence/deaths in 2020	18,440/16,170	27,600/11,010	104,610/53,200	57,600/ 47,050	42,810/ 30,160

Types of GI cancers, common risk factors for each type of GI cancers, and expected incidence/deaths in 2020. Data from https://www.cancer.org

Esophageal cancer: ESCC manifests from chronic inflammation and irritation of the cells lining the esophagus [7]. Smoking, frequent consumption of alcohol and/or hot temperature drinks, and a diet heavy in smoked or pickled foods are linked to an increased incidence of ESCC [8]. EAC develops from differentiation of normal mucosal esophageal cells into the premalignant Barrett's esophagus that overtime transitions into esophageal adenocarcinoma [9]. The risk factors associated with EAC are gastroesophageal reflux disease (GERD), smoking, and obesity [9–11].

Similar to EAC, gastric adenocarcinoma develops from chronic inflammation known as gastritis. The most significant risk factor that contributes to gastritis is infection from the bacterium, *Helicobacter pylori*. *H. pylori*-induced inflammation, depending on virulence of pathogen, alters the gastric epithelium and causes gastric lesions and ulceration [12]. These injuries can cause the glandular gastric tissue to become dysplastic and eventually cancerous [13].

Pancreatic cancer's risk factors are not well understood. PC lacks a strong risk factor as compared to other GI cancers. Studies have shown that there is an association between chronic and acute pancreatitis and a subsequent development of PC. Pancreatitis causes precancerous lesions called pancreatic intraepithelial neoplasia (PanIN) to form in the head of the pancreas. PanIn lesions are present in pancreas affected with invasive pancreatic ductal adenocarcinoma. Environmental risk factors for chronic pancreatitis include heavy consumption of alcohol, greater than five drinks per day [14, 15].

HCC is due to cirrhosis induced by infection from either *hepatitis B*, *hepatitis C*, or alcoholic liver disease [16]. Cirrhosis is the profound scarring of the liver that severely limits liver function. Risk factors for HCC can be often high-risk behavior such as unsterile intravenous drug use that could lead to the infection of *hepatitis B* or *hepatitis C* or heavy alcoholic drinking. Aflatoxin exposure due to consumption of food with *Aspergillus flavus* or *Aspergillus parasiticus* mold growth is another risk factor in the development of HCC as it causes cirrhosis with severe acute exposure or chronic low-level exposure [17]. Risk factors for the liver cancer type cholangiocarcinoma is the consumption of improperly cooked fish which may cause a parasitic infestation of liver flukes (a type of flatworm) [18]. Diagnosis of the bile duct inflammatory disease, primary sclerosing cholangitis, is another risk factor for the development of cholangiocarcinoma [19].

In CRC, a considerable proportion of anal squamous cell carcinoma incidence can be directly attributed to precancerous lesions caused by infection from the human papillomavirus virus (HPV) [20]. HPV transmission is made via receptive anal intercourse [21]. Colorectal cancers share risk factors strongly associated with lifestyle such as heavy red and processed meat consumption, high BMI, and high alcohol intake.

3.5 CRC Screening

Routine screening or testing depending on symptoms or family history help to identify the risk of getting CRC or the disease at an early stage. The recommendations of US Multi-Society Task Force of Colorectal Cancer representing the 1. American

Table 3.2 CRC screening methods. The standard and recommended tests for CRC by tier and the frequency for testing

Tier	Recommended test	Recommended frequency
1	Colonoscopy	10 years
	Fecal immunochemical test	Annual
2	CT colonography	5 years
	Fecal DNA test-FIT	3 years
	Flexible sigmoidoscopy	5 or 10 years
3	Capsule colonoscopy	3 years

College of Gastroenterology, 2. American Gastroenterological Association, and 3. American Society for Gastrointestinal Endoscopy clearly outline the guidelines for CRC screening. Screening tests are categorized in in three tiers depending on specific features, performance and costs, etc. The tests include colonoscopy (for every 10 year), fecal immunochemical test (every year), and capsule colonoscopy [22]. Details are in Table 3.2.

3.6 COVID-19

The COVID-19 outbreak began in early December 2019 [23]. The virus was traced back to individuals who visited the Huanan Seafood Wholesale Market in Wuhan City of Hubei Province [24]. Originally the virus was reported to the World Health Organization (WHO) as cases of pneumonia, only to later be identified as a novel strain of the coronavirus. Since then, the virus has quickly spread over much of the world. As of September 2020, more than 200 countries have reported cases of the coronavirus, with total cases estimated to be over 28.3 million and over 911,000 deaths (https://www.cnn.com/interactive/2020/health/coronavirus-maps-and-cases/). In the United States, the trend in the weekly number of COVID-19 cases is depicted in Fig. 3.1.

The main method of transmission between persons is through respiratory droplets from someone actively carrying the virus when they cough or sneeze. The possibility of asymptomatic transmission is still controversial [25]; however fomites have been found to live on surfaces up to 96 hours, and this may significantly contribute to transmission of the virus [26]. The incidence of COVID-19 has been highest among the adult population with the median age of patients between 34 and 59 years [27–30]. Additionally, COVID-19 is more likely to infect those with chronic comorbidities and immunosuppression.

The symptoms of COVID-19 can vary from a mild fever and cough to severe respiratory distress. The most common symptoms include fever, dry cough, chest pain, fatigue, dyspnea, and muscle aches. Other symptoms can include nausea, vomiting, diarrhea, and dizziness [28, 29]. This wide variety of symptoms makes it difficult to distinguish COVID-19 from other respiratory infections. In some patients, the disease can progress to severe respiratory distress and organ failure. This is due to a rise in inflammatory cytokines such as IL2, IL7, IL10, MCP1, and

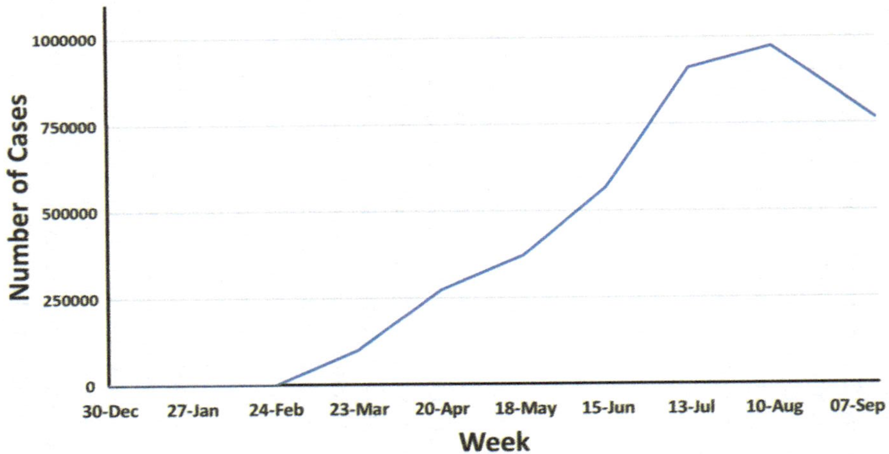

Fig. 3.1 COVID-19 case rates in the United States: In the United States, the COVID-19 cases have been rising quickly since March 2020. Data from the World Health Organization to display that the case rates have slowly started to decline since the end of July, but there is still a long way to go until cases are back to 0. Data from the World Health Organization

TNF alpha [30, 31]. With such an array of presentations, healthcare resources are being used up to care for COVID-19 patients, and as a result, other patient care is being put on the backburner.

3.7 Impact of COVID on Cancer Patients

The novelty of the coronavirus, as well as its quick transmission, has made it difficult to contain viral infection in many countries including the United States. In order to safely care for patients and employees, healthcare facilities are limiting the number of patients they see and are reducing unnecessary procedure for an indefinite period of time [32, 33]. Additionally, hospitals are avoiding transferring patients to hospitals, reducing patient stays in outpatient clinics, and using telecommunication whenever possible [34]. Balancing the continuity of care for cancer patients while at the same time restricting non-COVID related activities in hospitals has become a daily struggle for many healthcare workers [35]. Cancer continues to be the second leading cause of death worldwide, so it is essential to diagnose and treat patients, while it is still in the early stages. Delayed treatment of patients can lead to detrimental outcomes. Safety measures such as masks, sanitizing between patients, maintaining 6 ft distance, and isolating COVID-positive patients have been reinforced to ensure limited spread of the virus in oncology units. It is also advised that surgeries used for staging and diagnosis be replaced with radiologic diagnostic testing whenever possible. However, necessary procedures such as tumor resection for early operable stages should be done with surgical techniques that limit the risk of exposure to caregivers [36].

Due to the COVID-19 pandemic, oncology societies have begun to provide specific recommendations for different tumor types in order to maintain essential cancer care. This involves delaying non-essential imaging in cancer survivors, as well as limiting how often currently treated patients receive therapy [37]. Limited capacity to treat patients has been a common obstacle healthcare facilities face, due mainly to the fact that healthcare resources are being allocated to treat COVID patients. There has been a shortage of hospital bed, ventilators, and healthcare workers. Entire hospitals wings are being taken over to care for severely ill patients, and consequently cancer prevention, screening, and diagnosis have been restricted.

GI cancers in particular have experienced a slowdown in screenings and treatment. As COVID swept across the world, many clinics suspended outpatient services such as endoscopies. Even with the resumption of some services, there is now a backlog of patients that doctors have to see; therefore, most patient's treatment timeline will be delayed. This is mostly due to the fact that primary care doctors have continued to refer patients to GI specialists in the same volume as pre-COVID times. Additionally, PPE shortages have made it difficult to conduct upper GI endoscopies due to the aerosolization of particles [38]. One study in North America showed that 71 out of 73 clinics had postponed endoscopic screening procedures. These numbers vary between countries, but nonetheless delays in screening could result in detrimental outcomes for some patients [39–41]. Research has shown that in colon cancer, delays of over 30–40 days are associated with decreased survival rates. Moreover, for rectal cancer, surgical delays over 7–8 weeks have resulted in lower survival rates [42]. The rate of newly identified cancers during the pandemic has also significantly decreased. In March 2020, the number of newly identified patients with colorectal cancer was around 900 patients per week. As of April 2020, that number is around 500 patients per week. This shows that there has been a decline in cancer screenings during that one-month period alone. Additionally, weekly numbers of six common cancers (breast, colorectal, lung, pancreatic, gastric, and esophageal) decreased by 46.4% combined, which further supports that screening rates are lower [43]. The current recommendations by the American Society for Gastrointestinal Endoscopy state that clinics should strongly consider rescheduling non-urgent endoscopy procedures. Also whenever possible, elective office visits should be held remotely via telemedicine (https://www.asge.org/home/joint-gi-society-message-covid-19).

3.8 Future Perspectives

With the reduction in gastrointestinal screening and diagnostic procedures all around the world due to COVID-19, there is an accumulating population that is at risk for gastrointestinal cancers. The risk of many gastrointestinal cancers going undiagnosed is very high and is continuing to increase with time [40]. It is vital that medical professionals implement safety protocols and provide a safe way for high-risk patients to receive routine checkups and screenings. Studies showed there was roughly an 80% drop in routine screening appointments in March and April when the pandemic hit (https://time.com/5884236/coronavirus-pandemic-cancer-care/). Canceling cancer screenings misses the opportunity to detect the risk or actual disease at an early stage. Medical professionals state that "canceling screening is a bigger concern than the pandemic" (https://time.com/5884236/coronavirus-pandemic-cancer-care/). Telemedicine has exponentially increased since the pandemic hit, and it is essential that patients utilize this new way of accessing healthcare [43]. While people are implementing social distancing, cancer does not halt.

3.9 Conclusion

The COVID-19 pandemic has grown quickly, and it continues to evolve as we move through 2020. As COVID patients fill up hospital wings and use up healthcare resources, many clinical procedures are being halted. Cancer patients are particularly being affected during this time period. All non-urgent procedures such endoscopy or colonoscopy are being rescheduled in order to minimize patient exposure to COVID-19. As a result, there have been a decline in newly diagnosed GI cancers over the past few months. This could be detrimental to the health and survival of GI cancer patients. It is of the utmost importance that a solution be found to both safely and effectively screen and treat for GI cancers or many patients may suffer as a result. While certain asymptomatic cancers lack screening tests to determine the risk at an early stage of the disease, standard and recommended tests are available for screening CRC. Furthermore, CRC is a slowly growing cancer, and early determination highly increases the outcomes in CRC patients. The hesitation of the public to go for routine screenings, as well as the limitations at clinical and surgical facilities to conduct these tests during the pandemic, can potentially impact the diagnosis and treatment of CRC. It should be the priority for the government, healthcare professionals, and organizations to design strategies to overcome the shortfalls and focus on increasing CRC screening and the treatment of cancer patients.

References

1. Arnold M, Abnet CC, Neale RE, Vignat J, Giovannucci EL, McGlynn KA, Bray F. Global burden of 5 major types of gastrointestinal cancer. Gastroenterology. 2020 Jul;159(1):335–49 e15. PubMed PMID: 32247694. Epub 2020/04/06.
2. Duarte HO, Gomes J, Machado JC, Reis CA. Gastric cancer: basic aspects. Helicobacter. 2018;23(Suppl 1):e12523. PubMed PMID: 30277636. Epub 2018/10/03.
3. Greten FR, Weber CK, Greten TF, Schneider G, Wagner M, Adler G, Schmid RM. Stat3 and NF-kappaB activation prevents apoptosis in pancreatic carcinogenesis. Gastroenterology. 2002;123(6):2052–63. PubMed PMID: 12454861. Epub 2002/11/28.
4. Jiang K, Al-Diffhala S, Centeno BA. Primary liver cancers-part 1: histopathology, differential diagnoses, and risk stratification. Cancer Control. 2018;25(1):1073274817744625. PubMed PMID: 29350068. PMCID: PMC5933592. Epub 2018/01/20.
5. Vogelstein B, Fearon ER, Hamilton SR, Kern SE, Preisinger AC, Leppert M, Nakamura Y, White R, Smits AM, Bos JL. Genetic alterations during colorectal-tumor development. N Engl J Med. 1988;319(9):525–32. PubMed PMID: 2841597. Epub 1988/09/01.
6. Manton KG, Akushevich I, Kravchenko J. Cancer mortality and morbidity patterns in the U. S. Population an interdisciplinary approach. New York: Springer Nature; 2009.
7. Arnold M, Soerjomataram I, Ferlay J, Forman D. Global incidence of oesophageal cancer by histological subtype in 2012. Gut. 2015;64(3):381–7. PubMed PMID: 25320104. Epub 2014/10/17.
8. Islami F, Boffetta P, Ren JS, Pedoeim L, Khatib D, Kamangar F. High-temperature beverages and foods and esophageal cancer risk--a systematic review. Int J Cancer. 2009;125(3):491–524. PubMed PMID: 19415743. PMCID: PMC2773211. Epub 2009/05/06.
9. Lagergren J, Bergstrom R, Lindgren A, Nyren O. Symptomatic gastroesophageal reflux as a risk factor for esophageal adenocarcinoma. N Engl J Med. 1999;340(11):825–31. PubMed PMID: 10080844. Epub 1999/03/18.
10. Green JA, Amaro R, Barkin JS. Symptomatic gastroesophageal reflux as a risk factor for esophageal adenocarcinoma. Dig Dis Sci. 2000;45(12):2367–8. PubMed PMID: 11258559. Epub 2001/03/22.
11. Brown LM, Devesa SS. Epidemiologic trends in esophageal and gastric cancer in the United States. Surg Oncol Clin N Am. 2002;11(2):235–56. PubMed PMID: 12424848. Epub 2002/11/12.

12. Jencks DS, Adam JD, Borum ML, Koh JM, Stephen S, Doman DB. Overview of current concepts in gastric intestinal metaplasia and gastric cancer. Gastroenterol Hepatol (N Y). 2018;14(2):92–101. PMCID: PMC5866308. Epub 2018/04/03.
13. Correa P, Piazuelo MB. The gastric precancerous cascade. J Dig Dis. 2012;13(1):2–9. PMCID: PMC3404600. Epub 2011/12/23.
14. Recavarren C, Labow DM, Liang J, Zhang L, Wong M, Zhu H, Wang J, Francis F, Xu R. Histologic characteristics of pancreatic intraepithelial neoplasia associated with different pancreatic lesions. Hum Pathol. 2011;42(1):18–24. PubMed PMID: 21056895. Epub 2010/11/09.
15. Yadav D, Hawes RH, Brand RE, Anderson MA, Money ME, Banks PA, Bishop MD, Baillie J, Sherman S, DiSario J, Burton FR, Gardner TB, Amann ST, Gelrud A, Lawrence C, Elinoff B, Greer JB, O'Connell M, Barmada MM, Slivka A, Whitcomb DC. North American Pancreatic Study G. Alcohol consumption, cigarette smoking, and the risk of recurrent acute and chronic pancreatitis. Arch Intern Med. 2009;169(11):1035–45. PubMed PMID: 19506173. PMCID: PMC6785300. Epub 2009/06/10.
16. Villanueva A. Hepatocellular Carcinoma. N Engl J Med. 2019;380(15):1450–62. PubMed PMID: 30970190. Epub 2019/04/11.
17. Williams JH, Phillips TD, Jolly PE, Stiles JK, Jolly CM, Aggarwal D. Human aflatoxicosis in developing countries: a review of toxicology, exposure, potential health consequences, and interventions. Am J Clin Nutr. 2004;80(5):1106–22. PubMed PMID: 15531656. Epub 2004/11/09.
18. Khan SA, Thomas HC, Davidson BR, Taylor-Robinson SD. Cholangiocarcinoma. Lancet. 2005;366(9493):1303–14. PubMed PMID: 16214602. Epub 2005/10/11.
19. Broome U, Olsson R, Loof L, Bodemar G, Hultcrantz R, Danielsson A, Prytz H, Sandberg-Gertzen H, Wallerstedt S, Lindberg G. Natural history and prognostic factors in 305 Swedish patients with primary sclerosing cholangitis. Gut. 1996;38(4):610–5. PubMed PMID: 8707097. PMCID: PMC1383124. Epub 1996/04/01.
20. de Martel C, Plummer M, Vignat J, Franceschi S. Worldwide burden of cancer attributable to HPV by site, country and HPV type. Int J Cancer. 2017;141(4):664–70. PubMed PMID: 28369882. PMCID: PMC5520228. Epub 2017/04/04.
21. Flejou JF. An update on anal neoplasia. Histopathology. 2015;66(1):147–60. PubMed PMID: 25283345. Epub 2014/10/07.
22. Rex DK, Boland CR, Dominitz JA, Giardiello FM, Johnson DA, Kaltenbach T, Levin TR, Lieberman D, Robertson DJ. Colorectal cancer screening: recommendations for physicians and patients from the U.S. Multi-Society Task Force on Colorectal Cancer. Am J Gastroenterol. 2017;112(7):1016–30. PubMed PMID: 28555630. Epub 2017/05/31.
23. Harapan H, Itoh N, Yufika A, Winardi W, Keam S, Te H, Megawati D, Hayati Z, Wagner AL, Mudatsir M. Coronavirus disease 2019 (COVID-19): a literature review. J Infect Public Health. 2020;13(5):667–73. PubMed PMID: 32340833. PMCID: PMC7142680. Epub 2020/04/29.
24. Lu H, Stratton CW, Tang YW. Outbreak of pneumonia of unknown etiology in Wuhan, China: the mystery and the miracle. J Med Virol. 2020;92(4):401–2. PubMed PMID: 31950516. PMCID: PMC7166628. Epub 2020/01/18.
25. Saichanapan J, Promsuwan K, Limbut W. Adsorption and determination of sibutramine in illegal slimming product using porous graphene ink-modified electrode. Talanta. 2020;212:120788. PubMed PMID: 32113551. Epub 2020/03/03.
26. Kramer A, Schwebke I, Kampf G. How long do nosocomial pathogens persist on inanimate surfaces? A systematic review. BMC Infect Dis. 2006;6:130. PubMed PMID: 16914034. PMCID: PMC1564025. Epub 2006/08/18.
27. Bai Y, Yao L, Wei T, Tian F, Jin DY, Chen L, Wang M. Presumed asymptomatic carrier transmission of COVID-19. JAMA. 2020;323(14):1406–7. PubMed PMID: 32083643. PMCID: PMC7042844. Epub 2020/02/23.
28. Wang D, Hu B, Hu C, Zhu F, Liu X, Zhang J, Wang B, Xiang H, Cheng Z, Xiong Y, Zhao Y, Li Y, Wang X, Peng Z. Clinical characteristics of 138 hospitalized patients with 2019 novel

coronavirus-infected pneumonia in Wuhan, China. JAMA. 2020;323(11):1061–9. PubMed PMID: 32031570. PMCID: PMC7042881. Epub 2020/02/08.

29. Huang C, Wang Y, Li X, Ren L, Zhao J, Hu Y, Zhang L, Fan G, Xu J, Gu X, Cheng Z, Yu T, Xia J, Wei Y, Wu W, Xie X, Yin W, Li H, Liu M, Xiao Y, Gao H, Guo L, Xie J, Wang G, Jiang R, Gao Z, Jin Q, Wang J, Cao B. Clinical features of patients infected with 2019 novel coronavirus in Wuhan, China. Lancet. 2020;395(10223):497–506. PubMed PMID: 31986264. PMCID: PMC7159299. Epub 2020/01/28.
30. Chang LM, Wei L, Xie L, Zhu G, Dela Cruz CS, Sharma L. Epidemiologic and clinical characteristics of novel coronavirus infections involving 13 patients outside Wuhan, China. JAMA. 2020;323(11):1092–3. PubMed PMID: 32031568. PMCID: PMC7042871. Epub 2020/02/08.
31. Singhal T. A review of coronavirus disease-2019 (COVID-19). Indian J Pediatr. 2020;87(4):281–6. PubMed PMID: 32166607. PMCID: PMC7090728. Epub 2020/03/14.
32. Fauci AS, Lane HC, Redfield RR. Covid-19 - navigating the uncharted. N Engl J Med. 2020;382(13):1268–9. PubMed PMID: 32109011. PMCID: PMC7121221. Epub 2020/02/29.
33. Liang W, Guan W, Chen R, Wang W, Li J, Xu K, Li C, Ai Q, Lu W, Liang H, Li S, He J. Cancer patients in SARS-CoV-2 infection: a nationwide analysis in China. Lancet Oncol. 2020;21(3):335–7. PubMed PMID: 32066541. PMCID: PMC7159000. Epub 2020/02/19.
34. National University Cancer Institute of Singapore Workflow T. A segregated-team model to maintain cancer care during the COVID-19 outbreak at an academic center in Singapore. Ann Oncol. 2020;31(7):840–3. PubMed PMID: 32243893. PMCID: PMC7174823. Epub 2020/04/04.
35. Persad G, Phillips J, Emanuel EJ. Allocating medical resources in the time of Covid-19. Reply N Engl J Med. 2020;382(22):e79. PubMed PMID: 32343503. Epub 2020/04/29.
36. Raymond E, Thieblemont C, Alran S, Faivre S. Impact of the COVID-19 outbreak on the management of patients with cancer. Target Oncol. 2020;15(3):249–59. PubMed PMID: 32445083. PMCID: PMC7243433. Epub 2020/05/24.
37. Ueda M, Martins R, Hendrie PC, McDonnell T, Crews JR, Wong TL, McCreery B, Jagels B, Crane A, Byrd DR, Pergam SA, Davidson NE, Liu C, Stewart FM. Managing Cancer care during the COVID-19 pandemic: agility and collaboration toward a common goal. J Natl Compr Cancer Netw. 2020;20:1–4. PubMed PMID: 32197238. Epub 2020/03/21.
38. Verma AM, Nagpal JK. Gastrointestinal cancer pathways may breakdown due to COVID-19. Frontline Gastroenterol. 2020;11(5):413. PubMed PMID: 32879723. PMCID: PMC7447284. Epub 2020/09/04.
39. Maida M. Screening of gastrointestinal cancers during COVID-19: a new emergency. Lancet Oncol. 2020;21(7):e338. PubMed PMID: 32615111. PMCID: PMC7324111. Epub 2020/07/03.
40. Lee YC, Fann JC, Chiang TH, Chuang SL, Chen SL, Chiu HM, Yen AM, Chiu SY, Hsu CY, Hsu WF, Wu MS, Chen HH. Time to colonoscopy and risk of colorectal cancer in patients with positive results from fecal immunochemical tests. Clin Gastroenterol Hepatol. 2019;17(7):1332–40 e3. PubMed PMID: 30391435. Epub 2018/11/06.
41. Forbes N, Smith ZL, Spitzer RL, Keswani RN, Wani SB, Elmunzer BJ. North American Alliance for the study of digestive manifestations of C. Changes in gastroenterology and endoscopy practices in response to the coronavirus disease 2019 pandemic: results from a North American Survey. Gastroenterology. 2020;159(2):772–4 e13. PubMed PMID: 32376410. PMCID: PMC7196540. Epub 2020/05/08.
42. Fligor SC, Wang S, Allar BG, Tsikis ST, Ore AS, Whitlock AE, Calvillo-Ortiz R, Arndt KR, Gangadharan SP, Callery MP. Gastrointestinal malignancies and the COVID-19 pandemic: evidence-based triage to surgery. J Gastrointest Surg. 2020;24(10):2357–73. PubMed PMID: 32607860. PMCID: PMC7325836. Epub 2020/07/02.
43. Kaufman HW, Chen Z, Niles J, Fesko Y. Changes in the number of US patients with newly identified cancer before and during the coronavirus disease 2019 (COVID-19) pandemic. JAMA Netw Open. 2020;3(8):e2017267. PubMed PMID: 32749465. PMCID: PMC7403918. Epub 2020/08/05.

Chapter 4
Role of NMR Metabolomics and MR Imaging in Colon Cancer

Pradeep Kumar and Virendra Kumar

Abstract Colon cancer is clinically challenging, heterogeneous, and among the most frequently diagnosed malignancies. The screening for colon cancer is carried out by using procedures such as colonoscopy, sigmoidoscopy, fecal occult blood test, and virtual colonoscopy. These screening methods have some limitations like invasiveness and low sensitivity and specificity. Nuclear magnetic resonance (NMR) metabolomics may play an important role in colon cancer by providing noninvasive metabolite signatures and understanding its metabolism. Metabolic reprogramming is one of the hallmarks of cancer, including deregulated uptake of glucose and amino acids, opportunistic modes of nutrient acquisition, and utilizing glycolysis and tricarboxylic acid (TCA) cycle intermediates providing selective advantage during initiation and progression of cancer. Oncometabolites refer to metabolites which show a marked increase in levels in cancers, like D-2-hydroxyglutarate, L-2-hydroxyglutarate, succinate, and fumarate. Magnetic resonance imaging (MRI) techniques, in particular, dynamic contrast-enhanced MRI (DCE-MRI) and diffusion-weighted imaging (DWI) have shown potential to study angiogenesis and water diffusion-based parameters, respectively. Additionally, these methods are not only useful for early diagnosis and therapy monitoring and staging of cancer but also for the identification of new therapeutic targets and designing new treatment strategies. In this chapter, we discuss the current state of NMR metabolic profiling and MRI in colon cancer.

Keywords Colon cancer · Metabolomics · NMR · MRI · Oncometabolites

---

P. Kumar · V. Kumar (✉)
Department of NMR and MRI Facility, All India Institute of Medical Sciences, New Delhi, India

G. P. Nagaraju et al. (eds.), *Colon Cancer Diagnosis and Therapy*,
https://doi.org/10.1007/978-3-030-63369-1_4

Abbreviations

1D	One dimensional
2D	Two dimensional
ADC	Apparent diffusion coefficient
ATP	Adenosine triphosphate
AUC	Area under the receiver operating characteristic curve
COSY	Correlation spectroscopy
CT	Computed tomography
DCE	Dynamic contrast enhanced
DNA	Deoxyribonucleic acid
DWI	Diffusion-weighted imaging
FDG	Fluorodeoxyglucose
Gd-EOB-DTPA	Gadolinium ethoxybenzyl diethylenetriamine pentaacetic acid
HRMAS	High-resolution magic angle spinning
MRI	Magnetic resonance imaging
NMR	Nuclear magnetic resonance
NOESY	Nuclear overhauser enhancement spectroscopy
OPLS-DA	Orthogonal partial least squares – discriminant analysis
PCA	Principal component analysis
PET	Positron emission tomography
PLS	Partial least squares
PLS-DA	Partial least squares – discriminant analysis
RNA	Ribonucleic acid
TCA cycle	Tricarboxylic acid cycle

4.1 Introduction

Colon cancer is one of the top five most common cancers diagnosed and cause of cancer-related deaths globally [4, 99]. Incidence of colon cancer is higher in developed countries compared to developing countries; however, recent data shows an increasing incidence and mortality in many low- and middle-income countries [17, 109]. Apart from geographical variations, colon cancer may show a wide variation in demographic and histological features [93]. In the Indian population, some differences in presentation of colon cancer compared to the West are younger age, more signet ring tumors, and more left-sided tumors [93]. Colon cancer is more common in men than in women, and its development is a slow progression from adenoma to carcinoma, involving an interplay of many factors like genetic and epigenetic mutations, diet, lifestyle, and presence of other conditions like diabetes [17, 93, 99].

The clinical investigations used for screening and diagnosis of colon cancer mainly include colonoscopy, computed tomography (CT) colonography (or virtual colonoscopy), sigmoidoscopy, fecal occult blood test, and fecal immunochemical test [13, 21, 129]. Screening for colon cancer is recommended for people above 45 years of age. Colonoscopy uses a colonoscope to look for polyps or cancer and requires sedation. CT colonography is usually advised as an alternative to colonoscopy for patients having contraindications for colonoscopy like risk of anesthesia or blockage in colon. Sigmoidoscopy is used for the rectum and lower part of the colon. Fecal occult blood test and fecal immunochemical test, guaiac and immunochemical tests, respectively, are performed to detect the presence of hemoglobin in stool. These fecal tests when performed every 2 or 3 years for individuals above 50 years may reduce the cases of colon cancer, about 15–33% [129]. These screening and diagnostic methods are either invasive or have limited sensitivity and specificity. For definitive diagnosis of colon cancer, biopsy is recommended. However, some other investigations like magnetic resonance imaging (MRI), positron emission tomography (PET), or PET-CT scan may also be included for diagnosis of colon cancer.

Colonoscopy and sigmoidoscopy are the most effective methods; however, they are invasive with potential risk of postoperative complications [13, 98, 108, 129]. Therefore, mainly due to limitations of the screening and diagnostic methods, only 40% of the patients with colon cancer are diagnosed and treated at early stage [129].

Clinical imaging modalities having potential role in screening, diagnosis, staging, treatment, and follow-up of colon cancer are CT, MRI, and PET-CT, and their use has significantly evolved over the last 20 years [30, 51, 75, 122]. CT is anatomical imaging while PET-CT is functional imaging. MRI is capable of providing anatomical and functional information with superior soft tissue contrast compared to other imaging modalities. Fluorodeoxyglucose (FDG)-PET-CT and functional MRI techniques may provide insights into tumor perfusion and metabolic and molecular phenotypes [115]. Functional imaging investigations provide data on tumor parameters which are not only helpful for clinical management but also to understand the underlying mechanisms of tumor physiology and progression, for example, response to chemotherapy [115].

Metabolomics is the study of small biomolecules in tissues and body fluids to identify metabolic changes associated with a disease. According to Daviss, metabolomics is the "systematic study of unique chemical fingerprints that specific cellular processes leave behind" [28]. The metabolome refers to the total metabolite pool of a biological system like a cell or biofluid [54, 89, 121]. Ideally, metabolomics aims toward identification and quantification of maximum number of metabolites in a given sample. The data from metabolomics studies could generate indispensable information not provided by genomics and proteomics studies which may also be used for systems biology approach [85, 86]. Metabolomics approaches are of two broad types, first, targeted, in which a particular metabolic mechanism or hypothesis is tested related to biochemical pathways, and second, untargeted, in which an attempt is made to detect and analyze as many metabolites as possible.

Nuclear magnetic resonance (NMR) spectroscopy is one of the preferred analytical methods of detection and quantification of metabolites for metabolomics studies of cancer [20, 116, 133, 134, 137]. NMR can be used to study atoms like ^{1}H, ^{13}C, and ^{31}P; however, ^1H (^1H-NMR) is the most commonly and extensively applied technique in cancer studies due to its high sensitivity and natural abundance. NMR spectrum acquired from a biological sample not only detects numerous metabolites but also allows determination of concentration of metabolites. Moreover, NMR requires very minimal sample preparation steps.

Metabolomics studies of colon cancer patients have reported the potential role of NMR metabolomics in detection and prognosis [84, 117]. With the currently available methods of investigations for screening and diagnosis of colon cancer, many of patients have to undergo invasive procedures. In this view, metabolomics provides an attractive noninvasive approach that serves not only as a clinical tool for better screening, diagnosis, and treatment monitoring and to distinguish between benign and aggressive metastatic forms of colon cancer but also a means to get insight into biochemical processes associated with malignancy. In the present chapter, we will describe the potential role of ^1H-NMR metabolomics and MRI in colon cancer.

4.2 NMR Metabolomics and MR Imaging

NMR and MRI can be used to study colon cancer. NMR is helpful for the detection of metabolites and metabolomics studies, while MRI provides structural and functional parameters. MR methods may be applied for in vitro experiments and preclinical and clinical studies of colon cancer. The imaging and metabolic information thus acquired may help to understand colon cancer initiation, progression, metastasis, and response to therapy.

A typical one dimensional (1D) ^1H-NMR experiment comprises a single pulse with solvent pre-saturation. Processing of NMR data comprises four main steps: Fourier transformation, phase correction, baseline correction, and calibration. At higher magnetic field strengths and optimum metabolic concentrations, well-resolved spectra can be obtained, and direct quantitation of the various metabolites from the assigned spectra can be achieved. However, the spectrum acquired from biological samples by 1D NMR experiment is often crowded with overlapping peaks and poses difficulty in the assignment of resonance peaks to molecules unambiguously, due to chemical species with similar resonance frequencies [16, 91, 123]. This problem can be overcome by two-dimensional (2D) NMR experiments, where the data is collected along two axes.

2D NMR spectroscopy allows molecules to be assigned based on the coupling between the nuclear dipoles. The 2D spectrum has two frequency axes (F_1 and F_2), which are obtained after Fourier transformation with respect to the time domain functions S (t_1, t_2). The 2D NMR experiment consists of a series of 1D experiment in which the time interval, t_1, is incremented at regular time intervals and free induction decay signals acquired for each experiment are recorded during the time interval, t_2, as in the 1D spectrum. 2D NMR methods reduce the spectral complexity for identifying metabolites. Different kinds of information can be obtained from a 2D NMR experiment based on the type of 2D NMR experiment, for example, correlation spectroscopy (COSY) and nuclear overhauser enhancement spectroscopy (NOESY). COSY and NOESY and 2D NMR experiments give information on the structure of the molecule by analyzing the connectivity between the nuclei based on the couplings between magnetic nuclei. These can be dipolar (through space) determined by NOESY or scalar (through bond) couplings determined by the COSY experiment [10, 41, 112].

4.3 Metabolomics Analysis

Biological samples are complex mixtures of many molecules; therefore, their NMR spectra contain numerous signals (resonance peaks), many of them remain unassigned to particular molecules in 1D NMR. Besides, metabolomics studies are carried out on a large number of samples. This poses a challenge for analysis and interpretation of NMR data. Therefore, bioinformatics and chemometrics methods are being adopted and developed for analyzing NMR metabolomics data. These methods consist of data reduction methods, pattern recognition, and clustering algorithms to identify differences among groups of samples. Such analysis may include binning and normalization of NMR data, principal component analysis (PCA), partial least squares (PLS), PLS-discriminant analysis (PLS-DA), or orthogonal PLS-discriminant analysis (OPLS-DA) [131, 132]. Few databases have been established to help in the identification of metabolites like Human Metabolome Database. Due to complexity of the data and computationally intensive statistics, there is work toward development of software tools for such analysis like MetaboAnalyst and Kyoto Encyclopedia of Genes and Genomes pathway analysis [8].

PCA is an unsupervised statistical analysis method which has been extensively used in metabolomics analysis of NMR data. PLS, OPLS, and OPLS-DA are supervised methods in which the relationship between two data matrices X and Y are sought. Among them X is the matrix consisting of the descriptor variables (such as the profile from NMR spectroscopy) and Y is the response variable(s), containing quantitative or qualitative variables [119, 131]. Such a procedure can also be employed in discriminate analysis where Y defines two distinct classes.

4.4 Metabolic Reprogramming and Oncometabolites in Colon Cancer

"Metabolic rewiring" is one of the hallmarks of cancer and provides selective advantage during initiation and progression of tumors [15, 32, 38, 95, 128]. Within the process of metabolic rewiring, Pavlova and Thompson describe six major changes observed: deregulated uptake of glucose and amino acids, opportunistic modes of nutrient acquisition, utilizing glycolysis and tricarboxylic acid (TCA)

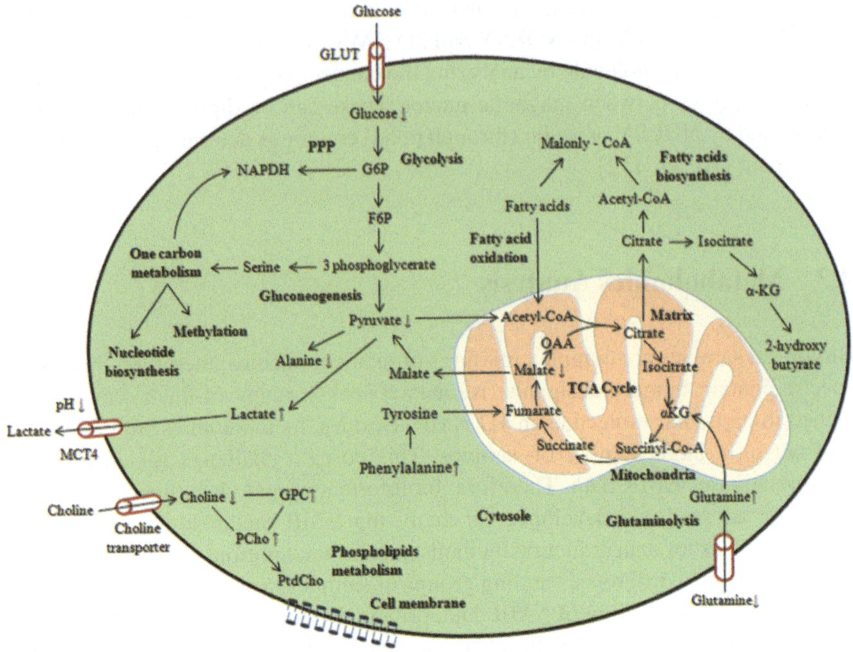

Fig. 4.1 Diagrammatic representation of metabolic reprogramming in colorectal cancer with alterations of levels of some of the metabolites involved (increase,↑; decrease, ↓). PPP pentose phosphate pathway, G6P glucose-6-phosphate, F6P fructose-6-phosphate, PC phosphocholine, GPC glycerophosphocholine, OAA oxaloacetate, TCA cycle tricarboxlylic acid cycle, PtdCho phosphatidylcholine, α-KG α-ketoglutarate, GLUT glucose transporter, MCT4 monocarboxylate transporter 4

cycle intermediates, increased nitrogen demand, alterations in metabolic-driven gene regulation, and metabolic interactions with the micro-environment [38, 95]. Figure 4.1 shows diagrammatic representation of some important metabolic pathways and alterations reprogrammed in cancer cells. One of the earliest reports on metabolic change associated with cancer cells was the over-utilization of glucose even in presence of oxygen by Otto Warburg, known as "Warburg effect" [127]. The FDG-PET is based on a high rate of uptake of glucose by cancer cells and is a validation of Warburg's observation. Rapidly proliferating cancer cells require biomolecules to support their growth, and some of the intermediates of glycolysis are utilized for this purpose [60]. For example, glucose-6-phosphate, fructose-6-phosphate, and glyceraldehyde-3-phosphate are converted to ribose-5-phosphate in the pentose phosphate pathway [60]. Glyceraldehyde-3-phosphate is utilized to synthesize phospholipids to generate biomembranes [60]. The pyruvate produced during aerobic glycolysis is converted to lactate by the enzyme lactate dehydrogenase-5 [37].

Oncometabolites refer to metabolites which show a marked alteration in their levels in cancers compared to levels in normal cells [32, 128, 135]. To differentiate metabolic reprogramming and oncometabolites, DeBerardinis and Chandel propose that "the term metabolic reprogramming be used to describe conventional metabolic pathways whose activities are enhanced or suppressed in tumor cells relative to benign tissues as a consequence of tumorigenic mutations and/or other factors" [32]. The term oncometabolites be "reserved metabolites for (i) there is a clear mechanism connecting a specific mutation in the tumor to accumulation of the metabolite, and (ii) there is compelling evidence for involvement of the metabolite in the development of malignancy" [32]. Currently, there are only few oncometabolites identified in cancer metabolism which include D-2-hydroxyglutarate, L-2-hydroxyglutarate, succinate, and fumarate [25, 32, 135]. D-2-hydroxyglutarate is a reduced form of TCA cycle intermediate α-ketoglutarate [32, 135]. It is found in trace amounts in normal tissues, however, rises to millimolar concentrations in tumors with mutations in isocitrate dehydrogenase 1 or 2 [25, 32, 128, 135]. Similarly, succinate and fumarate are intermediates of TCA cycle; however, some tumors accumulate high levels of these metabolites [25, 32, 128, 135].

Glutamine is the important nutrient other than glucose required by cells for their growth. Glutamine provides carbon intermediates for synthesis of macromolecules, and being a nitrogen containing molecule, supporting amino acid pool and nucleotide biosynthesis [3, 31, 38]. Additionally, it also participates in cell-signaling and gene expression [31]. Cancer cells channelize glutamine to enter the TCA cycle in a process termed anaplerosis [61]. Like the Warburg effect of glucose, this glutamine metabolic phenotype is common to numerous different cancer types including colon cancer [61, 76]. Mitochondria take up glutamine, and there it is converted to α-ketoglutarate by either glutamate dehydrogenase or amino acid transaminases [3, 31, 32, 38, 95]. Another anaplerotic substrate is oxaloacetate, which enters into TCA cycle, produced by carboxylation of pyruvate catalyzed by pyruvate carboxylase [95]. Glutaminase-1 and glutamate dehydrogenase are upregulated in colon cancer and correlate with tumor carcinogenesis and poor prognosis [49, 67, 110].

Reprogrammed fatty acid metabolism is another important hallmark of various cancers [6, 9, 57, 101]. Cancer cells rewire fatty acid metabolism by various mechanisms including alterations in fatty acid transport, de novo lipogenesis, and β-oxidation to generate adenosine triphosphate (ATP) [57]. This is in contrast to normal cells, which preferentially use circulating fatty acids derivative from diets, and de novo lipogenesis is restricted to hepatocytes and adipocytes [104]. De novo lipogenesis is the process of synthesis of fatty acids from molecules like glucose or glutamine. However, cancer cells may continue de novo lipogenesis even in the presence of exogenous lipid sources [57]. Citrate or acetate can be converted to acetyl-CoA for fatty acid synthesis [9, 101]. The conversion of citrate and acetate to acetyl-CoA is catalyzed by enzyme adenosine triphosphate (ATP)-citrate lyase andacetyl-CoA synthetase 2, respectively [57, 101]. Upregulation of de novo lipogenesis allows cancer cells to redirect fatty acids for various purposes like signaling lipids and synthesis of phospholipids and cholesterol and to be stored as lipid droplets to generate energy [23, 27, 57, 101, 136]. Elevated levels of lipid droplets have been reported in colon cancer cells facilitating prostaglandin E2synthesis from arachidonic acid [1, 81]. Lipid biogenesis pathways have been associated with colon cancer epithelial mesenchymal invasion, progression, and metastasis cascade [26, 103].

Colon adenocarcinoma and several other cancers have been reported to reprogram one carbon metabolism [5, 46, 68, 83, 105, 125, 138]. Proliferating cells require constant supply of substrates for nucleotide synthesis for which one carbon unit is necessary to synthesize purine and pyrimidine nucleotides [125]. Therefore, cancer cells have a large demand for one-carbon units for synthesis of deoxyribonucleic acid (DNA) and ribonucleic acid (RNA). One carbon metabolism can be divided into three pathways: the folate cycle, methionine cycle, and trans-sulfuration pathway [125]. In the folate cycle, serine, glycine, and threonine donate carbon to convert tetrahydrofolate to 5-methyl tetrahydrofolate and homocysteine to methionine [125]. Methionine is converted to S-adenocylmethionine by adenylation. S-adenocylmethionine has been reported to be the most upregulated metabolite in colon cancer across all tumor stages [102]. Phosphoglycerate dehydrogenase redirects 3-phosphoglycerate from glycolysis into the serine biosynthetic pathway in colorectal tumors compared to adjacent normal tissue and is correlated with advanced stage and size [53, 66, 71, 73].

A complex relationship arising from cross-communication between metabolic pathways, gut microbiota, diet, genetics and other environmental factors affects colon cancer initiation, progression, and invasion [14, 39, 87, 118]. The role of bacterial metabolites, especially butyrate, has been studied in relation to colon cancer [39, 87, 118]. Butyrate is a short-chain fatty acid, and it is produced when dietary fiber is fermented in the colon. However, with the currently available data, the role of butyrate is not clearly understood, and the butyrate paradox remains open for further studies.

4.5 Metabolic Profiling in Biofluids and Tissue Samples in Colon Cancer

Changes in the metabolites and their levels observed in biofluids (e.g., blood, urine) and tissues samples are a result of underlying physiological and pathological changes. In colon or colorectal cancer, blood, urine, and fecal samples are most widely used for metabolomics studies (Table 4.1). In particular urine is frequently used by metabolomics researchers [12], because it is easy to collect in large volumes and may provide diagnostic information for many cancer types [70, 114], including colon cancer [97]. For many of such studies, NMR spectroscopy is a method of choice because it involves minimal interference with original samples with high reproducibility and avoid separation or derivatization steps [111].

Metabolomics studies of tissues in patients with colorectal cancer have revealed changes in lactate, amino acids, fatty acids carboxylic acids, and urea cycle metabolites compared to normal tissues [117, 124]. Metabolomics profile of serum from colorectal cancer patients showed abnormal, tumor-associated proline metabolism,

Table. 4.1 Altered metabolite levels (increase,↑; decrease, ↓) identified in colorectal tissue and blood, urine, and fecal samples in colorectal patients

Metabolite	NMR-based metabolomics study			
	Blood	Urine	Fecal	Tissue
3 hydroxybutyrate	↑			
Acetate	↑	↑		↑
Formate	↑			
Phenylalanine	↑	↓		
Proline	↑		↑	
Glycoprotein	↑			
Lactate	↑		↑	↑
Pyruvate	↓			
Alanine	↓	↓	↑	
Glutamine	↓	↑	↓	↑
Creatinine		↓		↑
Choline		↓		
Dimethyl sulfone		↓		
Asparagine		↓		
Isocitrate		↓		
Hippurate		↓		
Cysteine		↓		
Taurine		↓		
Short-chain fatty acids			↓	
Glucose			↓	↓
Succinate			↑	
Isoleucine			↑	
Valine			↑	
Leucine			↑	↑
Glutamate			↑	↑
Dimethylglycine			↑	↑
Glycine			↓	
Myo-inositol				↑
Scyllo-inositol				↑
Phosphocholine				↑
Malate				↓
Phoshoethanolamine				↑
Glycerophosphocholine				↑

glycolysis, fatty acid metabolism, arginine metabolism, and oleamide metabolism [35]. Fecal metabolomics study showed increased glycolysis and glutaminolysis and nutrient malabsorption and disrupted bacterial ecology in patients with colorectal cancer [63].

4.5.1 Blood Samples

Blood is the medium for the circulation of many small biomolecules. Therefore, it may be assumed that the effect of many pathologies is evident as an alteration of metabolite levels in the blood. Usually, it is preferred to collect blood samples in the morning after overnight fasting otherwise required by specific design and objectives of the study. However, it should be noted that many factors other than disease may be associated with changes in metabolic profile like environmental factors.

In a multi-centric study of metastatic colorectal cancer using NMR metabolomics, Bertini et al. [11] segregated patients with metastatic colorectal cancer from healthy subjects with a cross-validated accuracy of 100%, using serum metabolomics profile. The study concluded that NMR metabolomic profiling of serum in patients with metastatic colorectal cancer provides a strong metabolomic signature which can be used as a tool to predict overall survival [11]. Specifically, the levels of 3-hydroxybutyrate, acetate, formate, glycerol, phenylalanine, proline, lipids, and glycoproteins were higher in patients with metastatic colorectal cancer compared to healthy subjects. However, the levels of metabolites like lactate, pyruvate, alanine, and glutamine were decreased in patients with metastatic colorectal cancer, and there was no change in glucose levels compared to healthy subjects. These findings of Bertini et al. were in contrast with other earlier studies that reported high levels of lactate [11].

Gu et al. [43] used NMR metabolomics of serum samples obtained from patients with colorectal polyps, colorectal cancer, and healthy controls. They reported activation of pyruvate and glycerolipid metabolism in patients with colorectal polyps and glycolysis, glycine, serine, and threonine metabolism in patients with colorectal cancer. These activations of metabolism may play an important role in promoting cellular proliferation in colorectal cancer. The metabolic rates of acetate/glycerol and lactate/citrate in colorectal polyp and colorectal cancer, respectively, were suggested as biomarkers [43]. Ghini et al. studied the effect of general anesthesia drugs, etomidate, and propofol on the blood plasma metabolic profile of patients with non-metastatic colorectal cancer and metastatic colorectal cancer with liver metastasis using NMR spectroscopy [40]. In the study, NMR-detectable metabolites were significantly decreased; hence, it is not suggested to use samples collected during anesthesia for metabolomics studies. Nevertheless, the study showed that plasma metabolomics could represent a valuable tool to monitor the effect of different anesthesia drugs and/or the individual metabolic response to anesthesia [40].

4.5.2 Urine Samples

Several studies have demonstrated a correlation between colorectal cancer and perturbed urinary metabolomics profiles [22, 97]. Aimed toward the early diagnosis of colorectal cancer to improve outcomes, an NMR metabolomics study of urine samples in patients with colorectal cancer was carried out by Wang et al. [126]. Metabolic signature profiles obtained from urine samples distinguished all colorectal stages from healthy controls and showed a distinctive urinary metabolomic profile of stage I and II colorectal cancer patients. The levels of following metabolites were increased, acetoacetate, glutamine, guanidoacetate, cis-aconitate, trans-aconitate, and homocysteine; however, levels of creatinine, choline, dimethyl sulfone, asparagine, alanine, methylamine, isocitrate, hippurate, cysteine, and phenylalanine were decreased in stage I and II colorectal cancer patients compared to healthy controls [126]. A total of 16 potential metabolic biomarkers were identified in stage I and II colorectal cancer, involved in amino acid metabolism, glycolysis, TCA cycle, urea cycle, choline metabolism, and gut microbiota metabolism pathway deregulation [126]. Further, in this study, the authors identified urinary metabolomic differences in early-stage colorectal cancer samples compared to esophageal cancer. This finding highlights the metabolic differences between upper and lower gastrointestinal cancers. Overlapping metabolites may be due to contributions resulting from common process of tumorigenesis and gut mircobiota [126].

A recent study by Kim et al. explored the potential role of urine NMR metabolomics for the early detection of colorectal cancer [55]. Metabolomics profile of advanced adenoma, stage 0 colorectal cancers, and colorectal cancer at various stages were studied [55]. For the diagnosis of pre-invasive colorectal neoplasia, sensitivity, 96.2%, and specificity, 95%, were reported [55]. OPLS-DA model was used to predict the grades with area under the receiver operating characteristic curve (AUC) for taurine, 0.823; alanine,0.783; and 3-aminoisobutyrate, 0.842 [55]. It is noteworthy to mention that development of predictor models based on metabolomics data may help in the clinical management of colorectal patients.

4.5.3 *Fecal Samples*

Metabolomics studies of the fecal sample are of particular interest in relation to colorectal cancer. A study conducted by Monleón et al. on colorectal cancer patients using NMR metabolic profiling using fecal water extract samples from cancer patients and healthy controls revealed that fecal water extracts have an abundance of some metabolites that can be used for detecting colorectal cancer and differentiate between colorectal patients and healthy controls [77]. The study reported low concentration of short-chain fatty acids (acetate and butyrate), which in agreement of earlier reports, could serve as an effective marker for colorectal cancer. Significant alterations in levels of proline and cysteine were also observed in samples from patients of colorectal cancer compared to healthy controls [77]. Lin et al. carried out a study on NMR metabolomics to profile fecal metabolites of colorectal cancer patients, including stage I to stage IV patients and healthy controls [63]. In particular, their result revealed some interesting findings that the fecal metabolomics profile of each stage of colorectal cancer was significantly different compared to healthy controls including those of early-stage (stage I and II) colorectal cancer patients

[63]. Lower levels of acetate, butyrate, propionate, glucose, glutamine, and increased levels of succinate, proline, alanine, dimethylglycine, valine, glutamate, leucine, isoleucine, and lactate were observed [63]. These alterations in metabolites were suggested to be associated with microbiota, malabsorption of nutrients, and increased glycolysis and glutaminolysis [63]. In addition, there were significant changes in the metabolic profile of stage I and II compared to stage III and IV indicated by alterations of levels of glucose, lactate, short-chain fatty acids, glutamate, and succinate. These observations indicate the possibility of noninvasive staging of colorectal cancer based on metabolomics data [63].

In a step forward to earlier studies, a parallel investigation of colonic tumor tissues and their normal adjacent tissue along with patient-matched feces was carried out using NMR metabolomics [64]. The study reported a set of overlapping discriminatory metabolites across feces and tumor tissues of colorectal cancer. Increased levels of lactate, glutamate, alanine, and succinate and decreased levels of butyrate were observed which could indicate the interaction of metabolic pathway alterations in glucose and glycolytic metabolism, TCA cycle, glutaminolysis, and short-chain fatty acids metabolism associated with colorectal cancer [64]. Metabolic changes apparent in the fecal samples and tissue showed a positive correlation. Acetate in feces correlated with glucose and myo-inositol in colorectal tumor tissues to meet the increased energy demand of proliferating cells [64]. Acetate showed the highest diagnostic performance among fecal metabolites (AUC, 0.843) in the training set and a good predictive ability in the validation set [64]. Overall, the study highlighted the potential role of NMR metabolomics of feces and colorectal tissue samples to cancer microenvironment and as a novel and noninvasive tool for colorectal cancer [64].

NMR metabolomics has been used to determine absolute concentrations of metabolites in fecal extracts samples from patients with colorectal cancer and healthy controls [59]. Over 80 metabolites were assigned in the NMR spectra using 2D NMR and literature values [59]. The concentration data showed an increase in branched-chain fatty acids, isovalerate, and isobutyrate plus valerate and phenylacetate and decrease in concentration of amino acids, sugars, methanol, and bile acids (deoxycholate, lithodeoxycholate, and cholate) [59]. In addition, the study reported a weak but significant link between NMR data and microbiota; however, there was no correlation between individual metabolite with individual microbial trait [59].

4.5.4 Tissues Samples

Tissue samples used for NMR metabolomics study of colorectal cancer are either collected at the time of biopsy or after surgery from the surgical specimen. The tissue samples thus obtained should be snap frozen in liquid nitrogen as soon as possible after collection to arrest any further metabolic changes or degradation of tissue which can affect the results of metabolic studies.

Tissue metabolic profiles of colorectal cancer have been reported by a number of studies using NMR spectroscopy [11, 18, 19, 54, 69, 78, 96, 100, 106, 113, 130]. Most widely used methods to carry out NMR metabolomics study on the tissue sample are, first, by extraction (e.g., perchloric acid extraction) of the metabolites from tissue and, second, on intact tissues without any pretreatment using high-resolution magic angle spinning (HRMAS) [65] [130].

Several studies have reported the use of HRMAS-NMR spectroscopy in colorectal cancer metabolomics [130]. Colorectal HT29, HCT116, and SW620 xenografts and human rectal cancer biopsies have been studied by HRMAS metabolomics [106]. The study revealed differences in metabolic profiles of different xenografts and rectal biopsies [106]. The metabolic profile of HT29 xenograft was most similar to the human rectal cancer tissue metabolic profile [106]. In addition, the study concluded that necrotic fraction can be assessed from NMR spectra [106].

The feasibility of metabolic characterization of intact, unaltered tissue by using HRMAS in human rectal adenocarcinoma specimens has been reported [54]. The results of the study found that HRMAS can be used for metabolic characterization of intact tissue and to differentiate between pathological features [54]. Chan et al. tested the hypothesis that metabolomics of colon mucosae could discriminate malignant from normal mucosae [19]. HRMAS-NMR spectroscopy and mass spectrometry were used to obtain metabolic profiles data, and OPLS-DA models generated from both the analytical techniques could discriminate normal from malignant samples [19]. Alterations in level of a number of metabolites were reported, including lactate, glycine, taurine, scyllo-inositol, phosphoethanolamine, and phosphocholine, and among these altered metabolites, many are associated with tumor metabolism like hypoxia, glycolysis, nucleotide biosynthesis, lipid metabolism, inflammation, and steroid metabolism [19].

HRMAS-NMR metabolomics study of healthy and neoplastic colorectal tissues was used to discriminate tumoral colorectal tissue [100]. The levels of taurine, acetate, lactate, and lipids were increased, whereas the levels of glucose, creatine, glutamate, myo-inositol, scyllo-inositol, and choline-containing compounds were decreased in colorectal cancer compared to healthy tissue [100]. Moreover, it was found that colorectal tissue collected at least 15 cm from the adenocarcinoma which was appearing normal showed a metabolic pattern quite similar to that of tumoral lesions [100]. The results of human colon cancer and normal adjacent tissue metabolic profiles studied by HRMAS revealed that cancer samples were clearly separated from normal adjacent mucosa by 100% accuracy [113]. Several metabolites were identified as potential biomarkers for colon cancer such as lactate, taurine, glycine, myo-inositol, scyllo-inositol, phosphocholine, glycerophosphocholine, creatine, and glucose [113]. The metabolic differences in normal colon mucosa between microsatellite instability and microsatellite stable colon tissue were also reported, which may be supportive information toward the early detection of cancer development [113]. Alterations in levels of myo-inositol, scyllo-inositol, and taurine in cancer samples may suggest an osmotic imbalance in cancer cells [100, 113]. From the analysis perspective, determination of the concentration of individual metabolites and multivariate analysis has been shown to of importance for metabolomics studies of colorectal cancer [18].

4.6 Magnetic Resonance Imaging in Colon Cancer

Seminal articles on hallmarks of cancer by Hanahan and Weinberg started to describe biological capabilities acquired by cancers during the multistep development process, which comprises sustaining proliferative signaling, evading growth suppressors, activating invasion and metastasis, enabling replicative immortality, inducing angiogenesis, resisting cell death, metabolic reprogramming, avoiding immune destruction, and deregulating cellular energetics [38, 44, 45, 95, 128]. Spatial and temporal heterogeneity and alterations in cell physiology are among the central characteristics of cancers [36]. These hallmarks provide clues to understand and investigate cancers using imaging [34, 52, 92].

MRI techniques comprise methods to generate contrast in images using different mechanisms, for example, dynamic contrast-enhanced (DCE)-MRI and diffusion-weighted imaging (DWI) [36, 47]. DCE-MRI utilizes the administration of an external contrast agent, and DWI generates contrast based on the diffusion of water in tissue [36]. Recently, there has been an interest in magnetic nanoparticles MRI in theranostics of colorectal cancer [62].

4.6.1 Diffusion-Weighted Imaging

DWI is becoming an increasingly established technique in oncology [90, 94]. There is growing interest in the application of DWI for the evaluation of colorectal cancer and is part of the routine clinical MRI protocol for the patients of colorectal cancer [7]. High-b-value DWI showed high sensitivity and specificity for detecting colorectal cancer [50]. DWI and CT have been found similar in detecting early colorectal cancer [107]. However, DWI is more sensitive in detecting advanced colorectal cancer compared to CT, indicating its clinical potential for preoperative staging and postoperative follow-up examinations [107].

A prospective study for the comparison of DWI with multi-detector CT in staging of colorectal cancer revealed that DWI is more accurate for detecting hepatic metastases [56]. The sensitivity and specificity reported for DWI were 100% and 100%, respectively, compared with 87.5% and 95.5% for multi-detector CT, respectively [56]. Colagrande et al. in a study comparing the role of DWI with unenhanced and gadolinium ethoxybenzyl diethylenetriamine pentaacetic acid (Gd-EOB-DTPA)-enhanced MRI in detecting hepatic metastases from colorectal cancer reported that DWI improved all statistical parameters in the unenhanced examinations resulting in an increase in specificity [24].

DWI has been found useful for preoperative detection of metastatic lymph nodes in colorectal cancer [88]. Detection of lymph node metastasis using DWI showed sensitivity, 79%; specificity, 95%; positive predictive value, 94%; and negative predictive value, 83% [88]. DWI found to be better than CT in patients with colorectal cancer and peritoneal metastases for estimation of the spread of peritoneal carcinomatosis, staging, and operability [33]. DWI had sensitivity, 97.8%; specificity, 93.2%; positive predictive value, 88.9%; and negative predictive value, 98.7% for detection of peritoneal carcinomatosis. In addition, DWI enabled better detection of inoperable distant metastases compared to CT and improved prediction of inoperability over CT with sensitivity, 90.6% compared to 25% for CT [33].

Apparent diffusion coefficient (ADC) is a quantitative parameter that can be derived from DWI. In metastatic colorectal cancer, ADC histogram analysis has been reported for potential in discriminating progressive from the non-progressive disease [58]. ADC of the primary tumor has been shown to be a potential biomarker to predict metastatic colon cancer [82]. ADC of advanced tumors was significantly different than of early tumors in colon cancer [82]. A 100% sensitivity and specificity was found in predicting lymph node metastasis by using a cutoff value of 1.179×10^{-3} mm^2/s for ADC determined from the primary tumor [82].

4.6.2 Dynamic Contrast-Enhanced MRI

DCE-MRI is one of the most important MRI techniques for examination of colorectal cancer which provide parameters to assess vasculature and perfusion [42, 120].

In pre-clinical studies of colon cancer, DCE-MRI has the potential to assess angiogenesis. DCE-MRI has been shown to detect the early anti-angiogenic activity of SU11248 which was measured as 42% decrease in vascular permeability in the tumor rim cells [74]. DCE-MRI has been reported to be an effective method in investigation of anti-angiogenic effects of bumetanide in a colon cancer model [72]. In a colon cancer mouse model, DCE-MRI has been used for quantitative assessment of tumor response after radiation therapy [2]. A human colorectal xenograft model with DLD-1 cancer cells producing tumors was irradiated and examined with baseline and follow-up DCE-MRI [2]. All the mice in good response group showed marked reductions in K(trans) after the first radiation [2].

Gd-EOB-DTPA-enhanced MRI has been found to be more accurate for evaluation of liver metastasis in colorectal cancer patients [80]. Mross et al. used DCE-MRI to assess the effect of vandetanib on tumor vasculature in patients with advanced colorectal cancer and liver metastases [79]. Vandetanib did not modulate tumor vasculature and tissue measured by DCE-MRI parameters [79]. DCE-MRI has shown potential role in prediction of response to preoperative chemotherapy with bevacizumab for colorectal liver metastases, and high relative decrease in K(trans) was found to be a favorable prognostic factor [29]. Hirashima et al. conducted a phase II trial to confirm the pharmacokinetic parameters of DCE-MRI as surrogate biomarkers of bevacizumab and FOLFIRI (leucovorin calcium,

5-fluorouracil, and irinotecan) regimen efficacy in colorectal cancer with liver metastasis [48]. ΔK(trans) and ΔK(ep) can predict response to chemotherapy at 1 week and confirmed the potential of these biomarkers as surrogate predictors of response and time to progression [48].

4.7 Challenges and Limitations of Metabolic Profiling and Imaging

NMR metabolomics and MR imaging have shown tremendous potential in preclinical and clinical research; however, further studies are required to establish these techniques and their use for routine clinical management. Metabolomics is a relatively new field, and its techniques and analysis methods are undergoing constant development. For metabolomics studies, standardization of sample collection and preparation, technical protocol for NMR data acquisition, and then robust and reproducible analysis methods for identification and quantification of metabolites or biomarkers are being developed. Availability, cost, and expertise required to perform metabolomics as a routine clinical test are also challenges. In addition, results of metabolomics studies need to be performed in a large number of samples for validation. Similarly, for imaging studies, variability between imaging scanners and image sequences made available by scanner vendor needs to be addressed. Another challenge is the measurement of error of a technique and kinetic parameters [36]. Test-retest reproducibility and natural variation of individual kinetic parameters are critical to establish and understand before proposing it as a biomarker for response to therapy [36]. Metabolomics and imaging biomarkers must undergo clinical trials and rigorous evaluations before transitioning into the clinic.

In this chapter, we have highlighted the potential role of NMR metabolomics and MR imaging in colon cancer. Integration of genomics, transcriptomics, and proteomics data with metabolomics data may provide a comprehensive view of cancer by possibly applying the systems biology approach. Such advancements in knowledge may help to achieve the goal of personalized medicine.

References

1. Accioly MT, Pacheco P, Maya-Monteiro CM, Carrossini N, Robbs BK, Oliveira SS, et al. Lipid bodies are reservoirs of cyclooxygenase-2 and sites of prostaglandin-E2 synthesis in colon cancer cells. Cancer Res. 2008;68:1732–40. https://doi.org/10.1158/0008-5472.CAN-07-1999.
2. Ahn SJ, Koom WS, An CS, Lim JS, Lee SK, Suh JS, et al. Quantitative assessment of tumor responses after radiation therapy in a DLD-1 colon cancer mouse model using serial dynamic contrast-enhanced magnetic resonance imaging. Yonsei Med J. 2012;53:1147–53. https://doi.org/10.3349/ymj.2012.53.6.1147.
3. Altman BJ, Stine ZE, Dang CV. From Krebs to clinic: glutamine metabolism to cancer therapy. Nat Rev Cancer. 2016;16:619–34. https://doi.org/10.1038/nrc.2016.71.

4. Arnold M, Sierra MS, Laversanne M, Soerjomataram I, Jemal A, Bray F. Global patterns and trends in colorectal cancer incidence and mortality. Gut. 2017;66:683–91. https://doi.org/10.1136/gutjnl-2015-310912.
5. Asante I, Chui D, Pei H, Zhou E, De Giovanni C, Conti D, et al. Alterations in folate-dependent one-carbon metabolism as colon cell transition from normal to cancerous. J Nutr Biochem. 2019;69:1–9. https://doi.org/10.1016/j.jnutbio.2019.02.008.
6. Baenke F, Peck B, Miess H, Schulze A. Hooked on fat: the role of lipid synthesis in cancer metabolism and tumour development. Dis Model Mech. 2013;6:1353–63. https://doi.org/10.1242/dmm.011338.
7. Barral M, Eveno C, Hoeffel C, Boudiaf M, Bazeries P, Foucher R, et al. Diffusion-weighted magnetic resonance imaging in colorectal cancer. J Visc Surg. 2016;153:361–9. https://doi.org/10.1016/j.jviscsurg.2016.08.004.
8. Barton RH, Nicholson JK, Elliott P, Holmes E. High-throughput 1H NMR-based metabolic analysis of human serum and urine for large-scale epidemiological studies: validation study. Int J Epidemiol. 2008;37:i31–40. https://doi.org/10.1093/ije/dym284.
9. Beloribi-Djefaflia S, Vasseur S, Guillaumond F. Lipid metabolic reprogramming in cancer cells. Oncogenesis. 2016;5:e189. https://doi.org/10.1038/oncsis.2015.49.
10. Bernini P, Bertini I, Luchinat C, Nincheri P, Staderini S, Turano P. Standard operating procedures for pre-analytical handling of blood and urine for metabolomic studies and biobanks. J Biomol NMR. 2011;49:231–43. https://doi.org/10.1007/s10858-011-9489-1.
11. Bertini I, Cacciatore S, Jensen BV, Schou JV, Johansen JS, Kruhoffer M, et al. Metabolomic NMR fingerprinting to identify and predict survival of patients with metastatic colorectal cancer. Cancer Res. 2012;72:356–64. https://doi.org/10.1158/0008-5472.CAN-11-1543.
12. Bouatra S, Aziat F, Mandal R, Guo AC, Wilson MR, Knox C, et al. The human urine metabolome. PLoS One. 2013;8:e73076. https://doi.org/10.1371/journal.pone.0073076.
13. Brenner H, Stock C, Hoffmeister M. Effect of screening sigmoidoscopy and screening colonoscopy on colorectal cancer incidence and mortality: systematic review and meta-analysis of randomised controlled trials and observational studies. BMJ. 2014;348:g2467. https://doi.org/10.1136/bmj.g2467.
14. Brown RE, Short SP, Williams CS. Colorectal cancer and metabolism. Curr Colorectal Cancer Rep. 2018;14:226–41. https://doi.org/10.1007/s11888-018-0420-y.
15. Cairns RA, Mak TW. The current state of cancer metabolism. Nat Rev Cancer. 2016;16:613.
16. Carr HY, Purcell EM. Effects of diffusion on free precession in nuclear magnetic resonance experiments. Phys Rev. 1954;94:630. https://doi.org/10.1103/PhysRev.94.630.
17. Center MM, Jemal A, Smith RA, Ward E. Worldwide variations in colorectal cancer. CA Cancer J Clin. 2009;59:366–78. https://doi.org/10.3322/caac.20038.
18. Chae YK, Kang W-Y, Kim SH, Joo JE, Han JK, Hong BW. Combining information of common metabolites reveals global differences between colorectal cancerous and normal tissues. Bull Kor Chem Soc. 2010;31:74. https://doi.org/10.5012/bkcs.2010.31.02.379.
19. Chan EC, Koh PK, Mal M, Cheah PY, Eu KW, Backshall A, et al. Metabolic profiling of human colorectal cancer using high-resolution magic angle spinning nuclear magnetic resonance (HR-MAS NMR) spectroscopy and gas chromatography mass spectrometry (GC/MS). J Proteome Res. 2009;8:352–61. https://doi.org/10.1021/pr8006232.
20. Chan EC, Pasikanti KK, Hong Y, Ho PC, Mahendran R, Raman Nee Mani L, et al. Metabonomic profiling of bladder cancer. J Proteome Res. 2015;14:587–602. https://doi.org/10.1021/pr500966h.
21. Chen C, Deng L, Wei S, Nagana Gowda GA, Gu H, Chiorean EG, et al. Exploring metabolic profile differences between colorectal polyp patients and controls using seemingly unrelated regression. J Proteome Res. 2015;14:2492–9. https://doi.org/10.1021/acs.jproteome.5b00059.
22. Cheng Y, Xie G, Chen T, Qiu Y, Zou X, Zheng M, et al. Distinct urinary metabolic profile of human colorectal cancer. J Proteome Res. 2012;11:1354–63. https://doi.org/10.1021/pr201001a.
23. Cohen S. Lipid droplets as organelles. Int Rev Cell Mol Biol. 2018;337:83–110. https://doi.org/10.1016/bs.ircmb.2017.12.007.

24. Colagrande S, Castellani A, Nardi C, Lorini C, Calistri L, Filippone A. The role of diffusion-weighted imaging in the detection of hepatic metastases from colorectal cancer: a comparison with unenhanced and Gd-EOB-DTPA enhanced MRI. Eur J Radiol. 2016;85:1027–34. https://doi.org/10.1016/j.ejrad.2016.02.011.
25. Collins RRJ, Patel K, Putnam WC, Kapur P, Rakheja D. Oncometabolites: a new paradigm for oncology, metabolism, and the clinical laboratory. Clin Chem. 2017;63:1812–20. https://doi.org/10.1373/clinchem.2016.267666.
26. Cruz-Gil S, Sanchez-Martinez R, Gomez de Cedron M, Martin-Hernandez R, Vargas T, Molina S, et al. Targeting the lipid metabolic axis ACSL/SCD in colorectal cancer progression by therapeutic miRNAs: miR-19b-1 role. J Lipid Res. 2018;59:14–24. https://doi.org/10.1194/jlr.M076752.
27. Currie E, Schulze A, Zechner R, Walther TC, Farese RV Jr. Cellular fatty acid metabolism and cancer. Cell Metab. 2013;18:153–61. https://doi.org/10.1016/j.cmet.2013.05.017.
28. Daviss B. Growing pains for metabolomics: the newest 'omic science is producing results – and more data than researchers know what to do with. Scientist. 2005;19:25–9.
29. De Bruyne S, Van Damme N, Smeets P, Ferdinande L, Ceelen W, Mertens J, et al. Value of DCE-MRI and FDG-PET/CT in the prediction of response to preoperative chemotherapy with bevacizumab for colorectal liver metastases. Br J Cancer. 2012;106:1926–33. https://doi.org/10.1038/bjc.2012.184.
30. de Geus-Oei LF, Vriens D, van Laarhoven HW, van der Graaf WT, Oyen WJ. Monitoring and predicting response to therapy with 18F-FDG PET in colorectal cancer: a systematic review. J Nucl Med. 2009;50(Suppl 1):43S–54S. https://doi.org/10.2967/jnumed.108.057224.
31. DeBerardinis RJ, Cheng T. Q's next: the diverse functions of glutamine in metabolism, cell biology and cancer. Oncogene. 2010;29:313–24. https://doi.org/10.1038/onc.2009.358.
32. DeBerardinis RJ, Chandel NS. Fundamentals of cancer metabolism. Sci Adv. 2016;2:e1600200. https://doi.org/10.1126/sciadv.1600200.
33. Dresen RC, De Vuysere S, De Keyzer F, Van Cutsem E, Prenen H, Vanslembrouck R, et al. Whole-body diffusion-weighted MRI for operability assessment in patients with colorectal cancer and peritoneal metastases. Cancer Imaging. 2019;19:1. https://doi.org/10.1186/s40644-018-0187-z.
34. Ellenbroek SI, van Rheenen J. Imaging hallmarks of cancer in living mice. Nat Rev Cancer. 2014;14:406–18. https://doi.org/10.1038/nrc3742.
35. Farshidfar F, Weljie AM, Kopciuk K, Buie WD, Maclean A, Dixon E, et al. Serum metabolomic profile as a means to distinguish stage of colorectal cancer. Genome Med. 2012;4:42. https://doi.org/10.1186/gm341.
36. Figueiras RG, Goh V, Padhani AR, Naveira AB, Caamano AG, Martin CV. The role of functional imaging in colorectal cancer. AJR Am J Roentgenol. 2010;195:54–66. https://doi.org/10.2214/AJR.10.4422.
37. Fisel P, Schaeffeler E, Schwab M. Clinical and functional relevance of the monocarboxylate transporter family in disease pathophysiology and drug therapy. Clin Transl Sci. 2018;11:352–64. https://doi.org/10.1111/cts.12551.
38. Fouad YA, Aanei C. Revisiting the hallmarks of cancer. Am J Cancer Res. 2017;7:1016–36.
39. Garrett WS. The gut microbiota and colon cancer. Science. 2019;364:1133–5. https://doi.org/10.1126/science.aaw2367.
40. Ghini V, Unger FT, Tenori L, Turano P, Juhl H, David KA. Metabolomics profiling of pre- and post-anesthesia plasma samples of colorectal patients obtained via Ficoll separation. Metabolomics. 2015;11:1769–78. https://doi.org/10.1007/s11306-015-0832-5.
41. Ghini V, Quaglio D, Luchinat C, Turano P. NMR for sample quality assessment in metabolomics. New Biotechnol. 2019;52:25–34. https://doi.org/10.1016/j.nbt.2019.04.004.
42. Goh V, Padhani AR. Imaging tumor angiogenesis: functional assessment using MDCT or MRI? Abdom Imaging. 2006;31:194–9. https://doi.org/10.1007/s00261-005-0387-4.
43. Gu J, Xiao Y, Shu D, Liang X, Hu X, Xie Y, et al. Metabolomics analysis in serum from patients with colorectal polyp and colorectal cancer by (1)H-NMR spectrometry. Dis Markers. 2019;2019:3491852. https://doi.org/10.1155/2019/3491852.

44. Hanahan D, Weinberg RA. The hallmarks of cancer. Cell. 2000;100:57–70. https://doi.org/10.1016/s0092-8674(00)81683-9.
45. Hanahan D, Weinberg RA. Hallmarks of cancer: the next generation. Cell. 2011;144:646–74. https://doi.org/10.1016/j.cell.2011.02.013.
46. Hanley MP, Rosenberg DW. One-carbon metabolism and colorectal cancer: potential mechanisms of chemoprevention. Curr Pharmacol Rep. 2015;1:197–205. https://doi.org/10.1007/s40495-015-0028-8.
47. Haris M, Yadav SK, Rizwan A, Singh A, Wang E, Hariharan H, et al. Molecular magnetic resonance imaging in cancer. J Transl Med. 2015;13:313. https://doi.org/10.1186/s12967-015-0659-x.
48. Hirashima Y, Yamada Y, Tateishi U, Kato K, Miyake M, Horita Y, et al. Pharmacokinetic parameters from 3-Tesla DCE-MRI as surrogate biomarkers of antitumor effects of bevacizumab plus FOLFIRI in colorectal cancer with liver metastasis. Int J Cancer. 2012;130:2359–65. https://doi.org/10.1002/ijc.26282.
49. Huang F, Zhang Q, Ma H, Lv Q, Zhang T. Expression of glutaminase is upregulated in colorectal cancer and of clinical significance. Int J Clin Exp Pathol. 2014;7:1093–100.
50. Ichikawa T, Erturk SM, Motosugi U, Sou H, Iino H, Araki T, et al. High-B-value diffusion-weighted MRI in colorectal cancer. AJR Am J Roentgenol. 2006;187:181–4. https://doi.org/10.2214/AJR.05.1005.
51. Iyer RB, Silverman PM, DuBrow RA, Charnsangavej C. Imaging in the diagnosis, staging, and follow-up of colorectal cancer. AJR Am J Roentgenol. 2002;179:3–13. https://doi.org/10.2214/ajr.179.1.1790003.
52. Jailkhani N, Ingram JR, Rashidian M, Rickelt S, Tian C, Mak H, et al. Noninvasive imaging of tumor progression, metastasis, and fibrosis using a nanobody targeting the extracellular matrix. Proc Natl Acad Sci U S A. 2019;116:14181–90. https://doi.org/10.1073/pnas.1817442116.
53. Jia XQ, Zhang S, Zhu HJ, Wang W, Zhu JH, Wang XD, et al. Increased expression of PHGDH and prognostic significance in colorectal cancer. Transl Oncol. 2016;9:191–6. https://doi.org/10.1016/j.tranon.2016.03.006.
54. Jordan KW, Nordenstam J, Lauwers GY, Rothenberger DA, Alavi K, Garwood M, et al. Metabolomic characterization of human rectal adenocarcinoma with intact tissue magnetic resonance spectroscopy. Dis Colon Rectum. 2009;52:520–5. https://doi.org/10.1007/DCR.0b013e31819c9a2c.
55. Kim ER, Kwon HN, Nam H, Kim JJ, Park S, Kim YH. Urine-NMR metabolomics for screening of advanced colorectal adenoma and early stage colorectal cancer. Sci Rep. 2019;9:4786. https://doi.org/10.1038/s41598-019-41216-y.
56. Koh FHX, Tan KK, Teo LLS, Ang BWL, Thian YL. Prospective comparison between magnetic resonance imaging and computed tomography in colorectal cancer staging. ANZ J Surg. 2018;88:E498–502. https://doi.org/10.1111/ans.14138.
57. Koundouros N, Poulogiannis G. Reprogramming of fatty acid metabolism in cancer. Br J Cancer. 2020;122:4–22. https://doi.org/10.1038/s41416-019-0650-z.
58. Lavdas I, Rockall AG, Daulton E, Kozlowski K, Honeyfield L, Aboagye EO, et al. Histogram analysis of apparent diffusion coefficient from whole-body diffusion-weighted MRI to predict early response to chemotherapy in patients with metastatic colorectal cancer: preliminary results. Clin Radiol. 2018;73:832 e9–e16. https://doi.org/10.1016/j.crad.2018.04.011.
59. Le Gall G, Guttula K, Kellingray L, Tett AJ, Ten Hoopen R, Kemsley EK, et al. Metabolite quantification of faecal extracts from colorectal cancer patients and healthy controls. Oncotarget. 2018;9:33278–89. https://doi.org/10.18632/oncotarget.26022.
60. Levine AJ, Puzio-Kuter AM. The control of the metabolic switch in cancers by oncogenes and tumor suppressor genes. Science. 2010;330:1340–4. https://doi.org/10.1126/science.1193494.
61. Li T, Le A. Glutamine metabolism in cancer. Adv Exp Med Biol. 2018;1063:13–32. https://doi.org/10.1007/978-3-319-77736-8_2.

62. Li Y, Xin J, Sun Y, Han T, Zhang H, An F. Magnetic resonance imaging-guided and targeted theranostics of colorectal cancer. Cancer Biol Med. 2020;17:307–27. https://doi.org/10.20892/j.issn.2095-3941.2020.0072.
63. Lin Y, Ma C, Liu C, Wang Z, Yang J, Liu X, et al. NMR-based fecal metabolomics fingerprinting as predictors of earlier diagnosis in patients with colorectal cancer. Oncotarget. 2016;7:29454–64. https://doi.org/10.18632/oncotarget.8762.
64. Lin Y, Ma C, Bezabeh T, Wang Z, Liang J, Huang Y, et al. (1) H NMR-based metabolomics reveal overlapping discriminatory metabolites and metabolic pathway disturbances between colorectal tumor tissues and fecal samples. Int J Cancer. 2019;145:1679–89. https://doi.org/10.1002/ijc.32190.
65. Lindon JC, Nicholson JK. Spectroscopic and statistical techniques for information recovery in metabonomics and metabolomics. Annu Rev Anal Chem (Palo Alto, Calif). 2008;1:45–69. https://doi.org/10.1146/annurev.anchem.1.031207.113026.
66. Liu AY, Scherer D, Poole E, Potter JD, Curtin K, Makar K, et al. Gene-diet-interactions in folate-mediated one-carbon metabolism modify colon cancer risk. Mol Nutr Food Res. 2013;57:721–34. https://doi.org/10.1002/mnfr.201200180.
67. Liu G, Zhu J, Yu M, Cai C, Zhou Y, Yu M, et al. Glutamate dehydrogenase is a novel prognostic marker and predicts metastases in colorectal cancer patients. J Transl Med. 2015;13:144. https://doi.org/10.1186/s12967-015-0500-6.
68. Locasale JW. Serine, glycine and one-carbon units: cancer metabolism in full circle. Nat Rev Cancer. 2013;13:572–83. https://doi.org/10.1038/nrc3557.
69. Ludwig C, Ward DG, Martin A, Viant MR, Ismail T, Johnson PJ, et al. Fast targeted multidimensional NMR metabolomics of colorectal cancer. Magn Reson Chem. 2009;47(Suppl 1):S68–73. https://doi.org/10.1002/mrc.2519.
70. M'Koma AE, Blum DL, Norris JL, Koyama T, Billheimer D, Motley S, et al. Detection of pre-neoplastic and neoplastic prostate disease by MALDI profiling of urine. Biochem Biophys Res Commun. 2007;353:829–34. https://doi.org/10.1016/j.bbrc.2006.12.111.
71. Ma L, Tao Y, Duran A, Llado V, Galvez A, Barger JF, et al. Control of nutrient stress-induced metabolic reprogramming by PKCzeta in tumorigenesis. Cell. 2013;152:599–611. https://doi.org/10.1016/j.cell.2012.12.028.
72. Malamas AS, Jin E, Zhang Q, Haaga J, Lu ZR. Anti-angiogenic effects of bumetanide revealed by DCE-MRI with a biodegradable macromolecular contrast agent in a Colon cancer model. Pharm Res. 2015;32:3029–43. https://doi.org/10.1007/s11095-015-1684-4.
73. Martinelli M, Scapoli L, Mattei G, Ugolini G, Montroni I, Zattoni D, et al. A candidate gene study of one-carbon metabolism pathway genes and colorectal cancer risk. Br J Nutr. 2013;109:984–9. https://doi.org/10.1017/S0007114512002796.
74. Marzola P, Degrassi A, Calderan L, Farace P, Nicolato E, Crescimanno C, et al. Early antiangiogenic activity of SU11248 evaluated in vivo by dynamic contrast-enhanced magnetic resonance imaging in an experimental model of colon carcinoma. Clin Cancer Res. 2005;11:5827–32. https://doi.org/10.1158/1078-0432.CCR-04-2655.
75. McKeown E, Nelson DW, Johnson EK, Maykel JA, Stojadinovic A, Nissan A, et al. Current approaches and challenges for monitoring treatment response in colon and rectal cancer. J Cancer. 2014;5:31–43. https://doi.org/10.7150/jca.7987.
76. Miyo M, Konno M, Nishida N, Sueda T, Noguchi K, Matsui H, et al. Metabolic adaptation to nutritional stress in human colorectal cancer. Sci Rep. 2016;6:38415. https://doi.org/10.1038/srep38415.
77. Monleon D, Morales JM, Barrasa A, Lopez JA, Vazquez C, Celda B. Metabolite profiling of fecal water extracts from human colorectal cancer. NMR Biomed. 2009;22:342–8. https://doi.org/10.1002/nbm.1345.
78. Moreno A, Arus C. Quantitative and qualitative characterization of 1H NMR spectra of colon tumors, normal mucosa and their perchloric acid extracts: decreased levels of myo-inositol in tumours can be detected in intact biopsies. NMR Biomed. 1996;9:33–45. https://doi.org/10.1002/(SICI)1099-1492(199602)9:1<33::AID-NBM391>3.0.CO;2-G.

79. Mross K, Fasol U, Frost A, Benkelmann R, Kuhlmann J, Buchert M, et al. DCE-MRI assessment of the effect of vandetanib on tumor vasculature in patients with advanced colorectal cancer and liver metastases: a randomized phase I study. J Angiogenes Res. 2009;1:5. https://doi.org/10.1186/2040-2384-1-5.
80. Muhi A, Ichikawa T, Motosugi U, Sou H, Nakajima H, Sano K, et al. Diagnosis of colorectal hepatic metastases: comparison of contrast-enhanced CT, contrast-enhanced US, superparamagnetic iron oxide-enhanced MRI, and gadoxetic acid-enhanced MRI. J Magn Reson Imaging. 2011;34:326–35. https://doi.org/10.1002/jmri.22613.
81. Mutoh M, Komiya M, Teraoka N, Ueno T, Takahashi M, Kitahashi T, et al. Overexpression of low-density lipoprotein receptor and lipid accumulation in intestinal polyps in Min mice. Int J Cancer. 2009;125:2505–10. https://doi.org/10.1002/ijc.24667.
82. Nerad E, Delli Pizzi A, Lambregts DMJ, Maas M, Wadhwani S, Bakers FCH, et al. The Apparent Diffusion Coefficient (ADC) is a useful biomarker in predicting metastatic colon cancer using the ADC-value of the primary tumor. PLoS One. 2019;14:e0211830. https://doi.org/10.1371/journal.pone.0211830.
83. Newman AC, Maddocks ODK. One-carbon metabolism in cancer. Br J Cancer. 2017;116:1499–504. https://doi.org/10.1038/bjc.2017.118.
84. Ni Y, Xie G, Jia W. Metabonomics of human colorectal cancer: new approaches for early diagnosis and biomarker discovery. J Proteome Res. 2014;13:3857–70. https://doi.org/10.1021/pr500443c.
85. Nicholson JK, Connelly J, Lindon JC, Holmes E. Metabonomics: a platform for studying drug toxicity and gene function. Nat Rev Drug Discov. 2002;1:153–61. https://doi.org/10.1038/nrd728.
86. Nicholson JK, Lindon JC. Systems biology: Metabonomics. Nature. 2008;455:1054–6. https://doi.org/10.1038/4551054a.
87. O'Keefe SJ. Diet, microorganisms and their metabolites, and colon cancer. Nat Rev Gastroenterol Hepatol. 2016;13:691–706. https://doi.org/10.1038/nrgastro.2016.165.
88. Ogawa M, Ichiba N, Watanabe M, Yanaga K. The usefulness of diffusion MRI in detection of lymph node metastases of colorectal cancer. Anticancer Res. 2016;36:815–9.
89. Oliver SG, Winson MK, Kell DB, Baganz F. Systematic functional analysis of the yeast genome. Trends Biotechnol. 1998;16:373–8. https://doi.org/10.1016/s0167-7799(98)01214-1.
90. Padhani AR, Liu G, Koh DM, Chenevert TL, Thoeny HC, Takahara T, et al. Diffusion-weighted magnetic resonance imaging as a cancer biomarker: consensus and recommendations. Neoplasia. 2009;11:102–25. https://doi.org/10.1593/neo.81328.
91. Pan Z, Raftery D. Comparing and combining NMR spectroscopy and mass spectrometry in metabolomics. Anal Bioanal Chem. 2007;387:525–7. https://doi.org/10.1007/s00216-006-0687-8.
92. Pate KT, Stringari C, Sprowl-Tanio S, Wang K, TeSlaa T, Hoverter NP, et al. Wnt signaling directs a metabolic program of glycolysis and angiogenesis in colon cancer. EMBO J. 2014;33:1454–73. https://doi.org/10.15252/embj.201488598.
93. Patil PS, Saklani A, Gambhire P, Mehta S, Engineer R, De'Souza A, et al. Colorectal cancer in India: An audit from a Tertiary Center in a low prevalence area. Indian J Surg Oncol. 2017;8:484–90. https://doi.org/10.1007/s13193-017-0655-0.
94. Patterson DM, Padhani AR, Collins DJ. Technology insight: water diffusion MRI--a potential new biomarker of response to cancer therapy. Nat Clin Pract Oncol. 2008;5:220–33. https://doi.org/10.1038/ncponc1073.
95. Pavlova NN, Thompson CB. The emerging hallmarks of cancer metabolism. Cell Metab. 2016;23:27–47. https://doi.org/10.1016/j.cmet.2015.12.006.
96. Piotto M, Moussallieh F-M, Dillmann B, Imperiale A, Neuville A, Brigand C, et al. Metabolic characterization of primary human colorectal cancers using high resolution magic angle spinning 1 H magnetic resonance spectroscopy. Metabolomics. 2009;5:292. https://doi.org/10.1007/s11306-008-0151-1.

97. Qiu Y, Cai G, Su M, Chen T, Liu Y, Xu Y, et al. Urinary metabonomic study on colorectal cancer. J Proteome Res. 2010;9:1627–34. https://doi.org/10.1021/pr901081y.
98. Ransohoff DF, Lang CA. Screening for colorectal cancer with the fecal occult blood test: a background paper. American College of Physicians. Ann Intern Med. 1997;126:811–22. https://doi.org/10.7326/0003-4819-126-10-199705150-00014.
99. Rawla P, Sunkara T, Barsouk A. Epidemiology of colorectal cancer: incidence, mortality, survival, and risk factors. Prz Gastroenterol. 2019;14:89–103. https://doi.org/10.5114/pg.2018.81072.
100. Righi V, Durante C, Cocchi M, Calabrese C, Di Febo G, Lecce F, et al. Discrimination of healthy and neoplastic human colon tissues by ex vivo HR-MAS NMR spectroscopy and chemometric analyses. J Proteome Res. 2009;8:1859–69. https://doi.org/10.1021/pr801094b.
101. Rohrig F, Schulze A. The multifaceted roles of fatty acid synthesis in cancer. Nat Rev Cancer. 2016;16:732–49. https://doi.org/10.1038/nrc.2016.89.
102. Ryall JG, Cliff T, Dalton S, Sartorelli V. Metabolic reprogramming of stem cell epigenetics. Cell Stem Cell. 2015;17:651–62. https://doi.org/10.1016/j.stem.2015.11.012.
103. Sanchez-Martinez R, Cruz-Gil S, Gomez de Cedron M, Alvarez-Fernandez M, Vargas T, Molina S, et al. A link between lipid metabolism and epithelial-mesenchymal transition provides a target for colon cancer therapy. Oncotarget. 2015;6(36):38719. https://doi.org/10.18632/oncotarget.5340.
104. Santos CR, Schulze A. Lipid metabolism in cancer. FEBS J. 2012;279:2610–23. https://doi.org/10.1111/j.1742-4658.2012.08644.x.
105. Satoh K, Yachida S, Sugimoto M, Oshima M, Nakagawa T, Akamoto S, et al. Global metabolic reprogramming of colorectal cancer occurs at adenoma stage and is induced by MYC. Proc Natl Acad Sci U S A. 2017;114:E7697–E706. https://doi.org/10.1073/pnas.1710366114.
106. Seierstad T, Roe K, Sitter B, Halgunset J, Flatmark K, Ree AH, et al. Principal component analysis for the comparison of metabolic profiles from human rectal cancer biopsies and colorectal xenografts using high-resolution magic angle spinning 1H magnetic resonance spectroscopy. Mol Cancer. 2008;7:33. https://doi.org/10.1186/1476-4598-7-33.
107. Shinya S, Sasaki T, Nakagawa Y, Guiquing Z, Yamamoto F, Yamashita Y. The efficacy of diffusion-weighted imaging for the detection of colorectal cancer. Hepato-Gastroenterology. 2009;56:128–32.
108. Siegel R, Naishadham D, Jemal A. Cancer statistics, 2013. CA Cancer J Clin. 2013;63:11–30. https://doi.org/10.3322/caac.21166.
109. Siegel RL, Miller KD, Jemal A. Cancer statistics, 2018. CA Cancer J Clin. 2018;68:7–30. https://doi.org/10.3322/caac.21442.
110. Song Z, Wei B, Lu C, Li P, Chen L. Glutaminase sustains cell survival via the regulation of glycolysis and glutaminolysis in colorectal cancer. Oncol Lett. 2017;14:3117–23. https://doi.org/10.3892/ol.2017.6538.
111. Srivastava A, Creek DJ. Discovery and validation of clinical biomarkers of cancer: a review combining metabolomics and proteomics. Proteomics. 2019;19:e1700448. https://doi.org/10.1002/pmic.201700448.
112. Takis PG, Ghini V, Tenori L, Turano P, Luchinat C. Uniqueness of the NMR approach to metabolomics. TrAC Trends Anal Chem. 2019;120:115300. https://doi.org/10.1016/j.trac.2018.10.036.
113. Tessem MB, Selnaes KM, Sjursen W, Trano G, Giskeodegard GF, Bathen TF, et al. Discrimination of patients with microsatellite instability colon cancer using 1H HR MAS MR spectroscopy and chemometric analysis. J Proteome Res. 2010;9:3664–70. https://doi.org/10.1021/pr100176g.
114. Theodorescu D, Wittke S, Ross MM, Walden M, Conaway M, Just I, et al. Discovery and validation of new protein biomarkers for urothelial cancer: a prospective analysis. Lancet Oncol. 2006;7:230–40. https://doi.org/10.1016/S1470-2045(06)70584-8.
115. Thoeny HC, Ross BD. Predicting and monitoring cancer treatment response with diffusion-weighted MRI. J Magn Reson Imaging. 2010;32:2–16. https://doi.org/10.1002/jmri.22167.

116. Tian Y, Nie X, Xu S, Li Y, Huang T, Tang H, et al. Integrative metabonomics as potential method for diagnosis of thyroid malignancy. Sci Rep. 2015;5:14869. https://doi.org/10.1038/srep14869.
117. Tian Y, Xu T, Huang J, Zhang L, Xu S, Xiong B, et al. Tissue Metabonomic phenotyping for diagnosis and prognosis of human colorectal cancer. Sci Rep. 2016;6:20790. https://doi.org/10.1038/srep20790.
118. Tilg H, Adolph TE, Gerner RR, Moschen AR. The intestinal microbiota in colorectal cancer. Cancer Cell. 2018;33:954–64. https://doi.org/10.1016/j.ccell.2018.03.004.
119. Trygg J, Holmes E, Lundstedt T. Chemometrics in metabonomics. J Proteome Res. 2007;6:469–79. https://doi.org/10.1021/pr060594q.
120. Turkbey B, Kobayashi H, Ogawa M, Bernardo M, Choyke PL. Imaging of tumor angiogenesis: functional or targeted? AJR Am J Roentgenol. 2009;193:304–13. https://doi.org/10.2214/AJR.09.2869.
121. Tweeddale H, Notley-McRobb L, Ferenci T. Effect of slow growth on metabolism of Escherichia coli, as revealed by global metabolite pool ("metabolome") analysis. J Bacteriol. 1998;180:5109–16. https://doi.org/10.1128/JB.180.19.5109-5116.1998.
122. Van Cutsem E, Verheul HM, Flamen P, Rougier P, Beets-Tan R, Glynne-Jones R, et al. Imaging in colorectal cancer: progress and challenges for the clinicians. Cancers (Basel). 2016;8:81. https://doi.org/10.3390/cancers8090081.
123. Vignoli A, Ghini V, Meoni G, Licari C, Takis PG, Tenori L, et al. High-throughput metabolomics by 1D NMR. Angew Chem Int Ed Engl. 2019;58:968–94. https://doi.org/10.1002/anie.201804736.
124. Wang H, Wang L, Zhang H, Deng P, Chen J, Zhou B, et al. (1)H NMR-based metabolic profiling of human rectal cancer tissue. Mol Cancer. 2013;12:121. https://doi.org/10.1186/1476-4598-12-121.
125. Wang H, Xi Q, Wu G. Fatty acid synthase regulates invasion and metastasis of colorectal cancer via Wnt signaling pathway. Cancer Med. 2016;5:1599–606. https://doi.org/10.1002/cam4.711.
126. Wang Z, Lin Y, Liang J, Huang Y, Ma C, Liu X, et al. NMR-based metabolomic techniques identify potential urinary biomarkers for early colorectal cancer detection. Oncotarget. 2017;8:105819–31. https://doi.org/10.18632/oncotarget.22402.
127. Warburg O, Wind F, Negelein E. The metabolism of tumors in the body. J Gen Physiol. 1927;8:519–30. https://doi.org/10.1085/jgp.8.6.519.
128. Ward PS, Thompson CB. Metabolic reprogramming: a cancer hallmark even warburg did not anticipate. Cancer Cell. 2012;21:297–308. https://doi.org/10.1016/j.ccr.2012.02.014.
129. Weitz J, Koch M, Debus J, Hohler T, Galle PR, Buchler MW. Colorectal cancer. Lancet. 2005;365:153–65. https://doi.org/10.1016/S0140-6736(05)17706-X.
130. Williams MD, Reeves R, Resar LS, Hill HH Jr. Metabolomics of colorectal cancer: past and current analytical platforms. Anal Bioanal Chem. 2013;405:5013–30. https://doi.org/10.1007/s00216-013-6777-5.
131. Wold S, Sjöström M, Eriksson L. PLS-regression: a basic tool of chemometrics. Chemom Intell Lab Syst. 2001;58:109–30. https://doi.org/10.1016/S0169-7439(01)00155-1.
132. Xia J, Mandal R, Sinelnikov IV, Broadhurst D, Wishart DS. MetaboAnalyst 2.0--a comprehensive server for metabolomic data analysis. Nucleic Acids Res. 2012;40:W127–33. https://doi.org/10.1093/nar/gks374.
133. Xie G, Lu L, Qiu Y, Ni Q, Zhang W, Gao YT, et al. Plasma metabolite biomarkers for the detection of pancreatic cancer. J Proteome Res. 2015;14:1195–202. https://doi.org/10.1021/pr501135f.
134. Xu Y, Zheng X, Qiu Y, Jia W, Wang J, Yin S. Distinct Metabolomic profiles of papillary thyroid carcinoma and benign thyroid adenoma. J Proteome Res. 2015;14:3315–21. https://doi.org/10.1021/acs.jproteome.5b00351.
135. Yang M, Soga T, Pollard PJ. Oncometabolites: linking altered metabolism with cancer. J Clin Invest. 2013;123:3652–8. https://doi.org/10.1172/JCI67228.

136. Zaidi N, Lupien L, Kuemmerle NB, Kinlaw WB, Swinnen JV, Smans K. Lipogenesis and lipolysis: the pathways exploited by the cancer cells to acquire fatty acids. Prog Lipid Res. 2013;52:585–9. https://doi.org/10.1016/j.plipres.2013.08.005.
137. Zang X, Jones CM, Long TQ, Monge ME, Zhou M, Walker LD, et al. Feasibility of detecting prostate cancer by ultraperformance liquid chromatography-mass spectrometry serum metabolomics. J Proteome Res. 2014;13:3444–54. https://doi.org/10.1021/pr500409q.
138. Zaytseva YY, Rychahou PG, Gulhati P, Elliott VA, Mustain WC, O'Connor K, et al. Inhibition of fatty acid synthase attenuates CD44-associated signaling and reduces metastasis in colorectal cancer. Cancer Res. 2012;72:1504–17. https://doi.org/10.1158/0008-5472.CAN-11-4057.

Chapter 5
Role of MicroRNA In Situ Hybridization in Colon Cancer Diagnosis

Shalitha Sasi, Sapna Singh, Tamanna Walia, Ramesh Chand Meena, and Suresh Thakur

Abstract Colon cancer or colorectal cancer (CRC) is a cancer of the large intestine and is the third most commonly diagnosed cancer in the world after lung cancer and breast cancer. The highest occurrence has been reported in Australia/New Zealand and the lowest in Africa. Asian countries have differing rates of incidence showing a striking correlation with the economic development. In India, the incidence rate of CRC is comparatively low and ranks the fifth most common cancer. However last few decades have seen a steady rise in the number of reported cases in India, which could be attributed to the rapid urbanization, changing lifestyles, and increasing environmental risk factors.

The symptoms of colon cancer are usually not evident until the disease has advanced. This often results in diagnosis only at the late stages and a high mortality rates. The first step to diagnosis is a fecal blood test (FOBT) and colonoscopy. FOBT checks the presence of hidden (occult) blood in stool samples that may be indicative of colon cancer or polyps in the colon.

CRC has been linked to the changes in genetic makeup; therefore many DNA-based markers have been in practice for diagnosis of CRC. Microsatellite instability analysis (MSI), mutation in KRAS/NRAS/BRAF gene in particular BRAF V600E, and germline mutation testing of familial adenomatous polyposis gene (APC) have been used most widely for CRC diagnosis.

S. Sasi
Biocon-Bristol Myers Squibb R&D Centre, Bengaluru, Karnataka, India

S. Singh
Safety and Analytical Research Centre (SARC) LLP, Bhat, Ahmedabad, Gujarat, India

T. Walia
Dr Rajendra Prasad Government Medical College, Kangra, Himachal Pradesh, India

R. C. Meena
Division of Molecular Biology, Defence Institute of Physiology and Allied Sciences (DIPAS), DRDO, Timarpur, Delhi, India

S. Thakur (✉)
NextGen In-vitro Diagnostics Pvt Ltd., Gurugram, Haryana, India

G. P. Nagaraju et al. (eds.), *Colon Cancer Diagnosis and Therapy*,
https://doi.org/10.1007/978-3-030-63369-1_5

Immunohistochemistry (IHC) and protein-based biomarkers like MMR protein, CEA, CA19.9, MUC2, CDX2, Ck7, Ck20, KIT (CD117), and DOG1 are also being used for the diagnosis.

In spite of availability of DNA and protein-based biomarkers, there is lacuna of superior biomarker for CRC that can not only differentiate different types of CRC but also can be useful as prognostic markers.

MicroRNAs (miRNAs) are small (22 nucleotide) RNA molecules that regulate RNA transcription and protein expression in the cell. There is growing evidence linking miRNAs to various physiological processes and diseases. Moreover, there are growing numbers of literature strings suggesting that miRNA plays a significant role in cancer development, proliferation, regression, and metastasis with miRNA profiles changing at each stage. MiRNA signatures can therefore serve as reliable biomarkers for disease diagnosis and monitoring the therapeutic interventions.

In this review we highlight the recent discoveries in the field of miRNA as a biomarker for early diagnosis of CRC and also summarize roles of various miRNAs for the diagnosis of different types of CRC with special attention of miRNA in situ hybridization (ISH) and its probable function as prognostic markers and therapeutic interventions, if any.

Keywords Colorectal cancer (CRC) · MicroRNA (miRNA) · In situ hybridization (ISH) · Biomarkers

5.1 Introduction

The human body comprises billions of cells, each specialized to perform a specific function in a coordinated fashion, within a fixed lifespan. Cell growth, cell division, and cell death are a part of the natural cell cycle that gives way to cell renewal and help maintain physiological homeostasis. Sometimes, genetic mutations can cause the cell to evade or become unresponsive to apoptotic signals, resulting in uncontrollable proliferation that can lead to cancer. These "atypical or dysplastic" cells divide rapidly using up oxygen and nutrients and thereby hampering the growth of normal cells. If the immune system fails to clear these cells, over a period of time, they can build up causing a tumor and also metastasize via the lymphatic system to other sites in the body.

There are many different types of cancers, and from a histopathological viewpoint, they can be classified according to their origin. The major categories include carcinomas, sarcomas, leukemia, lymphomas, myelomas, and mixed type cancers. Carcinoma originates from the epithelial lining of organs and is the most common type of cancer. Sarcomas originate in supportive and connective tissues (such as bones, tendons, cartilage, muscle, and fat) and are more prevalent in young adults. Leukemia, lymphoma, and myeloma can be characterized as "liquid tumors" that develop in blood cells, lymphatic system, and plasma cells, respectively.

5.2 What Is Colon Cancer?

Colon cancer is a cancer that starts in the large intestine, which is the lower part of the digestive tract. Colon cancer is also referred to as colorectal cancer (CRC), a combined term for colon cancer and rectal cancer (lower most part of the large intestine). It is one of the most common types of cancers and the fourth leading cause of cancer-related mortality worldwide. Colon cancer is more prevalent in older adults and among the African-America race. Although it occurs sporadically in most cases, inherited genetic mutations can be a causative factor [24]. Other risk factors might include long-standing ulcerative colitis, food habits, smoking, alcohol consumption, low physical activity, obesity, and environmental factors [33, 36].

Colon cancer typically begins as small polyp (noncancerous clumps of cells) which if left untreated can become cancerous. These polyps do not show any symptoms, and most of the cases are diagnosed after metastasis. This presents a serious clinical problem and demands for awareness and timely screening, as well as the development of diagnostic tools for early detection.

5.3 Types of Colon Cancer

5.3.1 Adenocarcinoma

Adenocarcinomas comprise the vast majority of the colon cancer cases. They arise from adenomatous polyps on the epithelial lining of the colon. The polyps grow gradually and can metastasize if it penetrates the bowel wall and enters into the lymph node. A site of metastasis is usually the liver, lungs, and brain (*www.cancer.gov*). The other less common but more aggressive forms of adenocarcinoma include mucinous adenocarcinoma and signet ring cell adenocarcinoma. The mucinous type comprises 10–15% of the CRC cases and is characterized by the presence of mucin. It is known to be more prevalent in younger females [41]. The signet ring cell subtype is very rare and is seen in less than 1% of the patients. It is usually present in older people and has poor prognosis [81].

5.3.2 Gastrointestinal Carcinoid Tumors

These are categorized as neuroendocrine tumors which arise from the amine precursor uptake and decarboxylation (APUD) cells present on the mucosa of the gastrointestinal tract [14]. The symptoms are usually vague and non-specific, and diagnosis is done by endoscopy.

5.3.3 *Primary Colorectal Lymphomas*

It is a type of extranodal non-Hodgkin's lymphoma in the large intestine. It is extremely rare comprising only 0.2% of the malignancies seen in colon [72]. Reports show higher incidence rate in the aged population, especially in men. Currently there are no definite treatment protocols available for colorectal lymphomas.

5.3.4 *Gastrointestinal Stromal Tumors*

GIST is another infrequent sarcoma (of the colon) that stems from the interstitial cells of Cajal (ICCs), found in the lining of the GI tract. Most of the GIST cases are observed in the stomach followed by small intestine. GISTs are often misdiagnosed, and correct diagnosis impacts the treatment protocol. Mutation in the c-KIT or PDGFRA genes is common in most cases, and the KIT protein is the conventional clinical marker for characterizing GIST [60].

5.3.5 *Leiomyosarcomas*

Primary LMS of colon is also very rare and accounts for 1–2% of the entire GI malignancies. They are soft tissue sarcomas that histologically resemble GISTs. They can be differentiated by testing negative for KIT protein expression but positive for smooth muscle actin and desmin [78].

5.4 Incidences of Colon Cancer in India and Worldwide

Colorectal cancer is the third most commonly diagnosed cancer in the world after lung cancer and breast cancer [7]. The highest occurrence has been reported in Australia/New Zealand and the lowest in Africa. Asian countries have differing rates of incidence showing a striking correlation with the economic development. In India, the incidence rate of CRC is comparatively low and ranks the fifth most common cancer after breast, cervix/uteri, lip/oral cavity, and lung cancer. Also, the prevalence of age-related colon cancer is on the lower side as recorded by all the cancer registries in the country [45]. A demographic study by Patil and colleagues stated that 35% of the CRC patients were below 40 years of age and 80% were below 60 years [53]. With regard to gender, the incidence of colon cancer was found to be 0.7 to 3.7/100,000 among men and 0.4 to 3/100,000 among women [32]. However, the last few decades have seen a steady rise in the number of reported cases in India, which could be attributed to the rapid urbanization, changing lifestyles and increasing environmental risk factors.

5.5 Diagnosis of Colon Cancer

The symptoms of colon cancer are usually not evident until the disease has advanced. This often results in diagnosis only at the late stages and a high mortality rates. However, the last few decades have seen the advent of better diagnostic tools and therapeutic strategies which has significantly lowered the mortality rate of colon cancer globally.

Some of the first signs or symptoms of colon cancer include persistent change in bowel habits, blood in stools, persistent abdominal discomfort (such as cramps, gas or pain), weakness, fatigue, and unexplained weight loss. Since these symptoms are usually vague and non-specific, the patient tends to visit a general practitioner. In most cases, these symptoms are produced by benign, self-limiting illness, contributing to the patient's delay in seeking help and the practitioner's delay in referring the patient to a specialist.

The first step to diagnosis is a fecal blood test (FOBT) and colonoscopy. FOBT checks the presence of hidden (occult) blood in stool samples that may be indicative of colon cancer or polyps in the colon. Colonoscopy remains as the gold standard for CRC investigation. Computed tomography (CT) colonography could be an alternative, especially in elderly patients with poor specific symptoms such as abdominal pain or weight loss [76]. Often, the suspected tissue region is biopsied during a colonoscopy which is then subjected to various molecular screening tests to classify and stage the cancer.

1. *Histopathology tests*: Certain stains and markers are used to dissect the morphology of the tissue sample (biopsy) which helps classify the type of cancer and determine the stage of the tumor. Immunohistochemistry tests verify the protein biomarker expression levels.
2. *Genetic tests*: Colorectal cancer cells are typically tested to see if they show high levels of gene changes called microsatellite instability (MSI) and changes in DNA mismatch repair gene. Moreover, patients with mutations in KRAS, NRAS, and BRAF genes do not respond to general anti-cancer drugs and will require targeted therapy.

Other imaging techniques like CT scan, PET scan, X-ray, and ultrasound may be employed to determine if the cancer has spread to other sites in the body.

5.6 Treatments Available for CRC

Treatment of colon cancer typically involves a combination of surgery, radiology, and chemotherapy and/or immunotherapy. The type of therapeutic intervention is decided based on the stage of the cancer and the patient's overall health condition.

According to American Joint Committee on Cancer (AJCC), pathological staging of cancer is based on TNM score, where *T* is the tumor size; *N*, the spread to nearby lymph nodes; and *M*, the metastasis to distant lymph nodes or organs. As per the TNM scaling, colon cancer can be characterized into four stages.

- *Stage I*: The tumor has grown into the submucosa (T1) or muscularispropria (T2) but has not spread to nearby lymph nodes (N0) or to distant sites (M0).
- *Stage II*: The tumor has grown into the outermost layers of the colon. The T score can be T3 (confined to the colon wall), T4a (grown through the wall of the colon or rectum but has not grown into other nearby tissues or organs), or T4b (attached to or has grown into other nearby tissues or organs). N0 and M0.
- *Stage III*: The tumor has spread to nearby lymph nodes. The score can be N1 or N2 based on the number of nearby lymph nodes. Any T and M0.
- *Stage IV*: Has spread to distant organs, such as the liver or lungs and/or distant lymph nodes. Score of M1a-c is given in line with the number or organs affected. Any T and N.

The major therapeutic strategies in colon cancer involve surgical resection and adjuvant chemotherapy. Removal of the tumor, surrounding healthy tissue, and nearby lymph nodes is the first line of treatment for stage I and II patients. Selected patients of stage II and stage III patients will require chemotherapy drugs. Capecitabine (Xeloda), fluorouracil (5-FU), irinotecan (Camptosar), oxaliplatin (Eloxatin), and trifluridine/tipiracil (Lonsurf) are some of the chemodrugs that are used alone or in combinations to increase efficacy. Treatment for stage IV metastatic cancers aims at controlling the symptoms and providing palliative care to increase survival. The therapeutic plan is usually a combination of surgery, radiation, chemotherapy, and immunotherapy based on the overall health condition of the patient [74].

Immunotherapy has particularly benefited the patients with mutations in genes involved in DNA mismatch repair (dMMR) pathway. These patients have shown positive response to anti-PD1, anti-PDL1, and/or anti-CTLA monoclonal antibodies [29]. However, the other subtypes of colon cancer do not show effective response to this line of treatment, summoning more R&D in immunotherapeutic interventions.

5.7 Diagnostics Markers for Colon Cancer

In the case of colon cancer, a number of molecular biomarkers are used to classify the tumor type, measure the progression of the disease, as well as decide the course of treatment. Genetic alterations, namely, microsatellite instability (MSI), chromosomal instability (CIN), and the CpG island methylator phenotype (CIMP), are common in CRC which in turn produce quantifiable modifications in DNA, RNA, proteins, or metabolites [40]. These specific changes serve as diagnostic biomarkers and are measured in the tumor biopsy, blood, or stool. In the case of metastasis, some of these markers are also beneficial to trace the primary site to colon.

5.7.1 DNA Markers

- Microsatellite instability – MSI ensues from mutations in the genes coding for dMMR proteins, viz., MLH1, MSH2, MSH6, and PMS2 [54]. Typically, a PCR test is conducted to check for germline mutations. MSI-positive patients show good prognosis and respond to irinotecan treatment.
- KRAS/NRAS – oncogenes involved in EGFR signalling and serve as predictors for anti-EGFR treatment. Mutations often lead to bad prognosis and poor survival [2].
- BRAF – another pro-proliferative gene involved in EGFR pathway. BRAF V600E is the most common BRAF mutations leading to poor prognosis [43]. MAPK/PI3K pathway inhibitors have been used for treating metastatic CRC.
- APC/MUTYH – mutations in these tumor suppressive genes is common in CRC. These mutations can also be inherited. Germline mutation testing is done to assess the risk of familial adenomatous polyposis [82].

5.7.2 Protein Markers

The protein markers in the sample are measured by immunohistochemistry technique. It is a highly specific and sensitive technique using tagged antibodies to probe the protein target.

- MMR proteins – involved in dMMR signalling pathway.
- Carcinoembryonic antigen (CEA) and CA19.9 – these are the most common diagnostic tests in the case of CRC. CEA highlights the apical poles of cells lining the glandular lumen, and CA19.9 marks the cells of colonic mucosa. CEA is used to differentiate colon cancer from other cancer types.
- MUC2 – reveals the levels of mucin2 protein to ascertain mucinous carcinomas.
- CDX2 – a transcription factor that regulates proliferation of epithelial cells and their differentiation into villus enterocytes. This nuclear marker can be used to establish colorectal origin of the tumor.
- Cytokeratin 7 and 20 – CK 20 positive and CK 7 negative confirms adenocarcinomas of the colon.
- KIT (CD117) and DOG1 – distinguishes GIST tumors from other types of colon cancers.

5.8 miRNA and Colorectal Cancer

MiRNA is an evolutionarily conserved class of short ~22 nucleotide RNAs that can regulate transcription and protein expression in cells. They were first discovered in 1993 by Lee et al. but gained importance only in the 2000s. They exert their functional effects by triggering mRNA degradation or interfering mRNA translation [11, 37]. MiRNAs are known to modulate up to 60% of the coding genes with a single miRNA targeting multiple mRNAs or a single mRNA being regulated by multiple miRNAs [17]. Hence, there is growing evidence linking miRNAs to various physiological processes and diseases. They are now known to play significant roles in cancer development, proliferation, regression, and metastasis with miRNA profiles changing at each stage [38]. MiRNA signatures can therefore serve as reliable biomarkers for disease diagnosis and monitoring therapeutic interventions.

5.8.1 miRNA Biogenesis

MiRNA genes can be located in the non-coding areas of the DNA or can be intragenic, i.e., overlapping with introns (or exons in fewer cases). In most cases, miRNA genes are seen as a cluster near one another. A typical miRNA cluster will consist of two or three miRNA genes. These clusters are transcribed as polycistrons, which are then processed into multiple pre-miRNAs. The biogenesis of miRNA is a complex process and can be classified into canonical and non-canonical pathways.

In the *canonical pathway*, RNA polymerase II/III transcribes the miRNA gene into a characteristic hairpin-structured pri-miRNA. The pri-miRNA is cleaved into a precursor pre-miRNA by the microprocessor complex consisting of the ribonuclease III enzyme Drosha and the RNA-binding protein DiGeorge Syndrome Critical Region 8 (DGCR8) [16]. These pre-miRNA is then transported to the cytoplasm by the Exportin5(XPO5)/RanGTP complex, which is then processed into mature miRNA by the RNase III endonuclease Dicer [49]. Finally, the two strands are separated and either the 5p or 3p associates with the RNA binding protein, trinucleotide repeat-containing gene 6A (TNRC6A), and Argonaute (AGO) family of proteins to form a miRNA-induced silencing complex (miRISC). The guide RNA is selected based on the thermodynamic stability at the 5′ end. The strand with the most unstable base pairing at the 5′ end gets incorporated into miRISC while usually acts as the guide strand (known as the passenger or miR* strand) gets degraded. In very rare cases, both the strands associate with AGO proteins, serving as functional miRNAs [50].

Many *non-canonical pathways* for miRNA biogenesis have been identified. These can be Drosha/DGCR8-independent or Dicer-independent pathways. The microprocessor-independent pathways involve pre-miRNA-like hairpins called "Mirtrons" formed from introns of mRNA during splicing small nucleolar RNAs (snoRNAs) or 7-methylguanosine (m7G)-capped pre-miRNA [5]. These RNAs are directly transported to the cytoplasm byExportin5/RanGTP orExportin1 by passing Drosha cleavage. On the other hand, the Dicer-independent miRNAs are processed by Drosha from endogenous short hairpin RNA (shRNA) transcripts and mature in an AGO2-dependent manner to complete their maturation [47]. All the non-canonical pathways eventually lead to the formation of the miRISC complex.

The miRISC recognizes the miRNA response elements (MRE) on target RNA molecules and degree of miRNA: MRE complementarity is known to determine mode of mRNA regulation [27]. A 100% complementarity is very rare in animals, and in most cases the partial complementarity induces translational repression. This could possibly explain how a single miRNA can regulate numerous genes [23]. Studies have shown that a complete match of miRNA/MRE leads to AGO2-dependent slicing of target mRNA. Besides gene silencing, several miRNAs have been found to be involved in translational activation via AGO2 and FXR1 proteins [75].

5.8.2 *miRNA Localization and Distribution*

The biogenesis route of miRNAs suggests the presence of mature miRNAs in the cytoplasm, associated with miRISCs to exert their functional effects on mRNAs. Various research groups have described miRNA distribution in the form of miRISC and miRISC-associated complexes in several other subcellular compartments, as well as extracellular fluids. However, miRNA expression, abundance, and distribution are largely dictated by cell type, cell cycle phase, and cell disease state [15].

Based on their findings, O'Brien and colleagues have proposed location-specific functional implications for mature miRNAs associated with miRISCs. Within the nucleus, miRISC is often found at sites of active transcription suggesting a role in chromatin activation, apart from nascent mRNA splicing. The miRISC associated with nuclear messenger ribonucleoprotein (mRNP) has been detected in the nucleus as well as certain cytoplasmic compartments. This might hint at the miRNA's role in mRNP degradation and transportation across the nuclear membrane. Cytoplasmic miRISC is spread across the cytosol suggesting cytoplasmic transportation via the microtubules. In the cytoplasm they mediate mRNA translational repression on the rough endoplasmic reticulum and are then shuttled to endosomes for mRNA deadenylation and decay. Once their job is done, they can be moved to the lysosome for degradation. The mitochondria also show positive for the presence of miRISC, suggesting its probable role in the regulation of mitochondrial genes [83, 84]. Furthermore, miRISC localization within the Golgi explains the presence of extracellular miRNA in circulation.

Circulating vesicular or vesicle-free miRISC has been identified in blood and other body fluids which suggest their role in intracellular communication. Circulating miRNAs could also be a result of cell apoptosis or necrosis. The molecules can be released encapsulated in the cell-free lipid carriers (micro-vesicles, exosomes, and apoptotic bodies) or bound to protein complexes, with Argonaute or high-density lipoproteins (HDL), which enables them to evade the RNase digestion and remain stable in the circulation [34, 62].

5.8.3 Role of miRNA in Cancer Diagnosis

MiRNAs are involved in a multitude of cellular processes, including the regulation of cell cycle, differentiation, proliferation, apoptosis, stress tolerance, energy metabolism, and immune response. There has been growing evidence linking the dysregulation if miRNAs to human cancer, as well as cancer drug resistance [65]. Several miRNAs have been described to modulate tumor genes which can either result in tumor development (oncoMirs) or tumor suppression. The mechanisms of dysregulation can be attributed to various factors such as chromosomal abnormalities, transcriptional control changes, epigenetic changes, and defects in the miRNA biogenesis machinery [55].

Efforts are underway to elucidate the miRNA expression profiles in different tumor types that can be exploited as cancer-specific biomarkers for early detection and disease prognosis. More recently, circulating miRNAs secreted into body fluids including blood, saliva, and urine have been identified as novel candidates for various diseases including cancer [62]. Studies show that the secreted miRNAs are quite stable and quantifiable making them ideal non-invasive biomarkers for clinical use. MiRNAs can also be used as predictors of therapeutic response as there is emerging evidence pointing toward the role of several miRNAs in chemodrug resistance [65].

The lack of robust molecular markers for early diagnosis makes CRC the second most fatal form of cancer. Studies focusing on miRNA aberrations have revealed several miRNA markers that can be used in diagnostic and prognostic applications. These include a various tissue-specific markers like miR-21, miR-29b, miR-34a, and miR-155 [25] as well as circulating blood miRNA markers such as miR-20b, miR-29b, and miR-155 [73]. Moreover, Pan et al. published data on the sensitivity and specificity of multiple miRNA panels to distinguish CRC from colorectal adenoma [52]. Recent studies also suggest miR-21 and miR-92a as prospective fecal miRNA markers that can be used for CRC screening [80].

5.8.4 Cell-Type and Tumor-Type Specific Expression of miRNA Biomarkers in Cancer

Genome-wide profiling has correlated unique miRNA expression signatures to specific tumor types, tumor grade, and therapeutic outcomes. Hence miRNAs are gaining importance as prospective biomarkers for cancer diagnostics, prognosis, and therapeutics. Various research groups have illustrated the change in expression of a selected miRNA panel in cancer patients versus healthy individuals, as well as in samples pre- and post-surgery [22]. There are also several proposed miRNA blood tests that are being developed for early detection of tumors in the lung and prostate and for triple negative breast cancer [46, 64, 66].

The first association of miRNA and cancer was reported in 2002 when Calin et al. showed that chromosomal deletion of miR-15 and miR-16 was a frequent event in B-cell chronic lymphocytic leukemia [9]. The miRNA loci were also observed to be located at fragile sites, breakpoint regions, or frequently altered regions (e.g., deletion or amplification) in the cancer genome [10]. Since then there has been a surge in the field of miRNA research aiming to understand the biology and their clinical relevance.

5.8.5 *Circulating miRNA Markers*

The discovery of circulating miRNA has definitely created a buzz in miRNA research. More groups are now focusing on decoding the correlation between cancer types and serum miRNA levels (Table 5.1). Despite the developments, several challenges lay ahead in validating circulating miRNAs as ideal clinical biomarkers.

The huge amount of data being generated points out a lot of discrepancy among results of various groups. The implementation of a common standard procedure and normalization scheme might prove beneficial in this scenario. It was exemplified by Singh and colleagues that the choice of substrate for miRNA isolation impacts results [67]. In addition, factors like vesicle purification, disease-specific changes in secretary mechanisms, therapeutic alterations in blood volume, cell death, and tumor necrosis can all have an impact on the RNA yield [8, 31]. The relation between tissue expression and cell-free circulating miRNAs is also unclear, and continuing research can shed more light on the biology of miRNA secretion.

5.8.6 *What Is miRNA ISH*

In situ hybridization (ISH) is a molecular technique used to map the localization of nucleic acids in cells or tissue sections while preserving the morphological context. ISH works on the principle of complementary base pairing using a labelled probe to detect target DNA and RNA within the cell. DNA ISH is generally used to identify chromosome locations and abnormalities like gene deletions, amplifications, and

Table 5.1 MicroRNA expression level and its association with cancer types

S. no.	MicroRNA	Cancer type	Expression
1	miR-221	Breast cancer, melanoma, thyroid, renal cell carcinoma	Downregulated
2	miR-375	Breast cancer, pancreatic cancer, esophageal cancer	Downregulated
3	miR-21	Esophageal cancer, lung cancer	Downregulated
4	miR-486	Non-small cell lung cancer	Upregulated/ downregulated
		Gastric cancer	Downregulated

Adopted from Filipów and Łaczmanski [22]

rearrangements. On the other hand, RNA ISH can be used to assess the localization and expression levels of mRNA or miRNA inside the cell/tissue. ISH is capable of capturing nucleic acid expression in different types of samples including frozen tissues, formalin-fixed paraffin-embedded (FFPE) tissues, cell suspension smears, as well as fine needle aspiration smears [1].

Studying the spatiotemporal expression of miRNA is crucial to elucidate their roles in physiological and pathophysiological processes. Hence, ISH becomes an ideal molecular tool to dissect necessary information at a cellular level. Multiple research groups have established ISH as a reliable method to look into the miRNA expression in different cell and tissue types. Owing to their small size, detection of less expressing miRNAs has been challenging, while ISH readily captures abundant miRNAs. However over the last few years, several improvements have been introduced into the miRNA in situ techniques. Variations in sample processing, probe hybridization, and detection steps have been investigated to increase the specificity and sensitivity of ISH assays. Thermal stability of the probes and probe accessibility are other important factors that can impact ISH signal [71]. Locked nucleic acids (LNAs) have been a revolutionary invention and have greatly replaced the conventional oligonucleotide probes when it comes to miRNA-ISH [48]. LNAs are bicyclic RNA analogs that possess a greater affinity toward RNA and higher thermal stability, which considerably improves the assay sensitivity. LNA-RNA complex has melting temperatures >70 °C adding to the stringency and specificity. Other strategies developed include the use of double-labelled probes to increase signal-to-noise ratio and EDC-based sample fixation. Introduction of 1-ethyl-3-[3-dimethylaminopropyl] carbodiimide hydrochloride (EDC) in the fixation step prevents the loss of free miRNAs into hybridization buffers [58].

Chromogenic in situ hybridization (CISH) and fluorescent in situ hybridization (FISH) are widely used for miRNA detection, both having their own advantages and limitations. The general protocol involves (1) tissue fixation for FFPE samples or cryo-preservation for frozen samples, (2) proteinase K treatment, (3) probe hybridization, (4) stringent washes, and (5) signal amplification and detection. CISH uses probes labelled with a chromogenic enzyme such as alkaline phosphatase (AP) and horseradish peroxidase (HRP) which is visualized by adding a color producing substrate. Alternatively, signal amplification can be achieved by multistep CISH which uses a biotin or digoxigenin (DIG)-labelled probe followed by an enzyme-tagged antibody step that binds to the probe, similar to immunohistochemistry (Fig. 5.1). FISH incorporates fluorescent labels allowing multiplexing and quantification of signals. In comparison, FISH is more robust, but one of the major drawback is that it cannot detect miRNAs with very low copy number [85].

FFPE tissues are the major resources of tumor samples worldwide, and miRNAs have been found to be intact in such samples [28]. This makes ISH a steadfast tool to characterize miRNA profiles across cancer types. ISH preserves the spatial information, unlike qRT-PCR and microarray, which can be used to examine the regulatory networks within a tumor micro-environment. Additionally, miRNA ISH can be combined with immunohistochemistry or mRNA-ISH to develop clinical tests for disease diagnosis and therapy.

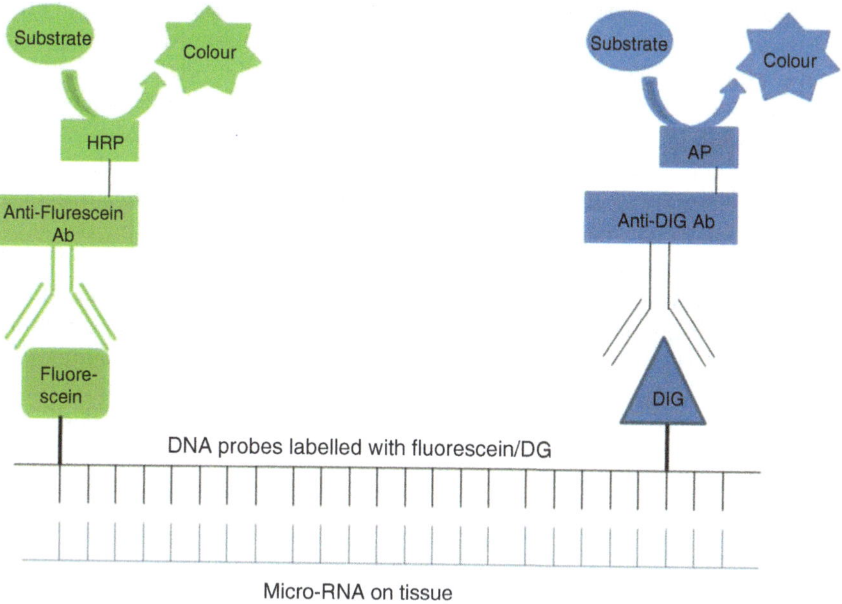

Fig. 5.1 Basic principle of chromogenic/flourescent in situ hybridization. Fluorescein/DIG-labelled DNA probes bind to the respective miRNA target(s) in tissue. In a subsequent step anti-fluorescein (HRP-conjugated)/anti-DIG (AP-conjugated)-labelled antibodies binds to the respective tags (Fluorescein/DIG). Final chromogenic visualization is done by adding respective substrate for HRP/AP. DIG Digoxigenin, HRP horseradish peroxidase, AP alkaline phosphatase

5.8.7 *Role of miRNA ISH in Cancer of Unknown Primary Origin and Poorly and Undifferentiated Tumor*

Of all the cancer cases worldwide, around 5% are reported to be cancers of unknown primary origin (CUPs). CUPs or occult cancers, as they are sometimes described, are metastasized malignant carcinomas whose primary site is unknown. In addition, cancers of unknown (and sometimes known) origin are often graded as poorly differentiated or undifferentiated carcinomas as cells display characteristics that are grossly different from normal cells or the cells of origin, making them unsuitable for targeted therapy. These grades of tumors are aggressive and result in poor prognosis of the patient. The development of more precise and accurate diagnostic tools to identify the primary tissue is key to the selection of an appropriate therapeutic intervention.

Clinically, a case of CUP is subjected to imaging of organs and histopathology analysis to determine the primary site. Histological assessments typically include cytogenetic stains and immunohistochemistry markers. Most of the available markers are helpful in identifying the type of carcinoma and the metastatic status but may not be able to speak of the tissue of origin. Recently, miRNA profiling has emerged as a probable classifier for the tissue of cancer origin. In this regard, several miRNA expression patterns have been evaluated in primary and metastatic tumors of different tissue types [21, 59]. Rosenfeld's group identified a 48-miRNA signature that could distinguish the tissue types with a >80% prediction accuracy. A study by Søkilde et al. stated that some histologies have a stronger and more homogeneous tissue-specific miRNA signature when compared to other tissues. MiRNA signatures in tumors such as adrenal, lymphoma, germ cell, prostate, gastrointestinal stromal tumor (GIST), and melanoma were found to be more consistent than ovary, lung, and colorectal where the cell heterogeneity is usually high [70].

ISH is a simple and cost-effective technique that can be used to analyze the miRNA fingerprint, providing an insight about the tissue of origin. The miRNA studies in FFPE samples showed high correlation with expression levels in frozen samples [6]. However, excessive fixation and tissue processing conditions can greatly affect the quality of miRNA. Therefore, standardization of protocols across labs will be necessary to avoid variability. Multiplex ISH probes can be designed to simultaneously look at miRNA as well as DNA rearrangements. In the clinic, miRNA ISH can be done as a complementary test along with the routine IHC investigations to verify the tumor type and tissue of origin.

5.8.8 Role of miRNA ISH in Colon Cancer

Several miRNAs have been identified in the carcinogenesis of colon cancer, regulating cell cycle, apoptosis, invasion, migration, and metastasis. Some function as tumor suppressors, while others are oncogenic. The oncomiRs act by inhibiting the expression of tumor-suppressing genes and have been reported to be upregulated in CRC. On the contrary, tumor suppressing miRNAs interfere with the expression of oncogenes and are usually downregulated in CRC. Multiple studies report differential miRNA expression patterns, as well as miRNA-mediated gene expression levels indifferent stages of colon cancer [19, 20, 30, 39, 51, 57]. MiRNA profiles have been screened in early-stage CRC tissues, precancerous lesions, and colonic intraepithelial neoplasia allowing development of appropriate miRNA panels for clinical diagnosis.

ISH makes for a cost-effective and reliable diagnostic tool to detect and quantify the miRNA expression. Multiplex ISH can be employed to analyze a series of miRNAs known to be dysregulated (against normal tissue) in a particular stage of colon cancer. Unlike PCR-based detection of miRNA where tissue is grinded before isolation of miRNA and therefore the expression lever exhibit both normal and cancer tissue, ISH can detect the expression of miRNA in spatial context that enables to see the differential expression of miRNA in normal vis-a-vis cancer tissue.

However, in order to develop clinical tests, it is important to conduct elaborate feasibility studies and protocol optimization to confirm specificity and sensitivity. Validation against known controls including diseased vs. normal tissues and edited cell lines is indispensable to make accurate diagnosis.

5.8.9 MiRNA Markers for Colon Cancer Diagnosis

Studies reveal that different signalling pathways control the progression of colon cancer from one stage to next. MiRNAs that participate in the tumor-related pathways such as Wnt, p53, EGFR/KRAS, TGF-β/SMAD, notch signalling, etc. have been mapped, and some key players have identified in different stages [4, 19].

Some of the commonly dysregulated miRNAs and the cellular effects are summarized in Table 5.2.

MiR-21 has been widely reported to be associated with colon cancers. The later stages show a rise in the expression of miR-21 [56], implying its potential as a clinical biomarker. Moreover, cases of lymph node metastases correlate with high miR-155 expression [63]. The tumor suppressor miRNAs miR-143 and miR-145 is usually downregulated in most colon cancers and has been linked to pathogenesis [61, 77]. Low levels of miR-145 have been particularly associated with large tumor size. Similarly Mir-106a, which is consistently over-expressed in CRC patients, has been postulated as a plausible marker for early detection and 5-FU treatment resistance [26, 65].

MiR-31 is another oncoMiR that has shown great clinical relevance. It has been seen to be upregulated in the advanced stages of colon cancer and poorly differentiated tumors [35, 61]. Studies also show that miR-31 plays a role in the development of colon cancer-associated fibroblasts (CAFs) and is known to contribute to cancer migration and invasiveness [79]. Recently, Anandappa et al. reported that metastatic CRC patients with low miR-31-3p expression showed better response to anti-EGFR treatment [3].

In a study by Makondi and group, miR-576-5p and miR-20a was identified as predictive markers for metastasis [42]. They also investigated miR-495, miR-449a, MiR-619, and miR-382 along with the other two as a panel for CRC progression to liver metastases.

5.9 Discussion

According to WHO, colorectal cancer is the third most prevalent cancer in the world and the second most fatal form of cancer after lung cancer. Although current data shows a lower prevalence of CRC in India, an increasing trend has been observed during the last few years owing to the rapid urbanization and change in lifestyle [68, 69]. Lifestyle modifications along with early diagnosis and timely therapeutic intervention remain prime in bringing down the mortality rate.

The carcinogenesis of colon cancer is a multistep molecular process involving several gene dysregulations that alter cellular function. The discovery of miRNAs has added a new perspective to gene regulation and the central dogma of molecular biology. The number of studies focusing on miRNAs has grown exponentially emphasizing its role in an array of cellular processes and diseases. There is growing

Table 5.2 MicroRNAs dysregulated in colon cancer and their proposed roles in disease progression [13, 18, 65]

MiRNA	Dysregulation	Direct/indirect targets	Cellular effects
MiR-21	Upregulated	PDCD4, TIAM1, SPRY2, PTEN, TGFBR2, CDC25A, hMSH2	Proliferation, apoptosis, invasion, migration, CSC maintenance, intravasation, cell cycle, chemo-resistance
MiR-92a	Upregulated	PTEN, SMAD2, SMAD4, TGFBR2	EMT, invasion, venous invasion, metastases, proliferation
MiR-96	Upregulated	TP53INP1, FOXO1, FOXO3A, UBE2N, XIAP, REV1, RAD51	Cell growth, proliferation, drug-sensitizing, apoptosis
MiR-135a/b	Upregulated	APC, hMLH1, hMSH2	Proliferation, gene dosage effects
MiR-155	Upregulated	PTPRJ, TP53INP1, MSH2, MSH6, MLH1, FOXO3a, HuR	Proliferation, invasion, stemness, angiogenesis, drug resistance, genome instability, ETM
MiR-224	Upregulated	SMAD4, p21, PHLPP1, PHLPP2, GSK-3β	Metastasis, proliferation, tumorigenicity, chemoradiosensitivity
MiR-192/215	Upregulated	SRPX2	Facilitates cell glycolysis
MiR-1273g-3p	Upregulated	CNR1	Promote cell proliferation, migration, and invasion
Let-7	Downregulated	KRAS	Proliferation
MiR-194	Downregulated	MAP4K4, AKT2	Proliferation, apoptosis, invasion, migration, cell cycle
MiR-143/145	Downregulated	IGF1R, CD44, KLF5, KRAS, BRAF	Proliferation, invasion, migration, apoptosis, angiogenesis, chemo-resistance
MiR-34a	Downregulated	E2F1, SIRT1, FMNL2, E2F5, SNHG7	Proliferation, invasiveness, metastasis, apoptosis, chemoresistance
MiR-126	Downregulated	PI3K, VCAM-1, CXCR4, VEGFA, IRS1, RhoA	Proliferation, invasion, migration, cell cycle, angiogenesis, hematopoiesis
MiR-27b	Downregulated	VEGF, Rab3D	Proliferation, colony formation, angiogenesis, EMT
MiR-7	Downregulated	EGFR, RAF-1	Proliferation
MiR-18a-3p	Downregulated	KRAS	Proliferation, anchorage-independent growth
MiR-26b	Downregulated	TAF12, PTP4A1, CHFR, ALS2CR2, FUT4	Proliferation, apoptosis, invasiveness, metastasis, migration, chemoresistance
MiR-101	Downregulated	COX-2, ZEB1	Proliferation, migration
MiR-144	Downregulated	mTOR	Proliferation
MiR-320a	Downregulated	β-catenin	Proliferation
MiR-330	Downregulated	CDC42	Proliferation
MiR-455	Downregulated	RAF1	Proliferation, invasion
MiR-149	Downregulated	FOXM1	Proliferation, migration, invasion

(continued)

Table 5.2 (continued)

MiRNA	Dysregulation	Direct/indirect targets	Cellular effects
MiR-155	Downregulated	CTHRC1	Suppress cell proliferation, promote cell cycle arrest, and apoptosis
MiR-205-5p	Downregulated	ZEB1	Inhibit epithelial to mesenchymal transition
MiR-18a	Downregulated	CDC42	Inhibit colorectal cancer cell growth and death
MiR-7	Downregulated	YY1	Resensitization to fas/FasL-apoptosis
miR-19b-1	Downregulated	ACSL/SCD	Inhibit invasion in colon cancer cells
MiR-30a	Downregulated	Metadherin	Inhibit cell migration and invasion
MiR-744	Downregulated	Notch1	Inhibit cell proliferation and invasion
MiR-383	Downregulated	PAX6	Inhibit cell proliferation and invasion
MiR-1271	Downregulated	Capn4	Suppress cell proliferation and invasion
MiR-186-5p	Downregulated	ZEB1	Inhibit cell proliferation, metastasis and epithelial to mesenchymal transition
MiR-511	Downregulated	HDGF	Reduce cell proliferation and invasion
MiR-374b	Downregulated	LRH-1	Inhibit cell proliferation and invasion
MiR-216a-3p	Downregulated	COX-2 and ALOX5	Suppress cell proliferation

interest in the application of miRNA signatures for diagnostic as well as therapeutic purposes. In the context of CRC, high-throughput genome-wide profiling and comprehensive screening technologies have enabled discovery of several miRNA–mRNA regulatory networks in pathogenesis and disease progression. Unique miRNA expression patterns have been identified in different stages of CRC that could be developed as diagnostic and prognostic indicators. From a clinical standpoint, an ideal diagnostic approach is to analyze a set of miRNAs that are usually dysregulated. This is important as a single miRNA is not specific enough to distinguish a particular cancer type or disease phase.

Coming to the molecular techniques used for miRNA detection, several platforms have been explored and implemented. Quantitative PCR, next-generation sequencing (NGS), and micro-arrays remain the most widely used high-throughput techniques. Northern blot is another traditional method that can be used to detect miRNAs but has low sensitivity and lacks quantitative ability. Other innovative technologies like DNA nano-switch using DNA scaffolds have also been described [12]. All these techniques require RNA isolation and suffer major setbacks in deducing the miRNA expression pattern with respect to tissue and cellular morphology.

Here, we have discussed the potential of ISH as a reliable molecular diagnostic tool for diagnosing CRC-related miRNA in a clinical setting. ISH is a simple complementarity hybridization technique that can be used on biopsy (frozen or FFPE) or fine needle aspiration samples to look into the expression patterns within a cell and in different cell types and stroma in a tissue. ISH will be able to pick up the upregulated oncoMiRs in the sample pointing toward the disease stage. Detection of the downregulated, low copy number miRNAs could be a major challenge. However, the sensitivity of ISH can be tweaked using LNA probes and signal amplification steps. Fluorescent ISH offers higher multiplexing capacity that can be employed to detect a panel of miRNAs. Moreover, multiplexing immunohistochemistry markers and miRNA ISH probes will present a superior clinical read-out, adding value to the existing diagnostic approaches.

Having said that, miRNA diagnostics is still in the early stages, and translation into clinic is seeing progression. Since data discrepancy has been observed among various studies, it is important to thoroughly validate the target miRNA panels. Consistency in sample processing and normalization methods across labs will be necessary to avoid technical deviations. Laying down some collective criteria for selection of control samples is also important for validation studies. For FFPE-ISH, reagents and protocol steps for tissue fixation and target retrieval may affect the RNA content. Another related challenge concerns the definition of biologically relevant cutoff miRNA levels for diagnostics. Quantification cutoff needs to be determined for specific miRNA in the primary and surrounding tissues in different stages of cancer.

Continuing research in miRNA will give more insights into this complex regulatory network. A deeper understanding of the biological role of each miRNA will help appropriate selection of miRNA panels for diagnostics. In a country like India where cancer burden is on the rise, screening for early detection markers for the common cancers including CRC should be compulsory in health checkups above 30 years of age. Finally, in situ hybridization (ISH) can be used as a sensitive and cost-effective method to implement miRNA-based CRC diagnostics and prognosis in clinics.

Adding to the existing dilemma, the outbreak of the COVID19 pandemic in January 2020 has overwhelmed the healthcare infrastructure posing great amount of ignorance for all other underlying conditions including CRC. Firstly, if contracted with SARS-CoV2, the patients will be at a higher risk of increased mortality rate. Secondly, the overcrowded intensive care during the pandemic can deprive the patients of proper hospital care and treatment. Marshall et al. have listed certain steps for the management of CRC patients in the wake of COVID19 [44]. Practicing personal hygeine and taking preventive measures along with timely diagnosis and treatment is essential to ensure patient health.

References

1. Acs B, Szekely N, Szasz AM, Lotz G, Szekely T, Istok R, Szekely E, Madaras L, Kulka J, Jaray B. Reliability of immunocytochemistry and fluorescence in situ hybridization on fine-needle aspiration cytology samples of breast cancers: a comparative study. Diagn Cytopathol. 2016;44:466–71. https://doi.org/10.1002/dc.23463.
2. Afrăsânie VA, Marinca MV, Alexa-Stratulat T, et al. KRAS, NRAS, BRAF, HER2 and microsatellite instability in metastatic colorectal cancer – practical implications for the

clinician. Radiol Oncol. 2019;53(3):265–74. Published 2019 Sep 24. https://doi.org/10.2478/raon-2019-0033.

3. Anandappa G, Lampis A, Cunningham D, Khan KH, Kouvelakis K, Vlachogiannis G, Hedayat S, Tunariu N, Rao S, Watkins D, Starling N, Braconi C, Darvish-Damavandi M, Lote H, Thomas J, Peckitt C, Kalaitzaki R, Khan N, Fotiadis N, Rugge M, Begum R, Rana I, Bryant A, Hahne JC, Chau I, Fassan M, Valeri N. miR-31-3p expression and benefit from anti-EGFR inhibitors in metastatic colorectal cancer patients enrolled in the prospective phase II PROSPECT-C trial. Clin Cancer Res. 2019;25(13):3830–8. https://doi.org/10.1158/1078-0432.CCR-18-3769.
4. Asadi M, Talesh ST, Gjerstorff MF, Shanehbandi D, Baradaran B, Hashemzadeh S, Zafari V. Identification of miRNAs correlating with stage and progression of colorectal cancer. Colorectal Cancer. 2019;8:2. https://doi.org/10.2217/crc-2018-0014.
5. Bhaskaran M, Mohan M. MicroRNAs: history, biogenesis, and their evolving role in animal development and disease. Vet Pathol. 2014;51(4):759–74. https://doi.org/10.1177/0300985813502820.
6. Boisen MK, Dehlendorff C, Linnemann D, et al. MicroRNA expression in formalin-fixed paraffin-embedded cancer tissue: identifying reference microRNAs and variability. BMC Cancer. 2015;15:1024. https://doi.org/10.1186/s12885-015-2030-2.
7. Bray F, Ferlay J, Soerjomataram I, Siegel RL, Torre LA, Jemal A. Global cancer statistics 2018: GLOBOCAN estimates of incidence and mortality worldwide for 36 cancers in 185 countries. CA Cancer J Clin. 2018;68:394–424. https://doi.org/10.3322/caac.21492.
8. Buschmann D, Kirchner B, Hermann S, et al. Evaluation of serum extracellular vesicle isolation methods for profiling miRNAs by next-generation sequencing [published correction appears in J Extracell Vesicles. 2019 Mar 08;8(1):1581487]. J Extracell Vesicles. 2018;7(1):1481321. Published 2018 Jun 4. https://doi.org/10.1080/20013078.2018.1481321.
9. Calin GA, Dumitru CD, Shimizu M, Bichi R, Zupo S, Noch E, Aldler H, Rattan S, Keating M, Rai K, et al. Frequent deletions and down-regulation of micro- RNA genes miR15 and miR16 at 13q14 in chronic lymphocytic leukemia. Proc Natl Acad Sci U S A. 2002;99:15524–9.
10. Calin GA, Sevignani C, Dumitru CD, Hyslop T, Noch E, Yendamuri S, Shimizu M, Rattan S, Bullrich F, Negrini M, Croce CM. Human microRNA genes are frequently located at fragile sites and genomic regions involved in cancers. Proc Natl Acad Sci U S A. 2004;101:2999–3004.
11. Cannell IG, Kong YW, Bushell M. How do microRNAs regulate gene expression. Biochem Soc Trans. 2008;36:1224–31.
12. Chandrasekaran AR, MacIsaac M, Dey P, Levchenko O, Zhou L, Andres M, Dey BK, Halvorsen K. Cellular microRNA detection with miRacles: microRNA- activated conditional looping of engineered switches. Sci Adv. 2019;5(3):eaau9443. https://doi.org/10.1126/sciadv.aau9443.
13. Chen B, Xia Z, Deng YN, et al. Emerging microRNA biomarkers for colorectal cancer diagnosis and prognosis. Open Biol. 2019;9(1):180212. https://doi.org/10.1098/rsob.180212.
14. Chung TP, Hunt SR. Carcinoid and neuroendocrine tumors of the colon and rectum. Clin Colon Rectal Surg. 2006;19(2):45–8. https://doi.org/10.1055/s-2006-942343.
15. de Rie D, Abugessaisa I, Alam T, Arner E, Arner P, Ashoor H, et al. An integrated expression atlas of miRNAs and their promoters in human and mouse. Nat Biotechnol. 2017;35:872–8. https://doi.org/10.1038/nbt.3947.
16. Denli AM, Tops BB, Plasterk RH, Ketting RF, Hannon GJ. Processing of primary microRNAs by the microprocessor complex. Nature. 2004;432:231–5. https://doi.org/10.1038/nature03049.
17. Di Leva G, Garofalo M, Croce CM. MicroRNAs in cancer. Annu Rev Pathol. 2014;9:287–314.
18. Ding L, Lan Z, Xiong X, et al. The dual role of microRNAs in colorectal cancer progression. Int J Mol Sci. 2018;19(9):2791. Published 2018 Sep 17. https://doi.org/10.3390/ijms19092791.
19. Du BB, Wu DW, Yang XF, Wang T, Shi XL, Lv YC, Zhou ZL, Liu Q, Zhang WS. The expression and significance of microRNA in different stages of colorectal cancer. Medicine. 2018;97:e9635. https://doi.org/10.1097/MD.0000000000009635.

20. Emami SS, Akbari A, Zare A, et al. MicroRNA expression levels and histopathological features of colorectal cancer. J Gastrointest Cancer. 2019;50:276–84. https://doi.org/10.1007/s12029-018-0055-x.
21. Ferracin M, Pedriali M, Veronese A, et al. MicroRNA profiling for the identification of cancers with unknown primary tissue-of-origin. J Pathol. 2011;225(1):43–53. https://doi.org/10.1002/path.2915.
22. Filipów S, Łaczmański Ł. Blood circulating miRNAs as cancer biomarkers for diagnosis and surgical treatment response. Front Genet. 2019;10:169. https://doi.org/10.3389/fgene.2019.00169.
23. Gunasekharan V, Laimins LA. Human papillomaviruses modulate microRNA 145 expression to directly control genome amplification. J Virol. 2013;87:6037–43. https://doi.org/10.1128/JVI.00153-13.
24. Hahn MM, de Voer RM, Hoogerbrugge N, Ligtenberg MJ, Kuiper RP, van Kessel AG. The genetic heterogeneity of colorectal cancer predisposition – guidelines for gene discovery. Cell Oncol (Dordr). 2016;39(6):491–510. https://doi.org/10.1007/s13402-016-0284-6.
25. Hibner G, Kimsa-Furdzik M, Francuz T. Relevance of microRNAs as potential diagnostic and prognostic markers in colorectal cancer. Int J Mol Sci. 2018;19:2944.
26. Huang Q, Ma Q. MicroRNA-106a inhibits cell proliferation and induces apoptosis in colorectal cancer cells. Oncol Lett. 2018;15(6):8941–4. https://doi.org/10.3892/ol.2018.8516.
27. Jo MH, Shin S, Jung SR, Kim E, Song JJ, Hohng S. Human Argonaute 2 has diverse reaction pathways on target RNAs. Mol Cell. 2015;59:117–24. https://doi.org/10.1016/j.molcel.2015.04.027.
28. Kakimoto Y, Tanaka M, Kamiguchi H, Ochiai E, Osawa M. MicroRNA stability in FFPE tissue samples: dependence on GC content. PLoS One. 2016;11(9):e0163125. Published 2016 Sep 20. https://doi.org/10.1371/journal.pone.0163125.
29. Kalyan A, Kircher S, Shah H, Mulcahy M, Benson A. Updates on immunotherapy for colorectal cancer. J Gastrointest Oncol. 2018;9(1):160–9. https://doi.org/10.21037/jgo.2018.01.17.
30. Kandimalla R, et al. Genome-wide discovery and identification of a novel miRNA signature for recurrence prediction in stage II and III colorectal cancer. Clin Cancer Res. 2018;24:3867–77. https://doi.org/10.1158/1078-0432.Ccr-17-3236.
31. Kawaguchi T, Komatsu S, Ichikawa D, et al. Circulating microRNAs: a next-generation clinical biomarker for digestive system cancers. Int J Mol Sci. 2016;17(9):1459. Published 2016 Sep 1. https://doi.org/10.3390/ijms17091459.
32. Kulkarni V, Darshan BB, Unnikrishnan B, Cheng K, Hui G, Theng AY, Yuien KS, Thapar K, Mithra P, Kumar N, Holla R, Kumar A. Colorectal cancer: how familiar are our future doctors with the cancer of tomorrow? Biomed Res Int. 2018;2018:7462101, 6 pages. https://doi.org/10.1155/2018/7462101.
33. Lakatos PL, Lakatos L. Risk for colorectal cancer in ulcerative colitis: changes, causes and management strategies. World J Gastroenterol. 2008;14(25):3937–47. https://doi.org/10.3748/wjg.14.3937.
34. Larrea E, Sole C, Manterola L, Goicoechea I, Armesto M, Arestin M, et al. New concepts in cancer biomarkers: circulating miRNAs in liquid biopsies. Int J Mol Sci. 2016;17:E627. https://doi.org/10.3390/ijms17050627.
35. Lei SL, Zhao H, Yao HL, Chen Y, Lei ZD, Liu KJ, Yang Q. Regulatory roles of microRNA-708 and microRNA-31 in proliferation, apoptosis and invasion of colorectal cancer cells. Oncol Lett. 2014;8:1768–74.
36. Lichtenstein P, Holm NV, Verkasalo PK, Iliadou A, Kaprio J, Koskenvuo M, Pukkala E, Skytthe A, Hemminki K. Environmental and heritable factors in the causation of cancer—analyses of cohorts of twins from Sweden, Denmark, and Finland. N Engl J Med. 2000;343:78–85. https://doi.org/10.1056/NEJM200007133430201.
37. Lin S, Gregory R. MicroRNA biogenesis pathways in cancer. Nat Rev Cancer. 2015;15:321–33. https://doi.org/10.1038/nrc3932.
38. Liu G, Li B. Role of miRNA in transformation from normal tissue to colorectal adenoma and cancer. J Cancer Res Ther. 2019;15:278–85.

39. Liu JX, Liu F, Li X, Song X, Zhou L, Jie JZ. Screening key genes and miRNAs in early-stage colon adenocarcinoma by RNA-sequencing. Tumor Biol. 2017;39:1010428317714899. https://doi.org/10.1177/1010428317714899.
40. Ludwig JA, Weinstein JN. Biomarkers in cancer staging, prognosis and treatment selection. Nat Rev Cancer. 2005;5:845–56. https://doi.org/10.1038/nrc1739.
41. Luo C, Cen S, Ding G, Wu W. Mucinous colorectal adenocarcinoma: clinical pathology and treatment options. Cancer Commun. 2019;39(1):13. Published 2019 Mar 29. https://doi.org/10.1186/s40880-019-0361-0.
42. Makondi PT, Wei P-L, Huang C-Y, Chang Y-J. Development of novel predictive miRNA/target gene pathways for colorectal cancer distance metastasis to the liver using a bioinformatic approach. PLoS One. 2019;14(2):e0211968. https://doi.org/10.1371/journal.pone.0211968.
43. Mármol I, Sánchez-de-Diego C, Pradilla Dieste A, Cerrada E, Rodriguez Yoldi MJ. Colorectal carcinoma: a general overview and future perspectives in colorectal cancer. Int J Mol Sci. 2017;18(1):197. Published 2017 Jan 19. https://doi.org/10.3390/ijms18010197.
44. Marshall JL, Yarden RI, Weinberg BA. Colorectal cancer care in the age of coronavirus: strategies to reduce risk and maintain benefit. Colorectal Cancer. 2020;9(1):CRC17. https://doi.org/10.2217/crc-2020-0010.
45. Mohandas KM. Colorectal cancer in India: controversies, enigmas and primary prevention. Indian J Gastroenterol. 2011;30(1):3–6.
46. Montani F, Marzi MT, Dezi F, Dama E, Carletti RM, Bonizzi G, Bertolotti R, Bellomi M, Rampinelli C, Maisonneuve P, Spaggiari L, Veronesi G, Nicassio F, Di Fiore PP, Bianchi F. miR-test: a blood test for lung cancer early detection. J Natl Cancer Inst. 2015;107:djv063.
47. O'Brien J, Hayder H, Zayed Y, Peng C. Overview of microRNA biogenesis, mechanisms of actions, and circulation. Front Endocrinol. 2018;9:402. https://doi.org/10.3389/fendo.2018.00402.
48. Obernosterer G, Martinez J, Alenius M. Locked nucleic acid-based in situ detection of microRNAs in mouse tissue sections. Nat Protoc. 2007;2:1508–14.
49. Okada C, Yamashita E, Lee SJ, Shibata S, Katahira J, Nakagawa A, et al. A high-resolution structure of the pre-microRNA nuclear export machinery. Science. 2009;326:1275–9. https://doi.org/10.1126/science.1178705.
50. Okamura K, Liu N, Lai EC. Distinct mechanisms for microRNA strand selection by Drosophila Argonautes. Mol Cell. 2009;36:431–44.
51. Ozawa T, et al. A microRNA signature associated with metastasis of T1 colorectal cancers to lymph nodes. Gastroenterology. 2018;154:844–8. https://doi.org/10.1053/j.gastro.2017.11.275.
52. Pan C, Yan X, Li H, Huang L, Yin M, Yang Y, Gao R, Hong L, Ma Y, Shi C, et al. Systematic literature review and clinical validation of circulating microRNAs as diagnostic biomarkers for colorectal cancer. Oncotarget. 2017;8:68317–28. https://doi.org/10.18632/oncotarget.19344.
53. Patil PS, Saklani A, Gambhire P, et al. Colorectal cancer in India: an audit from a tertiary center in a low prevalence area. Indian J Surg Oncol. 2017;8(4):484–90. https://doi.org/10.1007/s13193-017-0655-0.
54. Peltomäki P. Role of DNA mismatch repair defects in the pathogenesis of human cancer. J Clin Oncol. 2003;21:1174–9.
55. Peng Y, Croce C. The role of microRNAs in human cancer. Signal Transduct Target Ther. 2016;1:15004. https://doi.org/10.1038/sigtrans.2015.4.
56. Qiu S, Meng FX, Liu N, et al. The expression of microRNA-21 in colorectal cancer. Chin J Lab Diagn. 2014;18:0091.
57. Rammer M, et al. MicroRNAs and their role for T stage determination and lymph node metastasis in early colon carcinoma. Clin Exp Metastasis. 2017;34:431–40. https://doi.org/10.1007/s10585-017-9863-9.
58. Renwick N, Cekan P, Masry PA, Mcgeary SE, Miller JB, Hafner M, Li Z, Mihailovic A, Morozov P, Brown M, Gogakos T, Mobin MB, Snorrason EL, Feilotter HE, Zhang X, Perlis CS, Wu H, Suarez-Farinas M, Feng H, Shuda M, Moore PS, Tron VA, Chang Y,

Tuschl T. Multicolor microRNA FISH effectively differentiates tumor types. J Clin Invest. 2013;123(6):2694–702. https://doi.org/10.1172/JCI68760.
59. Rosenfeld N, Aharonov R, Meiri E, et al. MicroRNAs accurately identify cancer tissue origin. Nat Biotechnol. 2008;26(4):462–9.
60. Sanchez-Hidalgo JM, Duran-Martinez M, Molero-Payan R, et al. Gastrointestinal stromal tumors: a multidisciplinary challenge. World J Gastroenterol. 2018;24(18):1925–41. https://doi.org/10.3748/wjg.v24.i18.1925.
61. Schee K, Boye K, Abrahamsen TW, et al. Clinical relevance of microRNA miR-21, miR-31, miR-92a, miR-101, miR-106a and miR-145 in colorectal cancer. BMC Cancer. 2012;12:505. https://doi.org/10.1186/1471-2407-12-505.
62. Schwarzenbach H, Nishida N, Calin G, et al. Clinical relevance of circulating cell-free microRNAs in cancer. Nat Rev Clin Oncol. 2014;11:145–56. https://doi.org/10.1038/nrclinonc.2014.5.
63. Shibuya H, Iinuma H, Shimada R, et al. Clinicopathological and prognostic value of microRNA-21 and microRNA-155 in colorectal cancer. Oncology. 2010;79:313–20.
64. Shin VY, Siu JM, Cheuk I, Ng EK, Kwong A. Circulating cell-free miRNAs as biomarker for triple-negative breast cancer. Br J Cancer. 2015;112:1751–9.
65. Si W, Shen J, Zheng H, et al. The role and mechanisms of action of microRNAs in cancer drug resistance. Clin Epigenet. 2019;11:25. https://doi.org/10.1186/s13148-018-0587-8.
66. Singh PK, Preus L, Hu Q, Yan L, Long MD, Morrison CD, Nesline M, Johnson CS, Koochekpour S, Kohli M, Liu S, Trump DL, Sucheston-Campbell LE, Campbell MJ. Serum microRNA expression patterns that predict early treatment failure in prostate cancer patients. Oncotarget. 2014;5:824–40.
67. Singh R, Ramasubramanian B, Kanji S, Chakraborty AR, Haque SJ, Chakravarti A. Circulating microRNAs in cancer: hope or hype? Cancer Lett. 2016;381:113–21. https://doi.org/10.1016/j.canlet.2016.07.002.
68. Sinha R, Anderson DE, McDonald SS, Greenwald P. Cancer risk and diet in India. J Postgrad Med. 2003;49(3):222–8.
69. Sinha R, Doval DC, Hussain S, et al. Lifestyle and sporadic colorectal cancer in India. Asian Pac J Cancer Prev. 2015;16(17):7683–8. https://doi.org/10.7314/apjcp.2015.16.17.7683.
70. Søkilde R, Vincent M, Møller AK, Hansen A, Høiby PE, Blondal T, Nielsen BS, Daugaard G, Møller S, Litman T. Efficient identification of miRNAs for classification of tumor origin. J Mol Diagn. 2014;16(1):106–15. https://doi.org/10.1016/j.jmoldx.2013.10.001.
71. Song R, Ro S, Yan W. In situ hybridization detection of microRNAs. Methods Mol Biol. 2010;629:287–94. https://doi.org/10.1007/978-1-60761-657-3_18.
72. Stanojevic GZ, Nestorovic MD, Brankovic BR, Stojanovic MP, Jovanovic MM, Radojkovic MD. Primary colorectal lymphoma: an overview. World J Gastrointest Oncol. 2011;3(1):14–8. https://doi.org/10.4251/wjgo.v3.i1.14.
73. Ulivi P, Canale M, Passardi A, Marisi G, Valgiusti M, Frassineti G, Calistri D, Amadori D, Scarpi E. Circulating plasma levels of miR-20b, miR-29b and miR-155 as predictors of bevacizumab efficacy in patients with metastatic colorectal cancer. Int J Mol Sci. 2018;19:307.
74. Vacante M, Borzì AM, Basile F, Biondi A. Biomarkers in colorectal cancer: current clinical utility and future perspectives. World J Clin Cases. 2018;6(15):869–81. https://doi.org/10.12998/wjcc.v6.i15.869.
75. Vasudevan S, Steitz JA. AU-rich-element-mediated upregulation of translation by FXR1 and Argonaute 2. Cell. 2007;128:1105–18. https://doi.org/10.1016/j.cell.2007.01.038.
76. Vega P, Valentín F, Cubiella J. Colorectal cancer diagnosis: pitfalls and opportunities. World J Gastrointest Oncol. 2015;7(12):422–33. https://doi.org/10.4251/wjgo.v7.i12.422.
77. Wang CJ, Zhou ZG, Wang L, et al. Clinicopathological significance of microRNA-31, -143 and -145 expression in colorectal cancer. Dis Markers. 2009;26(1):27–34. https://doi.org/10.3233/DMA-2009-0601.
78. Yang J. Primary leiomyosarcoma in the colon: a case report. Medicine (Baltimore). 2018;97(7):e9923. https://doi.org/10.1097/MD.0000000000009923.
79. Yang X, Xu X, Zhu J, et al. miR-31 affects colorectal cancer cells by inhibiting autophagy in cancer-associated fibroblasts. Oncotarget. 2016;7(48):79617–28. https://doi.org/10.18632/oncotarget.12873.

80. Yau TO, Tang C, Harriss EK, et al. Faecal microRNAs as a non-invasive tool in the diagnosis of colonic adenomas and colorectal cancer: a meta-analysis. Sci Rep. 2019;9:9491. https://doi.org/10.1038/s41598-019-45570-9.
81. Yun SO, Cho YB, Lee WY, et al. Clinical significance of signet-ring-cell colorectal cancer as a prognostic factor. Ann Coloproctol. 2017;33(6):232–8. https://doi.org/10.3393/ac.2017.33.6.232.
82. Zhang L, Shay JW. Multiple roles of APC and its therapeutic implications in colorectal cancer. J Natl Cancer Inst. 2017;109(8):djw332. https://doi.org/10.1093/jnci/djw332.
83. Zhang X, Zuo X, Yang B, Li Z, Xue Y, Zhou Y, et al. MicroRNA directly enhances mitochondrial translation during muscle differentiation. Cell. 2014a;158:607–19. https://doi.org/10.1016/j.cell.2014.05.047.
84. Zhang X, Lu X, Lopez-Berestein G, Sood A, Calin G. In situ hybridization-based detection of microRNAs in human diseases. Microrna Diagn Ther. 2014b;1(1):12–23. https://doi.org/10.2478/micrnat-2013-0002.
85. Zhang D, Xie L, Jin Y. In situ detection of microRNAs: the art of microRNA research in human diseases. J Cytol Histol. 2015;Suppl 3(1):013. https://doi.org/10.4172/2157-7099.S3-013.

[illegible]

Chapter 6
Role of Epigenetics in Colorectal Cancer

Beiping Miao, Sonal Gupta, Manisha Mathur, Prashanth Suravajhala, and Obul Reddy Bandapalli

Abstract In 2018 alone, colorectal cancer (CRC) accounted for 10.2% among all cancer cases. It is known to be a consequence of accumulated alterations in the genome. Several studies on genetics have improved our understanding of CRC. While genetics play its role as the first code of genome, role of epigenetics in CRC as the second code of genome has been highlighted in the last decades. We focus on the essential factors like DNA methylation drivers-writer, reader, eraser and non-coding RNA, miRNA and long non-coding RNAs associated with CRC.

Keywords Colorectal cancer · Epigenetics · DNA methylation regulators · miRNA · lncRNA

B. Miao
Hopp Children's Cancer Center (KiTZ), Heidelberg, Germany

Division of Pediatric Neuro Oncology, German Cancer Research Center (DKFZ), German Cancer Consortium (DKTK), Heidelberg, Germany

S. Gupta
Department of Biotechnology and Bioinformatics, Birla Institute of Scientific Research (BISR), Statue Circle, Jaipur, Rajasthan, India

Department of Paediatrics, Sawai Man Singh Medical College, Jaipur, Rajasthan, India

M. Mathur
Advance Milk Testing Research Laboratory, Post Graduate Institute of Veterinary Education and Research (RAJUVAS), Jaipur, Rajasthan, India

P. Suravajhala
Department of Biotechnology and Bioinformatics, Birla Institute of Scientific Research (BISR), Statue Circle, Jaipur, Rajasthan, India

O. R. Bandapalli (✉)
Hopp Children's Cancer Center (KiTZ), Heidelberg, Germany

Division of Pediatric Neuro Oncology, German Cancer Research Center (DKFZ), German Cancer Consortium (DKTK), Heidelberg, Germany

Medical Faculty, University of Heidelberg, Heidelberg, Germany
e-mail: o.bandapalli@kitz-heidelberg.de

G. P. Nagaraju et al. (eds.), *Colon Cancer Diagnosis and Therapy*,
https://doi.org/10.1007/978-3-030-63369-1_6

Abbreviations

CRC	Colorectal cancer
LncRNA	Long non-coding RNA
MBD1	Methyl-CpG binding domain protein 1
miRNA	MicroRNA
ncRNAs	Non-coding RNAs
PVT1	Plasmacytoma variant translocation 1
TET	Ten-eleven translocation methylcytosine

6.1 Introduction

Colorectal cancer (CRC) ranks the third most frequently diagnosed malignancy all over the world, with an overall incidence of 10.2% among all cancer cases in 2018. The incidence is increasing particularly in developed countries [1, 2]. The disease is the consequence of alterations accumulated in genome associated with tumor suppressor, oncogenes, and DNA damage repair genes. Around 90% of CRCs are sporicidal, and only less than 10% are hereditary [3]. Several genes have been discovered successfully from familial CRC screening project, such as APC, PTEN, MSH2, and MLH1 [4]. The Main findings mostly belong to protein regions, which only accounts for less than 2% of the whole genome [5]. It is estimated by the Encyclopedia of DNA Elements (ENCODE) that about 80% of human genome has some kind of functionality [6]. There is no doubt exploring the non-coding region is essential if the cancer needs to be fully understood. Within the last three decades of study, it is widely accepted that the non-coding regulatory regions of genome also contribute greatly to cancer initiation and progression, so-called epigenetics since it controls the gene expression without altering DNA sequences. The CRC has been shown to be one of the most epigenetic factor-related cancers. Many driving factors such as DNA methylations, non-coding RNAs, have been explored. In this chapter we will introduce these epigenetic factors in detail.

6.2 Drivers of DNA (De)methylation

In mammals, DNA methylation occurs by covalent modification of cytosine at the fifth carbon (C^5) in CpG dinucleotides within the genome [7]. The essential role of methylation in the cancer etiology has been emphasized with ample evidence since its discovery in 1983 [8]. Cancers can be promoted through different methylation level alterations at different genomic regions.

There are three main phases of methylation: de-novo methylation (write), maintenance (read), and demethylation (erase). The three phases need to be well coordinated in order to keep homeostasis; any disruption of this state would lead to deleterious consequences. There are two major active "writers" (de novo DNA methylation enzymes) DNMT3A and DNMT3B. Additional DNMT3L is catalytically inactive but could accompany DNMT3A and DNMT3B to regulate their activities. In general, DNA methylation takes place when methyl groups are added to the appropriate bases on the genome by the action of "writer."

Whether the genes are expressed or not based on how the methylation mark signal is read and interpreted by different types of readers. The proteins recognize and bind to the methylated regions (MBP) [9]. There are three main reader families discovered: the first is the family of "MBD-containing proteins" with 11 members [9, 10], the second "methyl-CpG-binding zinc fingers" with at least 8 members [11, 12], and the third one is "set and RING-associated (SRA) domain proteins." Alteration in normal methylation pattern may change the way methylation marks are written, read, and interpreted in different disease states, which is a typical hallmark of cancer. This unique characteristic of DNA methylation "readers" has identified them as attractive therapeutic targets.

Active DNA demethylation is carried out by ten-eleven translocation (TET) methylcytosine dioxygenases (erasers), which precede DNA demethylation [13]. All the oxidized forms can promote DNA demethylation during replication [14, 15]. TET was found to hydroxylate the methyl group of mC and convert it to 5-hydroxymethyl cytosine (hmC) [16].

6.3 Alterations of Drivers in CRC

DNA methylation level needs to be maintained very precisely in order to keep homeostasis; any disruption of the above enzymes leads to deleterious consequence. In CRC, studies have investigated altered activity of enzymes drives aberrant methylation in CRC.

Regarding "writers" (DNMTs), it is known that DNMTs are overexpressed in CRC [17]; there are not so many mutations in CRC [18], which is contradictory to the fact that CRC has the feature of global hypo methylation [19]. These findings suggest that DNMT mutation or overexpression is unlikely to drive the aberrant promoter methylation in CRC, and such a model would also not explain the non-random pattern of promoter methylation observed in CRCs. Nevertheless, it is reported that mutation-induced DNMT1 inactivation in colon cancers result in DNA methylation [18]. Mice predisposed to develop fewer polyps in a DNMT1 heterozygous background [20]. Knockdown of DNMT1 through an antisense to DNA methyltransferase also blocks tumorigenesis and induces hypomethylation [21]. Deletion of the DNMT1 gene in a colon cancer cell line (HCT116) induces slower growth and reduces methylation levels around 20% [22].

Several members of "readers" were found involving the etiology of CRC. For example, in advanced CRC, MBD1 may be a tumor suppressor gene and affect the development and metastasis; reduced expression of MBD1 may lead to metastatic colorectal cancer [23]. MBD2 has been shown to block genes in colorectal cancer [24], whose expression can be restored by knocking out MBD2 in mice [25]; MeCP2 was also found to play a role in colorectal tumorigenesis and also as a global transcription repressor [26]. In Wnt-driven colon cancer cell lines, Kaiso mediates the silencing of the tumor suppressor genes CDKN1A, HIC1, and Rb [27, 28]. Mutations of MBD4 were found in around 30% of microsatellite unstable colorectal tumors [29]. Higher SETDB1 expression showed poor survival rate [30]; besides, Keli et al. found the SETDB1 inhibited the TP53 expression in CRC [31].

However, like DNMTs, mutations in TETs are rare in CRC. The first investigation to explore the TET mRNA levels and link them with prognosis was done in 2015 [32]. Somatic mutations in all three TET proteins were found in colorectal cancer (CRC) [33]. Interestingly, besides mutation, downregulation of TET [34] and CIMP-high/TET1-methylated CRCs have a globally higher incidence of promoter methylation compared with CIMP-high/TET1 non-methylated tumors. It is also reported that genetic deregulation of TET DNA demethylases by oncogenic BRAFV600E was responsible for CIMP-cancer initiation in the colon [35]. The other member TET2 was found to be responsible for loss of nuclear localization in CRC. The nuclear expression of TET2 was not found, while TET3 was present. Blocking the nuclear export with inhibitor enhances the 5hmC level in CRC cells that may be due to the consequence of regulating TET2 [36].

6.4 Non-coding RNAs

Non-coding RNAs (ncRNAs) are transcripts that cannot translate into proteins. As we know that, less than 2% of human genome encodes proteins, while around 75% of human genome is transcribed into ncRNA [37] with plenty of functions. Except housekeeping ncRNAs like ribosomal RNAs (rRNAs) and transfer RNAs (tRNAs), the regulatory ncRNAs draw more attention in cancer etiology, including microRNAs (miRNA, 17-22 nucleotides), PIWI-interacting RNA (piRNAs, 26–33 nucleotides), circular RNAs (circRNAs, average 300 ± 150 nucleotides), siRNAs (20–27 nucleotides), and long non-coding RNAs (lncRNAs, over 200 nucleotides) [38].

6.5 Small Non-coding RNAs in CRC

Collective evidence has shown that small non-coding RNA especially miRNA has a vital role in cancer progression, as oncogenes, tumor suppressors, or bidirectional roles.

The first report of differentially expressed miRNAs in CRC compared to healthy control was downregulation of miR-143 and miR-145 [39]. miR-193a-3p, miR-23a, and miR-338-5p were upregulated in more advanced stages of CRC, demonstrating as a classifier for CRC detection [40]; MiR-21 is the most commonly upregulated miRNA in CRC, normally counted as oncogenic miRNAs [41]. MiR-21 promotes cell proliferation, invasion, intravasation, and metastasis in CRC by targeting various tumor suppressor genes, such as PDCD4 (programmed cell death 4), CCL20 [chemokine (C-C motif) ligand 20], CDC25A (cell division cycle 25 homolog A), and PTEN (phosphatase and tensing homolog) [42, 43]. MiR-210 is found to be frequently upregulated in CRC tissues, and overexpression of mir-210 in CRC cells promotes migration and invasion through the repression of its target VMP1. Several investigations reported miR-31 upregulation in CRC. One of the most known oncogenic miRNA clusters in CRC is the miR-17-92 cluster consisting of six members (miR-17, miR-18a, miR-19a, miR-19b, miR-20a, and miR-92a) all with well-established oncogenic functions, all reported to be upregulated in CRC [44].

Some other miRNAs are found to be downregulated and are known to be tumor suppressors. For example, miR-143 and miR-145 are downregulated in colon cancer, which results in chronic inflammation and neoplastic progression [45]. Introducing the miR-34 into colon cell lines makes the cells become senescence-like state meaning that miR-34 plays an important role in cell cycle regulation [46].

What is more, some special miRNAs play bidirectional roles in the development of CRC. Members of the miR-200 family are classic example in colon cancer progression. On one hand in CRC with DICER1 deficiency, members of the miR-200 family are significantly downregulated thereby contributing to tumor initiation and metastasis [47]. Several studies have shown that all members of the miR-200 family have a central role in EMT [48].

On the other hand, over expression of other miR-200 family members were found to promote cancer progression. It is reported that oxidative stress induces the expression of miR-141 and miR-200a and thus promotes tumor growth in vivo by targeting p38α directly [49]. Tania et al. found that high levels of miR-200a and miR-200c were associated with better overall survival, while high levels of miR-429 correlated with longer overall and disease-free survival (DFS), and low miR-429 levels were identified as an independent prognostic marker [49]. These findings clearly indicate that the miR-200 family has huge potential for both prognostic and therapeutic management of CRC.

6.6 Long Non-coding RNAs in CRC

Long non-coding RNAs are the most diverse class of non-protein coding RNAs: their length is generally greater than 200 nucleotides, often reaching up to 100 kb. They include transcripts that may be derived from introns or inter-genes, which regulate gene expression through different mechanisms like acting as signals, decoys, guides, and scaffolds [50].

With the help of microarray, RNA sequencing, and real-time PCR [51], over the last few years, several research teams have reported on the involvement of lncRNAs in CRC genesis and progression, which convincingly suggested the involvement of lncRNAs in a wide spectrum of biological processes, such as cell cycle regulation, stemness, differentiation, and apoptosis [43].

LncRNAs can also be oncogenes or tumor suppressors based on the involved vital signalling pathways of CRC. One of the most known cancer-related lncRNAs is metastasis-associated lung adenocarcinoma transcript 1 (MALAT1), located on chromosome 11q13.1 and 8000 nt [52]. Point mutations of MALAT1 were detected in CRC cell lines and tissues [53]. BRAF-activated non-protein coding RNA (BANCR) seems to be closely associated with V600E BRAF in CRC [54]. In this year, a system experiment was done through transcriptome sequencing of normal, primary, and metastasis tissues leading to the identification of 148 differentially expressed RNAs associated with metastasis. Of which RAMS11 shows great interest since its close relation with poor disease-free survival and aggressive phenotypes. Similarly, they found that RAMS11 activates topoisomerase II alpha (TOP2α) by recruiting chromobox protein 4(CBX4), thereby implicating RAMS11 as biomarker and therapeutic target for CRC [55]. Another paper found long non-coding RNA SNHG14 enhances colorectal cancer metastasis through targeting EZH2-regulated EPHA7 [56].

BANCR overexpression increases cell migration of CRC cell lines, whereas its knockdown inhibits it. BANCR induces EMT by regulating the expression of epithelial and mesenchymal markers thus contributing to CRC migration [57]. It is found that CCAT2 is involved metastatic progression and chromosomal instability in CRC and also activates Wnt signalling, while CCAT2 itself is a Wnt downstream target, suggesting the existence of a positive feedback loop [58]. The long isoform of colon cancer-associated transcript 1 (CCAT1-L) is upregulated and positively related to tumor stage and progression in CRC [59].

Recently Zuo et al. [60] found that vitamin D treatment enhanced MEG3 expression and knockdown of VDR abolished the effect of MEG3 on glycolysis. These results indicate that vitamin D-activated MEG3 suppresses aerobic glycolysis in CRC cells by downregulating c-Myc.

The position where a long non-coding RNA-plasmacytoma variant translocation 1 (PVT1) located is the well-known cancer-related region- 8q24 [61]. Reduction of PVT1 in CRC cells leads to a significant inhibition of proliferation and invasion by activating TGF-β and apoptotic signalling [62]. Overexpression of PVT1 is necessary for high MYC protein levels in 8q24-amplified CRC cells. PVT1 and MYC protein expression correlate in primary tumors [63]. Olorunseun et al. found that PVT1 has the potential to be a diagnostic and therapeutic biomarker in CRC [64].

6.7 Merge Function of lncRNA and miRNA in CRC

lncRNA may induce the expression of the respective miRNAs' targets as molecular sponges for a miRNA. Collective evidences have showed that action plays vital roles in CRC development [65], for example, long intergenic non-protein-coding RNA 1567 (LINC01567) which is upregulated in CRC stem cells that can target miRNA-93 to regulate the proliferation and tumorigenesis [66]. LncRNA MALAT1 may regulate HMGB1 by sponging miR-129-5p, thereby inducing CC development [67]. Several projects also showed that PVT1 can promote CRC tumorigenesis by stabilizing miR-16-5p [61] or sponging miR-26b [68]. This sponge action of LncRNA on miRNA sheds light for CRC treatments that may be further applied to clinical aims.

References

1. Bray F, et al. Global cancer statistics 2018: GLOBOCAN estimates of incidence and mortality worldwide for 36 cancers in 185 countries. CA Cancer J Clin. 2018;68(6):394–424.
2. Arnold M, et al. Global patterns and trends in colorectal cancer incidence and mortality. Gut. 2017;66(4):683–91.
3. Puccini A, et al. Colorectal cancer: epigenetic alterations and their clinical implications. Biochim Biophys Acta Rev Cancer. 2017;1868(2):439–48.
4. Shao WH, et al. A hereditable mutation of MSH2 gene associated with lynch syndrome in a five generation Chinese family. Cancer Manag Res. 2020;12:1469–82.
5. Weinhold N, et al. Genome-wide analysis of noncoding regulatory mutations in cancer. Nat Genet. 2014;46(11):1160–5.
6. Consortium EP. An integrated encyclopedia of DNA elements in the human genome. Nature. 2012;489(7414):57–74.
7. Bird A. DNA methylation patterns and epigenetic memory. Genes Dev. 2002;16(1):6–21.
8. Feinberg AP, Vogelstein B. Hypomethylation distinguishes genes of some human cancers from their normal counterparts. Nature. 1983;301(5895):89–92.
9. Mahmood N, Rabbani SA. DNA methylation readers and cancer: mechanistic and therapeutic applications. Front Oncol. 2019;9:489.
10. Meehan RR, et al. Identification of a mammalian protein that binds specifically to DNA containing methylated CpGs. Cell. 1989;58(3):499–507.
11. Hudson NO, Buck-Koehntop BA. Zinc finger readers of methylated DNA. Molecules. 2018;23(10):2555.
12. Prokhortchouk A, et al. The p120 catenin partner Kaiso is a DNA methylation-dependent transcriptional repressor. Genes Dev. 2001;15(13):1613–8.
13. He YF, et al. Tet-mediated formation of 5-carboxylcytosine and its excision by TDG in mammalian DNA. Science. 2011;333(6047):1303–7.
14. Otani J, et al. Cell cycle-dependent turnover of 5-hydroxymethyl cytosine in mouse embryonic stem cells. PLoS One. 2013;8(12):e82961.
15. Hashimoto H, et al. Recognition and potential mechanisms for replication and erasure of cytosine hydroxymethylation. Nucleic Acids Res. 2012;40(11):4841–9.
16. Williams K, et al. TET1 and hydroxymethylcytosine in transcription and DNA methylation fidelity. Nature. 2011;473(7347):343–8.
17. Tse JWT, et al. Aberrant DNA methylation in colorectal cancer: what should we target? Trends Cancer. 2017;3(10):698–712.
18. Kanai Y, et al. Mutation of the DNA methyltransferase (DNMT) 1 gene in human colorectal cancers. Cancer Lett. 2003;192(1):75–82.
19. Wong JJ, Hawkins NJ, Ward RL. Colorectal cancer: a model for epigenetic tumorigenesis. Gut. 2007;56(1):140–8.
20. Subramaniam D, et al. DNA methyltransferases: a novel target for prevention and therapy. Front Oncol. 2014;4:80.

21. MacLeod AR, Szyf M. Expression of antisense to DNA methyltransferase mRNA induces DNA demethylation and inhibits tumorigenesis. J Biol Chem. 1995;270(14):8037–43.
22. Rountree MR, et al. DNA methylation, chromatin inheritance, and cancer. Oncogene. 2001;20(24):3156–65.
23. Qi L, Ding Y. Screening of tumor suppressor genes in metastatic colorectal cancer. Biomed Res Int. 2017;2017:2769140.
24. Park HY, et al. Differential promoter methylation may be a key molecular mechanism in regulating BubR1 expression in cancer cells. Exp Mol Med. 2007;39(2):195–204.
25. Sansom OJ, et al. Deficiency of Mbd2 suppresses intestinal tumorigenesis. Nat Genet. 2003;34(2):145–7.
26. Pancione M, et al. Epigenetic silencing of peroxisome proliferator-activated receptor gamma is a biomarker for colorectal cancer progression and adverse patients' outcome. PLoS One. 2010;5(12):e14229.
27. De La Rosa-Velazquez IA, et al. Epigenetic regulation of the human retinoblastoma tumor suppressor gene promoter by CTCF. Cancer Res. 2007;67(6):2577–85.
28. Lopes EC, et al. Kaiso contributes to DNA methylation-dependent silencing of tumor suppressor genes in colon cancer cell lines. Cancer Res. 2008;68(18):7258–63.
29. Riccio A, et al. The DNA repair gene MBD4 (MED1) is mutated in human carcinomas with microsatellite instability. Nat Genet. 1999;23(3):266–8.
30. Huang J, et al. Enhanced expression of SETDB1 possesses prognostic value and promotes cell proliferation, migration and invasion in nasopharyngeal carcinoma. Oncol Rep. 2018;40(2):1017–25.
31. Chen K, et al. Histone Methyltransferase SETDB1 promotes the progression of colorectal cancer by inhibiting the expression of TP53. J Cancer. 2017;8(16):3318–30.
32. Rawluszko-Wieczorek AA, et al. Clinical significance of DNA methylation mRNA levels of TET family members in colorectal cancer. J Cancer Res Clin Oncol. 2015;141(8):1379–92.
33. Seshagiri S, et al. Recurrent R-spondin fusions in colon cancer. Nature. 2012;488(7413):660–4.
34. Ichimura N, et al. Aberrant TET1 methylation closely associated with CpG Island Methylator phenotype in colorectal cancer. Cancer Prev Res (Phila). 2015;8(8):702–11.
35. Noreen F, et al. DNA methylation instability by BRAF-mediated TET silencing and lifestyle-exposure divides colon cancer pathways. Clin Epigenetics. 2019;11(1):196.
36. Huang Y, et al. Loss of nuclear localization of TET2 in colorectal cancer. Clin Epigenetics. 2016;8:9.
37. Djebali S, et al. Landscape of transcription in human cells. Nature. 2012;489(7414):101–8.
38. Chen H, Xu Z, Liu D. Small non-coding RNA and colorectal cancer. J Cell Mol Med. 2019;23(5):3050–7.
39. Michael MZ, et al. Reduced accumulation of specific microRNAs in colorectal neoplasia. Mol Cancer Res. 2003;1(12):882–91.
40. Yong FL, Law CW, Wang CW. Potentiality of a triple microRNA classifier: miR-193a-3p, miR-23a and miR-338-5p for early detection of colorectal cancer. BMC Cancer. 2013;13:280.
41. Volinia S, et al. A microRNA expression signature of human solid tumors defines cancer gene targets. Proc Natl Acad Sci U S A. 2006;103(7):2257–61.
42. Asangani IA, et al. MicroRNA-21 (miR-21) post-transcriptionally downregulates tumor suppressor Pdcd4 and stimulates invasion, intravasation and metastasis in colorectal cancer. Oncogene. 2008;27(15):2128–36.
43. Ragusa M, et al. Non-coding landscapes of colorectal cancer. World J Gastroenterol. 2015;21(41):11709–39.
44. Koga Y, et al. MicroRNA expression profiling of exfoliated colonocytes isolated from feces for colorectal cancer screening. Cancer Prev Res (Phila). 2010;3(11):1435–42.
45. Wang CJ, et al. Clinicopathological significance of microRNA-31, −143 and −145 expression in colorectal cancer. Dis Markers. 2009;26(1):27–34.
46. Tazawa H, et al. Tumor-suppressive miR-34a induces senescence-like growth arrest through modulation of the E2F pathway in human colon cancer cells. Proc Natl Acad Sci U S A. 2007;104(39):15472–7.

47. Iliou MS, et al. Impaired DICER1 function promotes stemness and metastasis in colon cancer. Oncogene. 2014;33(30):4003–15.
48. O'Brien SJ, et al. The role of the miR-200 family in epithelial-mesenchymal transition in colorectal cancer: a systematic review. Int J Cancer. 2018;142(12):2501–11.
49. Korpal M, et al. Direct targeting of Sec23a by miR-200s influences cancer cell secretome and promotes metastatic colonization. Nat Med. 2011;17(9):1101–8.
50. Wang KC, Chang HY. Molecular mechanisms of long noncoding RNAs. Mol Cell. 2011;43(6):904–14.
51. Xu MD, Qi P, Du X. Long non-coding RNAs in colorectal cancer: implications for pathogenesis and clinical application. Mod Pathol. 2014;27(10):1310–20.
52. Ji P, et al. MALAT-1, a novel noncoding RNA, and thymosin beta4 predict metastasis and survival in early-stage non-small cell lung cancer. Oncogene. 2003;22(39):8031–41.
53. Xu C, et al. MALAT-1: a long non-coding RNA and its important 3′ end functional motif in colorectal cancer metastasis. Int J Oncol. 2011;39(1):169–75.
54. Davies H, et al. Mutations of the BRAF gene in human cancer. Nature. 2002;417(6892):949–54.
55. Silva-Fisher JM, et al. Long non-coding RNA RAMS11 promotes metastatic colorectal cancer progression. Nat Commun. 2020;11(1):2156.
56. Di W, et al. Long noncoding RNA SNHG14 facilitates colorectal cancer metastasis through targeting EZH2-regulated EPHA7. Cell Death Dis. 2019;10(7):514.
57. Guo Q, et al. BRAF-activated long non-coding RNA contributes to colorectal cancer migration by inducing epithelial-mesenchymal transition. Oncol Lett. 2014;8(2):869–75.
58. Ling H, et al. CCAT2, a novel noncoding RNA mapping to 8q24, underlies metastatic progression and chromosomal instability in colon cancer. Genome Res. 2013;23(9):1446–61.
59. Nissan A, et al. Colon cancer associated transcript-1: a novel RNA expressed in malignant and pre-malignant human tissues. Int J Cancer. 2012;130(7):1598–606.
60. Zuo S, et al. Long non-coding RNA MEG3 activated by vitamin D suppresses glycolysis in colorectal cancer via promoting c-Myc degradation. Front Oncol. 2020;10:274.
61. Wu H, et al. lncRNA PVT1 promotes tumorigenesis of colorectal cancer by stabilizing miR-16-5p and interacting with the VEGFA/VEGFR1/AKT Axis. Mol Ther Nucleic Acids. 2020;20:438–50.
62. Takahashi Y, et al. Amplification of PVT-1 is involved in poor prognosis via apoptosis inhibition in colorectal cancers. Br J Cancer. 2014;110(1):164–71.
63. Tseng YY, et al. PVT1 dependence in cancer with MYC copy-number increase. Nature. 2014;512(7512):82–6.
64. Ogunwobi OO, Mahmood F, Akingboye A. Biomarkers in colorectal cancer: current research and future prospects. Int J Mol Sci. 2020;21(15):5311.
65. Shuwen H, et al. Competitive endogenous RNA in colorectal cancer: a systematic review. Gene. 2018;645:157–62.
66. Yu X, et al. Long intergenic non-protein-coding RNA 1567 (LINC01567) acts as a "sponge" against microRNA-93 in regulating the proliferation and tumorigenesis of human colon cancer stem cells. BMC Cancer. 2017;17(1):716.
67. Wu Q, et al. LncRNA MALAT1 induces colon cancer development by regulating miR-129-5p/HMGB1 axis. J Cell Physiol. 2018;233(9):6750–7.
68. Zhang R, et al. Long noncoding RNA plasmacytoma variant translocation 1 (PVT1) promotes colon cancer progression via endogenous sponging miR-26b. Med Sci Monit. 2018;24:8685–92.

Chapter 7
Exosomal Biomarkers in Colorectal Cancer

S. Priya and P. K. Satheeshkumar

Abstract Colorectal cancer (CRC) is the third most diagnosed cancer in the world which affects the large intestine or rectum. It is a multifactorial disease that gradually develops with the cumulative effects of genetic and epigenetic alterations, which changes the normal colon mucosal layer into invasive form. Recent research interest in CRC relies on the identification of specific biomarkers for early disease diagnosis, adopting better treatment modalities and analysing treatment efficacies. Developments in the omics techniques have identified number of biomarkers. The short oligonucleotides such as microRNA (miRNA) and long noncoding RNA (lncRNA) have proved as better biomarkers among diverse types. Exosomes are 30–150 nm sized membrane bound vesicles formed from endosomes and released to the extracellular space. The differentially expressed proteins, miRNAs, lncRNAs and circular RNAs found in the exosomal vesicles associated with body fluids that could serve as promising biomarkers for CRC. They exhibit entirely different roles in the tumorigenesis and prevention process when compared to the cellular and extracellular biomarkers. In the near future, exosomes will represent a promising non-invasive source of biomarkers for CRC.

Keywords Colorectal cancer · MiRNA · LncRNA · Tumorigenesis · Exosomes

S. Priya (✉)
Biochemistry Section, Agro-Processing and Technology Division, CSIR- National Institute for Interdisciplinary Science and Technology (CSIR-NIIST),
Pappanamcode, Trivandrum, Kerala, India
e-mail: priyasulu@niist.res.in

P. K. Satheeshkumar
Centre for Advanced Studies in Botany, Institute of Science, Banaras Hindu University, Varanasi, Uttar Pradesh, India

G. P. Nagaraju et al. (eds.), *Colon Cancer Diagnosis and Therapy*,
https://doi.org/10.1007/978-3-030-63369-1_7

Abbreviations

circRNA	Circular RNA
CRC	Colorectal cancer
Exo-miRNA	Exosomal microRNA
KRAS	Kirsten rat sarcoma
lncRNA	Long noncoding RNA
MMR	Mismatch repair
MSI	Microsatellite instability
SiRNA	Small-interfering RNA
TSPAN1	Tetraspanin1

7.1 Introduction

7.1.1 Cancer

Cancer is a common name used for a number of diseases with almost same identifiable symptom, the uncontrolled cell division. Cancer affects almost all parts of our body. Depending on the cell type and the organ type, there are many names used to indicate it. Cancer was one of the most prevalent killers of the twentieth century and is continuing to be so even in the present century. The known history of cancer dates back to 3000 BC in an ancient Egyptian text book on surgery. The name cancer came from Hippocrates (460–370 BC), the great Greek Physician, who used the words "carsinos" and "carcinoma" to indicate different tumours. The words literally mean, the "crab", probably due to the finger like projections from the ulcer-forming tumours. Scientific reports indicate that cancer was present in the past with the evidence in the fossilised bones and in the mummies of Egypt, where the cancer-mediated bony skull destructions was noticed.

Cancer is a deviation from a cell's normal life cycle. In the body cells maintain an orderly means of cell division. Once they are old/damaged, well-defined mechanisms are in place to replace the old cells with functional new cells. Cancer occurs when a cell falls out of its normal cycle and starts dividing uncontrollably. It makes a crowd of cells and forms a tumour. All cancers need not to form a tumour as in leukaemia (blood cancer). Some of the cancers are fast growing, while others grow slowly. Metastasis is the phenomenon in which the cancer cells are moved from its place of origin through the circulatory system to different parts of the body and attaches to a new place and multiply there. Metastatic form of cancer is more dreadful in terms of less treatment success and high mortality rate. The physical and physiological disturbances of the newly formed cells impose on the surrounding cells leading to the complications and pathology of cancer. Even though there were reports on the occurrence of cancer in the past, the disease becomes so prevalent during the twentieth century. It may be possible that either the evolution of modern scientific methods which had more accurate procedures to detect the disease or the changes in the overall physical environment in the beginning of the twentieth century cause a surge in the number of cancer incidences. There is a sharp increase in the recent past with regard to the number of cases reported, and it is concluded that the changing environment and food habits are the two major culprits behind it. As of now, there are more than 14 million new cases of cancers that are registered worldwide.

Cancer is considered as a curable disease if detected at an early stage of its appearance. Being a complex disease, the treatment is purely based on the cell type, organ, position, and the stage of progression and is highly specific to different cancers. In general, there are three major methods including radiation, chemotherapy and surgery and a combination of any two or three. Radiation and surgery are the primary line of treatment, which used to complement each other in varying order at different occasions. Chemotherapy is the method of choice once the metastasis starts to occur. Chemotherapy using highly specific hormones and antibodies are preferred at an advanced stage of the disease.

7.1.2 Colorectal Cancer (CRC) and the Symptoms Associated

Colorectal cancer is a gastrointestinal malignancy that develops in the colon or rectum. Even though there can be a differentiation as colon or rectal cancer depending on the origin, due to the high similarity in their biological and clinical features, they are considered under the common term. In a majority of patients, the diagnosis is late due to the asymptomatic nature of the disease. The prognosis thus become difficult till the cancer grows and spread substantially. The symptoms associated with CRC depend on the stage of the disease and the part where it occurs. Stage 1 CRC may or may not have symptoms. Even if it is there, it can be confused with the symptoms of stomach infections, ulcer, haemorrhoids or irritable bowel syndrome or Crohn's disease. It includes abdominal pain, cramps, constipation, diarrhoea, excess gas, changes in stool colour and shape, bleeding from the rectum and blood in the stool. The symptoms will change when CRC becomes stage 4 (metastasis) which include excessive fatigue, unexplained weakness, vomiting, anaemia, jaundice, unemptied bowel, weight loss, etc.

7.1.3 CRC: Prevalence

Colorectal cancer gained worldwide attention in the last few decades due to its increasing prevalence, mainly owing to the sedentary lifestyle and changes in the food habits. The job requirements of the present century pose a serious threat to the well-being of the humans, especially those who are involved in the office jobs, where the movements are highly restricted. Adding to this problem is the social life addiction among the new generation which forces them to adopt an unhealthy food habit. Colorectal cancer is the third most observed cancer in men and second most prevalent cancer among women. According to a new study, colorectal cancer is the third most frequent cancer around the world which affects a total of nearly 1.85 million persons each year after the lung cancer and breast cancer [1]. The study estimates that there will be a substantial increase among the patients (2.2 million new case in a year) by the end of 2030. Even though the occurrence of disease is more common in the developed countries, the recent trends show that even the developing countries started reporting an increase in the incidence mainly due to the adoption of a western lifestyle.

The susceptibility to the disease increases with age. According to a recent study, by the American Cancer Society, the prevalence of CRC among different age group is as follows. While the probability for occurrence of the disease can be any time irrespective of the age, there can be a difference in the rate of incidence among different age groups. While the rate stand as low as 2 per 100,000 individuals in an age group of 25–39, the rate reaches as big as up to 212 per 100,000 in the age group 65–85 [2]. The figures are in between among the age groups 40–49 (10.3–18.5 per 100,000) and 50–64 (34.3–62.5 per 100,000). According to the same study, human development index (HDI) found to be an appropriate factor to look in to the prevalence among different countries. The countries with higher HDI seem to be more vulnerable to the disease. For example, countries like New Zealand and Australia tops the list with maximum occurrence of the disease as 36.7 cases per 100,000 followed by Europe 28.8–32.1 cases per 100,000. The low HDI countries like Africa and South central Asia report an incident rate of 6.4–9.2 cases per 100,000 and 4.9 cases per 100,000, respectively. HDI was also used to predict the cumulative risk of developing CRC among different populations. It was shown that the Europeans are at the higher risk (1.17–1.55% between 0 and 74 years), compared to the South central Asian population where the risk index was only 0.24% between 0 and 74 years. Another study indicated an increase of around 10% between 2016 and 2018, proposing a serious concern about the increasing incidences of CRC among different populations [3]. In a report of WHO which analyse the figures related to the mortality rate in CRC, it was clearly indicated that there is a considerable increase of about 33% between 2000 and 2016, with the estimated death tally of 0.794 million in 2016 compared to 0.595 million in 2000 [4].

7.1.4 CRC: Major Reasons for the Occurrence

Colorectal cancer results from a number of both external and internal factors. While the family history is considered as a strong factor, most of the CRC occur sporadically (75%). The major factors controlling the origin of CRC are the induction and accumulation of mutations in the genes involved in tumour suppression, activation of pre-existing mutations, and susceptibility alleles (precancerous or induced by prior inflammation) and other conditions leading to chronic and lingering inflammation (inflammatory bowel disease, ulcerative colitis, Crohn's disease, etc.) in the colorectal region. Genetic changes that give rise to CRC include the mutations that occur in the genes adenomatous polyposis coli (APC-in around 81%), tumour protein 53 (TP53 in around 60%), and Kirsten rat sarcoma (KRAS-in around 43%). While these gene mutations account for most of the CRC (96%), the reason for the remaining percentage (4%) of the disease is the inflammation-mediated changes. These mutations occurring in the CRC follow a specific order always leading to the transition of adenoma to carcinoma to metastatic tumour [5]. The role played by the family history is proved with around 10–30% of CRC. The mutations initiate tumour development, and the subsequent changes in the intracellular environment cause severe DNA damage through a number of harmful by-products including reactive oxygen species and reactive nitrogen intermediates. The pro-inflammatory cytokines released by the activated immune cells as a result of inflammation further accelerate the DNA damage in the cancers where the inflammation plays role of an inducer [6]. Several inherited disorders such as familial adenomatous polyposis, Gardner syndrome, Lunch syndrome, Turcot syndrome, etc. can also increase the risk of CRC.

There are two factors, the inadequacies in the mismatch repair (MMR) and the microsatellite instability (MSI), which have been used to categorise CRC into two subsets. The mismatch repair system involves correcting the errors occur during DNA replication in cells which involve the activity of six DNA repair genes (MLH1, MSH2, PMS1, MSH6, PMS2 and MSH3). Microsatellites are the DNA sequences in the heterochromatic regions characterised by the presence of a large part of repetitive DNA sequence, which are highly prone to mutations and replication errors. If the errors happen during replication is not corrected, it may lead to the formation of small loops in the DNA, causing MSI-H. If the MMR is functional, the rate of mutation and microsatellite loops are minimised in the CRC (MSI-L). The subset dMMR-MSI-H indicates the CRC which has a defective MMR system due to the mutation of any one of the genes involved in MMR. In pMMR-MSI-L, the MMR is functional, and the number of microsatellite loops is also low. About 15% of CRC come under the category of dMMR-MSI-H against the pMMR-MSI-L, which accounts for the remaining 85% [7].

Change in the epigenome is another important factor contributing the occurrence of CRC. Methylation of cytosine residues on the DNA is the addition of a methyl group to the fifth carbon atom of cytosine. Methylation acts as an essential feature to control the transcription activity of many functional genes by regulating the polymerase interaction with the promoter region, which is methylated. Hypomethylation of genes in the repetitive DNA sequence and hypermethylation in the functional genes (mainly the tumour suppressors) have been reported in many cancer types. The "CpG island methylator phenotype" (CIMP) is a distinct group of tumours among CRC [8]. In general, the reasons for CRC can be categorised into two preventable and non-preventable, which are summarised in Fig. 7.1.

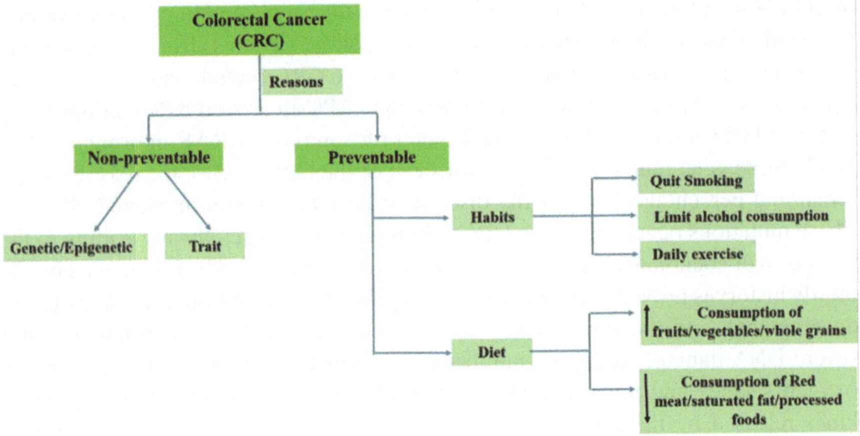

Fig. 7.1 *Major reasons for CRC:* The reasons can be divided into preventable and non-preventable. Genetic/epigenetic changes and trait are non-preventable reasons. Preventable reasons include habit and diet changes

7.1.5 CRC: Preventive Measures

Leading a healthy lifestyle is the best way to prevent CRC. Dietary intake rich in fruits, vegetables, whole grains with lot of vitamins, minerals, fibre and antioxidants can prevent the disease to a greater extent. Limiting the usage of saturated fat and red meat is also necessary. Maintaining the body weight by healthy eating and daily work out, limit alcohol usage and quit smoking are other ways in the preventive measures. There are some evidence indicating that regular use of aspirin or similar drugs reduced the risk of colon cancer but the dosage and time is not clear. Moreover it has complications in ulcer and gastrointestinal bleeding problems.

7.1.6 CRC: Screening and Treatment Methodologies

Screening for CRC among the suspects is done through mainly two methods, the invasive methods, such as colonoscopy, double contrast barium enema, computed tomographic colonography and flexible sigmoidoscopy, and the non-invasive techniques such as immunochemical tests, occult blood tests and exfoliated DNA tests. While the faecal-based non-invasive techniques are less sensitive, the invasive methods detect the CRC at an early stage [9]. The stool DNA testing using the molecular markers is considered as the most appropriate method to detect CRC. The classical treatment regime includes the neoadjuvant and adjuvant therapy. The neoadjuvant therapy includes the use of therapeutics which are given before the main treatment (surgery), and the adjuvant therapy is the treatment modalities along with or after the main cancer treatment. Neoadjuvant therapy found to increase the life span of CRC patients by supporting the treatment to a greater extent. There are many chemotherapeutic agents, mainly 5-fluorouracil (5-FU), oxaliplatin (FOLFOX) or irinotecan (FOLFIRI), which are used alone or in combination depending on the type and stage of CRC [10]. The targeted therapies using monoclonal antibodies are also introduced recently against the epidermal growth factor receptor (EGFR) and vascular endothelial growth factor (VEGF), which are involved in the cell proliferation and angiogenesis respectively. If the cancer is diagnosed at an early stage, a survival rate of 5 years is observed in 90% of the CRC patients. Those with localised cancer at an early stage survive better than those with metastatic tumours.

7.1.7 CRC: Biomarkers

The gold standard screening test, colonoscopy, has less patient compliance due to the expense and risk associated with it. The non-invasive faecal occult blood test has limitations like less sensitivity leading to false results. Therefore an alternate less expensive, non-invasive and accurate screening procedures are necessary for the CRC screening. Here comes the importance of biomarker-based disease prediction and therapy selection. Epidermal growth factor receptor (EGFR) pathway is the main biomarker for the diagnosis and treatment of CRC. Progress in omics techniques has expanded the number of biomarkers.

7.1.7.1 Biomarkers Identified by Proteomic Approaches

Proteomic analysis have identified the upregulation of actin beta-like 2 (ACTBL2) and dipeptidase 1 (DPEP1) in CRC tissues. LC/MS analysis of blood samples have identified five proteins, viz. leucine-rich alpha-2-glycoprotein 1, EGFR, inter-alpha-trypsin inhibitor heavy-chain family member 4, hemopexin and superoxide dismutase 3 in CRC. MS/MS technique have identified the downregulation of the protein serine/threonine kinase 4 (STK4 or MST1) in CRC. Serum analysis by HPLC/MS has identified the macrophage mannose receptor 1 (MRC1), S100 calcium-binding protein A9 (S100A9), SERPINA1 (alpha-1-antitrypsin, A1AT), SERPINA3 (alpha-1-antichymotrypsin, AACT) and SERPINC1 (antithrombin-3, AT-III) in CRC. Apolipoprotein E (APOE), angiotensinogen (AGT) and vitamin D-binding protein (DBP) are three identified survival biomarkers on treatment with the VEGF inhibitor bevacizumab in metastatic CRC. Proteosome subunit alpha type 1 (PSA1), leucine aminopeptidase 3 (LAP3), annexin A3 (ANXA3), and maspin (serpin B5), olfactomedin 4, CD11b and integrin alpha-2 are the overexpressed immunogenic proteins in CRC identified by proteomic analysis. Interferon-induced protein with tetratricopeptide repeats 1 (IFIT1), FAST kinase domains 2 (FASTKD2), phosphatidylinositol-5-phosphate 4-kinase type-2 beta (PIP4K2B), AT-rich interactive domain-containing protein 1B (ARID1B) and solute carrier family 25 member

33 (SLC25A33) were overexpressed in the tumour tissue in response to chemoradiotherapy. Carcinoembryonic antigen (CEA), a high-molecular-weight glycoprotein, is the prognostic biomarker in CRC clinical practice. Increased urinary levels of PGE-M, the metabolite of prostaglandin E2 is correlating the risk of CRC. Elevated expression of heat shock protein 47 (hsp47) in CRC is also identified as one promising biomarker [11].

7.1.7.2 Genetic and Epigenetic Biomarkers

Researches indicated that three major pathways are involved in the colon carcinogenesis, viz. chromosomal abnormalities, microsatellite instability pathways and methylation pathway due to epigenetic modification. The microsatellite instability status is also one biomarker: mutations of MMR, BRAF and Raf genes. *BRAF* gene is the regulator of MAPK pathway and is located downstream of *KRAS*. The conversion of Val (600) to glutamic acid accounts for more than 80% of *BRAF* mutations in CRC. Mutations of *KRAS* gene (encode for small GTPase transductor protein that regulates cellular growth and differentiation) lead to continuous activation of differentiation signal transduction. *PIK3CA* is a protooncogne encoding phosphatidylinositol-3-kinase, and mutation in the exon 20 of *PIK3CA* is a predictive therapeutic marker in CRC. Microsatellite instability (MSI) caused by the inactivation of four MMR genes (*MSH2*, *MLH1*, *MSH6* and *PMS2*) occurs in 15% of CRC. It is considered as a prognostic marker in CRC which can be assessed by five markers (*BAT25*, *BAT26*, *D2S123*, *D5S346* and *D17S2720*). DNA methylation in the CpG islands in the promoter region of tumour suppressor gene is one of the most explored CRC biomarkers. These epigenetic changes can affect the cellular pathways in many ways like DNA repair system, apoptosis, angiogenesis, cell cycle regulation and metastasis suppression. The five methylated CRC-specific genes which were significantly higher in cancer compared to normal are *SEPT9*, *TWIST1*, *IGFBP3*, *GAS7*, *ALX4* and *miR137*. Methylated thrombomodulin (*THBD*) and methylated syndecan 2 (*SDC2*) are two other blood biomarkers showed more 70% specificity in CRC. Mutation of APC (the suppressor gene adenomatous polyposis coli) is also responsible for CRC, and hypermethylation of APC is an important biomarker for early CRC [12].

7.1.7.3 MicroRNAs as Biomarkers

Cancer cells secrete some microRNAs (miRNAs) to the systemic circulation, which are also predictive biomarkers. miRNAs are small noncoding RNA sequences that can control the expression of genes at the post-transcriptional level which are controlling a number of cellular processes such as proliferation, apoptosis, differentiation, invasion and metastasis. The miRNAs isolated from blood, saliva and stool could be valuable biomarker for early detection, prognostic and treatment response predictors in CRC. Mir-21 is the most studied miRNA in CRC. High-level expressions of miR-92a, miR-141, let-7a, miR-1229, miR-1246, miR-150, miR-21, miR-223, miR-23a and miR-378 were identified as diagnostic biomarkers. High expression levels of miR-141, miR-320, miR-596 and miR-203 are majorly for prognosis and tumour recurrence, and miR-106a, miR-484 and miR-130b are associated with predictive biomarkers. Low-level expressions of miRNAs are also prognostic in nature such as miR-106a, miR-484 and miR-130b. Upregulation of hsa-miR-183-5p and hsa-miR-21-5p and the downregulation of hsa-miR-195-5p and hsa-miR-497-5p were associated with CRC by mediating the *MMR* pathway and transforming growth factor β, *WNT*, *RAS*, *MAPK* and *PI3K* signaling pathways. Plasma miR-141 is a novel biomarker par with CEA in detecting CRC. let-7a, miR-1229, miR1246, miR-150, miR-21, miR-223 and miR-23a are 7 miRNAs were identified to be suitable biomarkers to detect CRC. miR-135b was elevated in the stool samples of CRC patients with a sensitivity of more than 70%. *miR-7, miR-17, miR-20a, miR-21, miR-92a, miR-96, miR-106a, miR-134, miR-183, miR-196a, miR-199a-3p* and *miR-214* were found to be elevated in with the advancement of TNM stages in CRC. *miR-9, miR-29b, miR-127-5p, miR-138, miR-143, miR146a, miR-222* and *miR-938* were found to be reduced by increasing the TNM stages. miR-193a-3p was predicted as tumour suppressive in early stages of CRC which is sensitive in anti-EGFR therapy. miR-181c is associated predicted as a recurrent biomarker in second stage of CRC. miR-17-3p and miR-221 are identified as equally expressing in all stages of CRC with more than 60% sensitivity. miR-17 and miR-21 are expressed in faeces in all stages of cancer. Plasma miR-29a and miR-92a are identified as potential non-invasive biomarkers for early detection of CRC. Identification of miRNAs specific to each stage of TNM is the best way to stage specific management of CRC [13, 14].

7.1.8 Exosomes: General Introduction

Exosomes are membrane bound extracellular vesicles formed from endosomes that are released to the extracellular space. They are characteristic vesicular structures, about 30–150 nm size which carry proteins, DNAs and RNAs that are considered as the markers of the cells of their origin. Irrespective of the parent cell of origin, exosomes have common properties like the presence of certain tetraspanins (CD9, CD63 and CD81), heat shock proteins (Hsp 60, Hsp 70 and Hsp 90), biogenesis-related proteins (Alix and TSG 101), membrane transport and fusion proteins (GTPases, annexins and Rab proteins), nuclear acids (mRNA, miRNA and long noncoding RNAs and DNAs) and lipids (cholesterol and ceramide). The biogenesis of exosomes from the endosomal limiting membrane is by (endosomal sorting complexes required for transport) ESCRT-dependent or ESCRT-independent machinery. They are found in tissues as well as released into many of the biological fluids such as blood, urine, saliva, cerebrospinal fluid, etc. One major function of exosomes is to remove the excess or unwanted constituents from the cells to maintain the cellular homeostasis. In 1983 Stahl and group first discovered these vesicles in maturing mammalian reticulocytes, and later Johnstone and group identified that they play an important role in selective removal of many plasma membrane proteins during the formation of erythrocyte from reticulocytes. Four years later, Rose Johnstone coined the term exosomes to these vesicles, and in 2013 Ames E Rothman, Randy W Schekaman and Thomas C Sudhof won Nobel Prize for their discovery in identifying these as the major transport system in our cells. The targeted accumulation of specific components in exosomes indicates their role in regulating intercellular communications. The biomolecules (the cellular cargos) encapsulated within the lipid bilayer of exosomes are mediating intracellular communications and can transfer these biomolecules between cells by membrane vesicle trafficking mechanisms. Exosomes are taken up by the recipient cells by endocytosis mediated by cell adhesion molecules, specific receptors or membrane lipids or carbohydrates. The proteins, metabolites and nucleic acids delivered by exosomes to the recipient cells are controlling many biological responses such as immune response, microbial pathogenicity, cancer progression, etc. Due to the growing clinical importance of exosomal biomarkers in the prognosis, diagnosis and treatment of many diseases, an International Society for extracellular vesicles was also formed for discussing the research progress in this area [15]. The structure of exosomes, its biogenesis from the endosomes and cellular uptake by the recipient cells are diagrammatically represented in Fig. 7.2.

7.1.9 Exosomes: Research and Business Opportunities

After 2000, there was a boom in exosome research and many high impact articles have come in front. The Swedish Scientist Jan Lotvall in 2007 showed that some cells use exosomes to transfer genetic materials (especially mRNA and miRNA to regulate the expression of genes) between each other [16]. In view of this, the biotech startup company Codiak tried to use this messenger system to transfer drugs into cells in the parts of the body where in normal way it is difficult to reach. Like Codiak, many other companies are now manipulating exosomes for array of therapies like RNA therapy, viral gene therapy or even CRISPR gene editing tools. Research suggests that the study of exosomes derived from stem cells can become a superior branch of regenerative medicine. Matthew J A Wood from Oxford demonstrated that the exosomes filled with siRNA reached the brain of mice, and it lowered the production of BACE1, the protein involved in Alzheimer's disease [17]. Evox Therapeutics, the startup company cofounded by Wood, is developing exosome-based systems to deliver drugs to the brain in partnership with the German giant Boehringer Ingelheim. Casey Maguire from Massachusetts General Hospital has made vexosome (exosomes packed with adenovirus used for gene therapy) for the hard reaching sensory cells of inner ear [18]. Proteins, mRNA and CRISPR/Cas9 gene editing systems could also be delivered using exosomes [19]. Human mesenchymal stem cells (MSCs) can treat lung disease in animal models by reducing inflammation and repairing lung tissues, and MSC-derived exosomes are

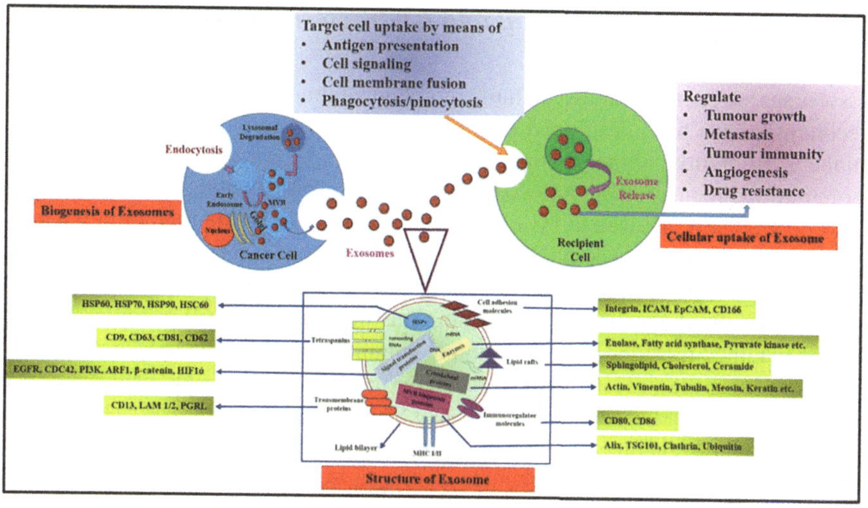

Fig. 7.2 *Biogenesis of exosomes, their cellular cargos and uptake by the recipient cells:* Biogenesis of exosomes begins with the formation of early endosome by the invagination of plasma membrane. The early endosomes mature into late endosomes and accumulate intraluminal vesicles (ILVs) in their lumen which are referred to as multivesicular bodies (MVBs). Bioactive molecules are packaged into the ILVs by means of endosomal sorting complex required for transport (ESCRT)-dependent and ESCRT-independent pathway. MVBs fuse with the plasma membrane resulting in the release of ILVs into the extracellular space as exosomes. Exosome membrane is enriched with sphingomyelin, cholesterol and ceramide as the lipid rafts. Moreover it contains tetraspanins, cell adhesion molecules, immune-regulating molecules and transmembrane proteins. The lumen of the vesicle contains proteins (cytoskeletal proteins, signal transduction molecules, enzymes, MVB biogenesis proteins, heat shock proteins), DNA, mRNA, miRNA and other non-coding RNAs. The exosomes released by the cancer cells are taken up by the recipient cells by endocytosis (different mechanisms like antigen presentation, cell signaling, cell membrane fusion, phagocytosis, pinocytosis, etc.). Once it get into the cells, exosomes release their cellular cargos which regulate number of cellular processes like proliferation, metastasis, immunity regulation, angiogenesis, inducing chemoresistance, etc. which alter the biological functions of the recipient cells

responsible for these effects [20]. Now, the US Food and Drug administration in partnership with industry is going to use these exosomes to treat bronchopulmonary dysplasia in new born babies. The exosomes derived from human MSCs and neural stem cells improved brain cell preservation and motor neuron movement in rodent and pig models of stroke, and the company ArunA biomedicals will start the clinical trial soon [21]. The stem cell biologist Raj Kishore from Temple University has received 11.6 million USD from NIH to study stem cell-derived exosomes in heart repair. The research areas with exosomes are not only restricted to human exosomes as there are many startups looking for new kinds of exosomes from bacteria, fungi, plants, animals, etc. Food-derived exosomes are also coming up now especially as drug delivery carriers. Mammalian milk is loaded with exosomes and the Swiss multinational healthcare company Roche gave 36 million USD to the company PureTech Health for exosomes extracted from cow milk.

7.1.10 Exosomes: Isolation and Characterization

Exosomes are found in almost all human biological fluids, and a number of isolation techniques have been developed for their separation. The most widely used technique is differential ultracentrifugation, while the yield is very low in this method. Solution sedimentation and low-speed centrifugation is another method where sucrose gradients are used to facilitate the isolation process. Immunoaffinity purification using antibodies specific to a particular exosomal surface antigen is another method for the purification. The emerging separation method involves the utilisation of microfluidic techniques, and using this method high level purity exosomes can be obtained less time, cost and sample volume. The physical characterization is by determining the size, shape, surface charge and density. Dynamic light scattering (DLS) and nanoparticle tracking analysis (NTA) are the methods used for this. A rarely adopted technique qNano (measures the particle size and concentration in a more accurate way) using the tunable resistive pulse sensing (TRPS) technology is also employed for size measurements. Transmission electron microscopy (TEM) can be utilised for visualisation of exosomes, but it only measures the membrane diameter and cannot extend to adhered molecules. Conventional fluorescent microscopy can be used for exosome visualisation if it is labelled with a fluorescent probe specific for exosome bilayer, proteins, nucleic acids or carbohydrates. Single particle interferometric reflectance (SPIR) imaging coupled with fluorescence microscopy can visualize individual exosomes with specific lipids, carbohydrates and proteins. Flow cytometry can also be used for analysing exosomes. Biochemical characterization of exosomes can be done by exploiting the specific RNA and marker proteins, and it can be used for the quality checking of isolated exosomes. Exoquick precipitation method yield exosomes with high purity when compared to chromatography and ultracentrifugation or with DynaBeads. The purity of isolated exosomes can be checked by the presence of marker proteins (Tsg101, Alix) and absence of possible contaminating proteins from the membrane structures such as Grp94, calnexin from endoplasmic reticulum and VDAC1 from mitochondria using western blot analysis [22].

7.1.11 Exosomes: Research Challenges

The extracellular vesicle diversity is the main challenge associated with exosome research. Like exosomes there are many vesicles and separation of these vesicles is a big task. Developing a fast and precise method for the isolation of exosomes is the most important challenge in the field. There is a variation in the size of exosomes (average size 100 nm), so the amount of drug loaded on exosomes will vary. This interrupts the consistency and reproducibility of the data especially in exosome-based therapies. The lack of tools required to identify the source and targets of exosomes is also one limitation in exosome research. Precise characterisation of exosomes from different sources is needed before it is used as a therapeutic carrier. Exosomes derived from cell cultures vary and show inconsistent properties when given to the donor, and mass production of exosomes through this method is not possible also. Lack of exclusive biomarkers and high-resolution visualisation techniques also the factors that limit the exosomes research [23].

7.1.12 Exosomes: Potential in Cancer Research

Exosomes are secreted under normal and diseased conditions, but the cellular information encapsulated within it will vary considerably under these two states. Researches indicated that tumour cells release exosomes at a faster rate, and these have important role in tumour development and metastasis. They offer a new dimension to biomarker route which can be identified by minimal invasive means. Among diverse cellular cargos, noncoding RNAs like miRNA and long noncoding RNA (lncRNA) which forms the viable source of biomarkers in cancer. The exosomes secreted by tumour cells may be tumour stimulative or suppressive properties. The tumour associated in exosomes can stimulate specific immune response which will help tumour growth, or they can stimulate termination of tumour by stimulating FAS ligand-mediated intrinsic apoptosis. Exosomes can play a role in every step of carcinogenesis process like initiation, growth, progression, drug resistance, etc. During the process of epithelial to mesenchymal transition, the cell lose the cell polarity and cell-cell contacts, and reports indicated that breast milk exosomes drive this process by the upregulation of TGFβ2. Circulating exosomes with proteins like CD24, EDIL3 and fibronectin are markers of early-stage breast cancers. In lung cancer-derived exosomes, EGFR, placental alkaline phosphatase and leucine-rich alpha 2 glycoprotein 1 were overexpressed. Cancer exosomes promote tumour growth by activating PI3K/AKT or MAPK/ERK signaling pathways. They can also manipulate the tumour microenvironment and promote angiogenesis though the transfer of mRNA, miRNA and proteins. In leukaemia cells, miR-92a enhanced cell migration and tube formation. The triple negative breast cancer derived exosomes can transfer miR-10b to the non-malignant cells and enhance cell invasion. Metastatic breast cancer exosome-derived miR-105 can target the tight junction protein zonulin 1, thereby promoting metastasis. The exosomes derived from pancreatic adenocarcinoma cells have a high expression of macrophage inhibitory factor, which induce the production of EMT inducer TGFβ [24]. Long noncoding RNAs (lncRNAs) are also involved in the regulation of gene expression, epigenetic modifications, etc. and the exosomal lncRNAs play a key role in cancer progression. lncRNA-ATB, the lncRNA activated by TGFβ, is involved in the EMT process by upregulating the ZEB1 and 2 and induced colonisation in the metastatic site by triggering STAT3 signaling by binding to IL-11. Metastasis-associated lung adenocarcinoma transcript-1 (MALT-1) is the first identified lncRNA in lung cancer metastasis. lncZFAS1 (zinc finger antisense 1) activated ZEB1, MMP14 and MMP16 in colon cancer to promote proliferation and migration. Increased levels of exo-lncZFAS1 are identified in gastric cancer in correlation with TNM stage. Exo-lncRNA HOTAIR is significantly overexpressed in the serum of patients with LSCC [25].

Another advantage of exosomes is its efficacy as effective drug carrier due to the presence of several targeted proteins over the surface for cellular communication. Thus the researchers and clinicians can exploit the exceptional properties of exosomes not only to understand the mechanistic aspects of tumour metastasis but also for other applications like early diagnosis of the disease, to monitor the effectiveness of the treatment modalities as well as for identification of targeted therapeutics. Exosomes carry MHC-peptide complexes that are recognised by T lymphocytes and could promote antitumour immune response. The drugs can be loaded into the exosomes by incubation, sonication or electroporation. Taxol filled exosomes treat cancers, evade multidrug resistance and are effective at 50-fold lower doses than conventional treatments. In 2017, Raghu Kalluri and Valerie LeBleu, cancer biologists from MD Anderson Cancer Center, University of Texas, have made success in delivering siRNA (that blocked the production of mutant KRas)-loaded exosomes to mice, better than siRNA-loaded lipid nanoparticles which suppressed the pancreatic cancer without any obvious immune reactions [26].

7.1.13 Exosomal Biomarkers in CRC: Types and Relevance

Exosomes carry molecular markers such as DNA, RNA and proteins. Moreover it contains significant amounts of mRNA, miRNA and lncRNA. Differentially expressed proteins and RNA have a key role in CRC initiation and progression. Studies indicated that the exosome-derived miRNA, lncRNA and proteins of CRC patients/cell lines differ significantly when compared to normal controls. Elaborating the relation between exosomes and CRC will help to identify novel biomarkers for this disease [27].

7.1.13.1 Exosomal Proteins as Biomarkers

Circulating tumour cells and exosomes from blood can be used as liquid biopsy samples to assess CRC [28]. Functionally different proteins are associated with exosomes which include tetraspanins (CD63, CD9, CD81), heat shock proteins (HSP70 and HSP90) and sorting proteins such as Alix and TSG101. EPCAM (epithelial cell adhesion molecule) is a transmembrane glycoprotein mediating calcium-dependent cell-cell adhesion in epithelial cells, and there was observed elevated levels of EPCAM from the exosomes isolated from CRC cells [29]. Glypican-1 is a member of the heparin sulphate proteoglycan expressed in cell membrane and ECM and is a modulator of growth factor signaling. This protein was overexpressed in the exosomes of patients before and after CRC surgery [30]. The transmembrane protein tetraspanin1 (TSPAN1) functions as an oncoprotein in many types of cancer and promotes EMT process, and it was identified in the plasma exosomes of CRC patients with more than 75% sensitivity when compared to normal controls [31]. Exosomes derived from the serum of CRC patients contain metastasis promoting extracellular matrix proteins SPARC and LRG1 which are considered as diagnosis and prognosis biomarker [32]. Heat shock protein 60 (Hsp60) in the plasma exosomes of patients is a promising candidate for CRC diagnosis [33]. Elevated levels of transmembrane protein CD147 and copine III (CPNE3) in the serum of CRC patients are effective diagnostic markers [34, 35].

7.1.13.2 Exosomal Nucleic Acids as Biomarkers

Apart from proteins, exosomes also carry circulating nucleic acids like mRNA, miRNA, lncRNA and DNA, and they are main source of circulating miRNAs. Exosomal miRNAs play a crucial role in the pathogenesis of CRC which can be exploited for the development of diagnostic strategies and early detection of the disease [36]. Overexpression of miR-21 was found in the exosomes released from three different CRC cell lines, and it is the first exo-miR reported in CRC. It is overexpressed in the metastatic tissues in the lung and liver and significantly correlated with the disease stage. The increased migration and invasive nature of CRC is due to the expression of miR-21 that targets the transcriptional regulator BRG1 [37]. Liver metastasis in CRC has been linked with the selective upregulation of serum exosomal miR-19a and miR-92a. miR-19a-5p expression is correlated with lymph node metastasis of CRC [38]. The exomiR-200 family members miR-141, miR-200c and miR-429 have protective effects against CRC [39 protection].

Microarray analysis of the exosomal miRNAs isolated from the serum samples of 88 colon cancer patients, 11 healthy controls, 5 colon cancer cells and 1 normal colon-derived cells showed the upregulation of 8 miRNAs (let-7a, miR-1224-5p, miR-1229, miR-1246, miR-150, miR-21, miR-223 and miR-23a) in CRC patients [40]. From the 369 peripheral blood sample exosome analysis, the elevated miR-27a and miR-130a were identified as the non-invasive biomarker for the early diagnosis and predicting prognosis of CRC [41]. Increased exosomal expression of miR-200c and miR-141 may be an indicator or biomarker candidate for the MET of CRC cells [42]. ExomiR-200b from CRC cells promoted the proliferation in recipient cells by lowering the expression of p27 [43]. Exo-miR-6869-5p decreased the CRC proliferation by inhibiting the production of IL-6 and TNF-α by the blocking the TL4/NF-ΚB signaling pathway [44 protection]. In CRC, exo-miR-193a has cell proliferation inhibition by targeting the cell cycle associated protein, caprin-1 [45]. Significantly higher level of exomiR-6803-5p, miR-17-5p and miR-92a-3p and lower levels of miR-548c-5p were observed in the sera of CRC patients [46–48]. Upregulated serum exosomal miR-320d is identified as a promising non-invasive diagnostic biomarker for distinguishing metastatic CRC from non-metastatic [49]. Decreased expression of exomiR-92b in plasma is a promising biomarker for early detection of CRC [50]. In CRC patients with liver metastasis serum, exosomal miR-122 upregulation is a novel potential diagnostic and prognostic biomarker

[51]. miR-424-5p expression was significantly upregulated in CRC tissues and cell lines and associated with prognosis of CRC patients. It promoted CRC cell proliferation and metastasis by directly inhibiting sodium voltage-gated channel beta subunit 4 [52]. Higher expressions of exomiR-23a and 301a were able to differentiate CRC from normal individuals [53]. The exo-miR-125a-3p from plasma of CRC patients was clearly upregulated, and its diagnostic power was utilised in combination with CEA [54]. Plasma exo-miR 125-b level (elevated) is useful in detecting the chemoresistance induced by modified fluorouracil, leucovorin and oxaliplatin in the firstline chemotherapy in advanced/recurrent CRC [55]. Serum exo-miR 150-5p (downregulation) is a non-invasive biomarker for CRC diagnosis/prognosis, and ZEB1 was identified as its downstream target [56]. Serum exosomal miRNAs miR-99b-5p and miR-150-5p (downregulation) associated with CRC are promising, sensitive, specific and non-invasive diagnostic biomarkers [57]. Homeodomain interacting protein kinase 2 (HIPK2) is a multifunctional signaling molecule and a tumour suppressor that mediate growth regulation and cellular apoptotic response. The exomiR-1229 was significantly elevated in the serum exosomes of CRC patients, and they can inhibit the protein expression of HIPK2, activating VEGF pathway and promoting angiogenesis [58]. Exosomes containing the oxygen-sensitive miRNAs 486-5p, 181a-5p and 30d-5p are circulating markers of high-risk locally advanced rectal cancer [59]. The downregulation of exosomal miR-548c-5p was observed in serum of CRC patients and may be a critical biomarker for diagnosis and prognosis [60].

The exosomes from the serum of CRC patients are also rich in lncRNAs which can act as potential biomarkers. LncRNA colorectal neoplasia differentially expressed-h (CRNDE-h), lncRNA breast cancer anti-oestrogen resistance 4 (BCAR4), mRNA keratin-associated protein 5-4(KRTAP5-4), mRNA melanoma antigen family A3 (MAGEA3), circular homeodomain-interacting protein kinase 3 (HIPK3) and lncRNA growth arrest specific 5 (GAS5) are certain upregulated lnRNAs in the CRC patients. The downregulated expression of lncRNA urothelial cancer associated 1 (UCA1) is also specific to CRC [61–64]. The lncRNA CRNDE-h was isolated from the serum exosomes of CRC patients, and its increased expression is a tumour marker for diagnosis and prognosis [65]. Exosomal circulating long noncoding RNA colon cancer-associated transcript 2 (CCAT2) is a potential biomarker for colorectal cancer [66].

Circular RNAs are noncoding RNAs characterised by covalently closed loop structures, and they are reported to be associated with initiation, progression and metastasis of tumours. They are abundant and stable in exosomes and exo-circular RNAs also considered as emerging diagnostic markers. Exo-hsa-circ-0004771 was significantly upregulated in CRC patients when compared to control [67]. The list of exosomal biomarkers in CRC are summarised in Table 7.1.

Table 7.1 List of selected exosomal biomarker molecules in CRC

Type of molecule	Name	Expression	Source of exosomes	Function	Reference
Protein	Epithelial cell adhesion molecule (EPCAM)	Upregulation	Cell line (HCT 116)	Diagnosis	[29]
	Glypican-1 (GPC1)	Upregulation	Plasma	Detection and therapy	[30]
	Tetraspanin1 (TSPAN1)	Upregulation	Plasma	Metastasis prediction	[31]
	Secreted protein acidic and rich in cysteine (SPARC)	Upregulation	Serum	Diagnosis and prognosis	[32]
	Leucine-rich alpha-2-glycoprotein 1 (*LRG1*)	Upregulation	Serum	Diagnosis and prognosis	[32]
	Heat shock protein 60 (Hsp60)	Upregulation	Serum	Diagnosis	[33]
	Cluster of differentiation 147 (CD147)	Upregulation	Serum	Diagnosis	[34]
	Copine III (CPNE3)	Upregulation	Serum	Diagnosis	[35]
miRNA	miR-21	Upregulation	Cell line (SW 480)	Metastasis prediction	[37]
	miR-19a and miR-92a	Upregulation	Serum	Metastasis prediction	[38]
	miR-141, miR-200c and miR-429	Downregulation	Serum	Prognosis and therapy	[39]
	let-7a, miR-1224-5p, miR-1229, miR-1246, miR-150, miR-21, miR-223 and miR-23a	Upregulation	Serum	Diagnosis	[40]
	miR-27a and miR-130a	Upregulation	Serum	Diagnosis and prognosis	[41]
	miR-200c and miR-141	Upregulation	Cell line (SW480 and SW 620)	Metastasis prediction	[42]
	ExomiR-200b	Upregulation	Cell line (HCT-116)	Diagnosis	[43]
	miR-6869-5p	Downregulation	Serum	Diagnosis	[44]
	miR-193a	Upregulation	Serum	Diagnosis	[45]
	miR-6803-5p	Upregulation	Serum	Diagnosis and prognosis	[46]
	miR-17-5p and miR-92a-3p	Upregulation	Serum	Diagnosis and prognosis	[47]
	miR-548c-5p	Upregulation	Serum	Diagnosis and prognosis	[48]
	miR-320d	Upregulation	Serum	Metastasis prediction	[49]
	miR-92b	Downregulation	Plasma	Prognosis	[50]

(continued)

Table 7.1 (continued)

Type of molecule	Name	Expression	Source of exosomes	Function	Reference
	miR-122	Upregulation	Serum	Prognosis and metastasis prediction	[51]
	miR-424-5p	Upregulation	Serum	Diagnosis	[52]
	miR-301a and miR-23a	Upregulation	Serum	Diagnosis	[53]
	miR-125a-3p	Upregulation	Plasma	Diagnosis	[54]
	miR 125-b	Upregulation	Serum	Therapeutic efficiency and recurrence prediction	[55]
	miR 150-5p	Downregulation	Serum	Diagnosis and prognosis	[56]
	miR-99b-5p and miR-150-5p	Downregulation	Serum	Diagnosis	[57]
	miR-1229	Upregulation	Serum	Angiogenesis prediction	[58]
	miR486-5p, miR181a-5p and miR30d-5p	Downregulation	Plasma	Metastasis prediction	[59]
	miR-548c-5p	Downregulation	Serum	Metastasis prediction	[60]
lncRNA	Neoplasia differentially expressed-h (CRNDE-h)	Upregulation	Serum	Prognosis	[61, 65]
	lncRNA breast cancer anti-oestrogen resistance 4 (BCAR4), mRNA keratin associated protein 5-4(KRTAP5-4), mRNA melanoma antigen family A3 (MAGEA3), circular homeodomain interacting protein kinase 3 (HIPK3)	Upregulation	Serum	Diagnosis	[62]
	Growth arrest specific 5 (GAS5)	Upregulation	Serum	Diagnosis	[63]
	Urothelial cancer associated 1 (UCA1)	Downregulation	Serum	Diagnosis	[64]
	Colon cancer-associated transcript 2 (CCAT2)	Upregulation	Serum	Diagnosis	[66]
CircRNA	hsa-circ-0004771	Upregulation	Serum	Diagnosis	[67]

7.2 Conclusion and Future Perspectives

The disease prevalence and thus the societal burdens due CRC are increasing day by day mainly due to the absence of confirmed methods for detection. The mode of progression of CRC, like any other cancer, is multifactorial, and the major complications associated are metastasis, chemoresistance and tumour reoccurrence.

Exosomes and their differentially expressed proteins/RNAs have a major role in these processes, and they can act as relevant biomarkers. The exosomal markers are superior because of their high sensitivity, specificity, stability, less interference (serum biomarkers have interference with number of proteins in it) and availability through non-invasive methods from number of biological fluids. Due to the exciting properties many exosome-based diagnostic kits are now used in labs with the approval from Food and Drug Administration.

Still there is long way to go with exosome-based biomarker approach that may be because of the problems associated like absence of quick and accurate methods for isolation, lack of purity (contamination with other extracellular vesicles) and heterogeneity in the exosomes from different sources. In spite of all these, exosomes provide a good platform for novel, non-invasive clinical tool for diagnosing and predicting CRC progression, metastasis, reoccurrence, chemosensitivity and chemoresistance. The future of exosome-based biomarker approach in CRC is bright and promising.

References

1. Arnold M, Sierra MS, Laversanne M, Soerjomataram, Jemal A, Bray F. Global patterns and trends in colorectal cancer incidence and mortality. Gut. 2017;66:683–91.
2. American Cancer Society. Colorectal cancer. Available online: https://www.cancer.org/cancer/colon-rectal-cancer.html, 2019.
3. International Agency for Research on Cancer. Cancer fact sheets. Available online: http://gco.iarc.fr/today/fact-sheets-cancers, 2019.
4. World Health Association. Mortality database. Available online: https://www.who.int/healthinfo/global_burden_disease/estimates/en/, 2019.
5. Robles AI, Traverso G, Zhang M, Roberts NJ, Khan MA, Joseph C, Lauwers GY, Selaru FM, Popoli M, Pittman ME, et al. Whole-exome sequencing analyses of inflammatory bowel disease-associated colorectal cancers. Gastroenterology. 2016;150:931–43.
6. Terzi'CJ, Grivennikov S, Karin E, Karin M. Inflammation and colon cancer. Gastroenterology. 2010;138:2101–21147.
7. Fleisher AS, Esteller M, Harpaz N, Leytin A, Rashid A, Xu Y, Liang J, Stine OC, Yin J, Zou TT, et al. Microsatellite instability in inflammatory bowel disease-associated neoplastic lesions is associated with hypermethylation and diminished expression of the DNA mismatch repair gene, hMLH1. Cancer Res. 2000;60:4864–8.
8. Toyota M, Ahuja N, Ohe-Toyota M, et al. CpG island methylator phenotype in colorectal cancer. Proc Natl Acad Sci U S A. 1999;96:8681–6.
9. Levin B, Lieberman DA, McFarland B, et al. Screening and surveillance for the early detection of colorectal cancer and adenomatous polyps, 2008: a joint guideline from the American Cancer Society, the US Multi-Society Task Force on Colorectal Cancer, and the American College of Radiology. CA Cancer J Clin. 2008;58:130–60.
10. Longley DB, Harkin DP, Johnston PG. 5-Fluorouracil: mechanisms of action and clinical strategies. Nat Rev Cancer. 2003;3:330–8.
11. Alves Martins BA, de Bulhões GF, Cavalcanti IN, Martins MM, de Oliveira PG, Martins AMA. Biomarkers in colorectal cancer: the roe of translational proteomics research. Front Oncol. 2019;9:1284.
12. Vacante M, Borzi AM, Basile F, Biondi A. Biomarkers in colorectal cancer: current clinical utility and future perspectives. World J Clin Cases. 2018;6:869–81.

13. Fadaka AO, Pretoriius A, Klein A. Biomarkers for stratification in colorectal cancer: MicroRNAs. Cancer Control. 2019;26:1073274819862784.
14. Yiu JA, Yiu CY. Biomarkers in colorectal cancer. Anticancer Res. 2016;36:1093–102.
15. Kalluri R, LeBleu VS. The biology, function and biomedical applications of exosomes. Science. 2020;367:pii: eaau6977.
16. Valadi H, Ekstrom K, Bossios A, Sjostrand M, Lee JJ, Lotvall JO. Exosome mediated transfer of mRNAs and microRNAs is a novel mechanism of genetic exchange between cells. Nat Cell Biol. 2007;9:654–9.
17. Alvarez-Erviti L, Seow Y, Yin H, Betts C, Lakhal S, Wood MJ. Delivery of siRNA to the mouse brain by systemic injection of targeted exosomes. Nat Biotechnol. 2011;29:341–5.
18. Gyorgy B, Sage C, Indzhykulian AA, Scheffer DI, Brisson AR, et al. Rescue of hearing by gene delivery to inner ear hair cells using exosome associated AAV. Mol Ther. 2017;25:379–91.
19. Wang Q, Yu J, Kadungure T, Beyene J, Zhang H, Lu Q. ARRMs as a versatile platform for intracellular delivery of macromolecules. Nat Commun. 2018;9:96020.
20. Willis GR, Fernandez-Gonzalez A, Anastas J, Vitali SH, Liu X, Ericsson M, Kwong A, Mitsialis SA, Kourembanas S. Mesenchymal stromal cell exosomes ameliorate experimental bronchopulmonary dysplasia and restore lung function through macrophage immunomodulation. Am J Respir Crit Care Med. 2018;197:104–16.
21. Webb RL, Kaiser EE, Jurgielewicz BJ, Spellicy S, Scoville SL, Thompson TA, Swetenburg RL, Hess DC, West FD, Stice SL. Human neuronal stem cell extracellular vesicles improve recovery in a porcine model of ischemic stroke. Stroke. 2018;49:1248–56.
22. Pegtel DM, Gould SJ. Exosomes. Annu Rev Biochem. 2019;88:487–514.
23. Ludwig N, Whiteside TL, Reichert TE. Challenges in exosome isolation and analysis in health and disease. Int J Mol Sci. 2019;20:pii:E4684.
24. Li X, Corberr AL, Taatizadeh E, Tasnim N, Little JP, Garnis C, Daugaard M, Guns E, Hoorfar M. Li ITS. APL Bioeng. 2019;3:011503.
25. Meng X, Pan J, Sun S, Gong Z. Circulating exosomes and their cargos in blood as novel biomarkers for cancer. Trasl Cancer Res. 2018;7:S226–42.
26. Kamerkar S, LeBleu VS, Sugimoto H, Yang S, Ruivo CF, Melo SA, Lee JJ, Kalluri R. Exosomes facilitate therapeutic targeting of oncogenic KRAS in pancreatic cancer. Nature. 2017;546:498–503.
27. Xiao Y, Zhong J, Zhong B, Huang J, Jiang L, Jiang Y, Yuan J, Sun J, Dai L, Yang C, Li Z, Wang J, Zhong T. Exosomes as potential sources of biomarkers in colorectal cancer. Cancer Lett. 2020;476:13–22.
28. Vafaei S, Fattahi F, Ebrahimi M, Janani L, Shariftabrizi A, Madjd Z. Common molecular markers between circulating tumor cells and blood exosomes in colorectal cancer: a systematic and analytical review. Cancer Manag Res. 2019;11:8669–98.
29. Manri C, Yokoi T, Nishida H. Size-selective harvesting of extracellular vesicles for strategic analyses towards tumor diagnoses. Appl Biochem Biotechnol. 2017;182:609–23.
30. Li J, Chen Y, Guo X, et al. GPC1 exosome and its regulatory miRNAs are specific markers for the detection and target therapy of colorectal cancer. J Cell Mol Med. 2017;21:838–47.
31. Lee C, Lm E, Moon P, Baek M. Discovery of a diagnostic biomarker for colon cancer through proteomic profiling of small extracellular vesicles. BMC Cancer. 2018;18:1058.
32. Zhong ME, Chen Y, Xiao Y, Xu L, Zhang G, Lu J, Qiu H, Ge W, Wu B. Serum extracellular vesicles contain SPAR and LRG1 as biomarkers of colon cancer and differ by tumour primary location. EBioMedicine. 2019;50:211–23.
33. Campanella C, Rappa F, Sciume C, Marino Gammazza A, Barone R, et al. Heat shock protein 60 levels in tissue and circulating exosomes in human large bowel cancer before and after ablative surgery. Cancer. 2015;121:3230–9.
34. Tian Y, Ma L, Gong M, Su G, Zhu S, et al. Protein profiling and sizing of extracellular vesicles from colorectal cancer patients via flow cytometry. ACS Nano. 2018;12:671–80.
35. Sun B, Li Y, Zhou Y, Ng KT, Zhao C, Gan Q, Gu X, Xiang J. Circulating exosomal CPNE3 as a diagnostic and prognostic biomarker for colon cancer. J Cell Physiol. 2019;244:1416–25.

36. Vautrot V, Chanteloup G, Elmallah M, Cordonnier M, Aubin F, Garrido C, Gobbo J. Exosomal miRNA: small molecules, big impact in colorectal cancer. J Oncol. 2019;2019:8585276.
37. Chiba M, Kimura M, Asari S. Exosomes secreted from human colorectal cancer cell lines contain mRNAs, microRNAs and natural antisense RNAs, that can transfer into the human hepatoma HepG2 and lung cancer A549 cell lines. Oncol Rep. 2012;28(5):1551–8.
38. Matsumura T, Sugimachi K, Iinuma H, Takahashi Y, Kurashige J, Sawada G, Ueda M, Uchi R, Ueo H, Takano Y, et al. Exosomal microRNA in serum is a novel biomarker of recurrence in human colorectal cancer. Br J Cancer. 2015;113:275–81.
39. O'Brien SJ, Carter JV, Burton JF, Oxford BG, Schmidt MN, Hallion JC, Galandiuk S. The role of miR-200 family in epithelial-mesenchymal transition in colorectal cancer: a systematic review. Int J Cancer. 2018;142:2501–11.
40. Ogata-Kawata H, Izumiya M, Kurioka D, Honma Y, Yamada Y, et al. Circulating exosomal miRNAs as biomarkers of colon cancer. PLoS One. 2014;9:e92921.
41. Liu X, Pan B, Sun L, Chen X, Zeng K, Hu X, Xu T, Xu M, Wang S. Circulating exosomal miR-27a and miR-130a act as novel diagnostic and prognostic biomarkers of colorectal cancer. Cancer Epidemiol Biomark Prev. 2018;27:746–54.
42. Tanaka S, Hosokawa M, Ueda K, Iwakawa S. Effects of decitabine on invasion and exosomal expression of miR-200c and miR-141 in oxaliplatin resistance colorectal cancer cells. Biol Pharm Bull. 2015;38:1272–9.
43. Zhang Z, Xing T, Chen Y, Xiao J. Exosome mediated miR-200b promotes colorectal cancer proliferation upon TGFβ1 exposure. Biomed Pharmacother. 2018;106:1135–43.
44. Yan S, Liu G, Jin C, et al. MicroRNA-6869-5p acts as a tumor suppressor via targeting TLR4/NF-κB signaling pathway in colorectal cancer. J Cell Physiol. 2018;233:6660–8.
45. Teng Y, Ren Y, Hu X, Mu J, Samykutty A, Zhuang X, et al. MVP mediated exosomal sorting of miR-193a promotes colon cancer progression. Nat Comun. 2017;8:14448.
46. Yan S, Jiang Y, Liang C, et al. Exosomal miR-6803-5p as potential diagnostic and prognostic marker in colorectal cancer. J Cell Biochem. 2018;119:4113–9.
47. Fu F, Jiang W, Zhou L, Chen Z. Circulating exosomal mir-17-5p and mir-92a-3p predict pathologic stage and grade of colorectal cancer. Transl Oncol. 2018;11:221–32.
48. Peng YZ, Gu RH, Yan B. Downregulation of exosome-encapsulated miR-548c-5p is associated with poor prognosis in colorectal cancer. J Extracell Vesicles. 2018;4:27031.
49. Tang Y, Zhao Y, Song X, Song X, Niu L, Xie L. Tumor derived exosomal miRNA-320d as a biomarker for metastatic colorectal cancer. J Clin Lab Anal. 2019;33:e23004.
50. Min L, Chen L, Liu S, Yu Y, Guo Q, Li P, Zhu S. Loss of circulatory exosomal miR-92b is a novel biomarker of colorectal cancer at early stage. Int J Med Sci. 2019;16:1231–7.
51. Sun L, Liu X, Pan B, Hu X, Zhu Y, Su Y, Guo Z, Zhang G, Xu M, Xu X, Sun H, Wang S. Serum exosomal miR-122 as a potential diagnostic and prognostic biomarker of colorectal cancer with liver metastasis. J Cancer. 2020;11:630–7.
52. Dai W, Zhou J, Wang H, Zhang M, Yang X, Song W. miR-424-5p promotes the proliferation and metastasis of colorectal cancer by directly targeting SCN4B. Pathol Res Pract. 2020;216:152731.
53. Karimi N, Ali Hosseinpour Feizi M, Safaralizadeh R, Hashemzadeh S, Baradaran B, Shokouhi B, Teimourian S. Serum overexpression of miR-301a and miR-23a in patients with colorectal cancer. J Chin Med Assoc. 2019;82:215–20.
54. Wang J, Yan F, Zhao Q, Zhan F, Wang R, Wang L, Zhang Y, Huang X. Circulating exosomal miR-125a-3p as a novel biomarker for early stage colon cancer. Sci Rep. 2017;7:4150.
55. Yagi T, Linuma H, Hayama T, Matsuda K, Nozawa K, et al. Plasma exosomal microRNA-125b as monitoring biomarker of resistance to mFOLFOX6-based chemotherapy in advanced and recurrent colorectal cancer patients. Mol Clin Ocol. 2019;11:416–24.
56. Zou SL, Chen YL, Ge ZZ, Qu YY, Cao Y, Kang ZX. Downregulation of serum exosomal miR-150-5p is associated with poor prognosis in patients with colorectal cancer. Cancer Biomark. 2019;26:69–77.

57. Zhao YJ, Song X, Niu L, Tang Y, Song X, Xie L. Circulating exosomal miR-150-5p and miR-99b-5p as diagnostic markers for colorectal cancer. Front Oncol. 2019;9:1129.
58. Hu HY, Yu CH, Zhang HH, Zhang SZ, Yu WY, Yang Y, Chen Q. Exosomal miR-1229 derived from colorectal cancer cells promotes angiogenesis by targeting HIPK2. Int J Biol Macromol. 2019;132:470–7.
59. Bjormetro T, Redalen KR, Meltser S, Thysyanthan NS, Samiappan R, Jegerschold C, Handeland KR, Ree AH. An experimental strategy unveiling exosomal microRNAs 486-5p, 181a-5p and 30d-5p from hypoxic tumor cells as circulating indicators of high risk rectal cancer. J Extracell Vesicles. 2019;8:1567219.
60. Peng ZY, Gu RH, Yan B. Downregulation of exosome encapsulated miR-548c-5p is associated with poor prognosis in colorectal cancer. J Cell Biochem. 2019;120:1457–63.
61. Liu T, Zhang X, Yang Y, Du L, Wang C. Increased expression of the long noncoding RNA CRNDE-h indicated a poor prognosis in colorectal cancer and is positively correlated with IRX5 mRNA expression. Onco Targets Ther. 2016;9:1437–48.
62. Dong L, Lin W, Qi P, Xu M, Wu X, et al. Circulating long RNAs in serum extracellular vesicles: their characterization and potential application as biomarkers for diagnosis of colorectal cancer. Cancer Epidemiol Biomark Prev. 2016;25:1158–66.
63. Liu L, Meng T, Yang XH, Sayim P, Lei C, Jin B, Ge L, Wang HJ. Prognostic and predictive value of long non-coding RNA GAS5 and mircoRNA-221 in colorectal cancer and their effects on colorectal cancer cell proliferation, migration and invasion. Cancer Biomark. 2018;22:283–99.
64. Barbagallo C, Brex D, Caponnetto A, Cirnigliaro M, Scalia M, et al. LncRNA UCA1, upregulated in CRC biopsies and downregulated in serum exosomes, controls mRNA expression by RNA-RNA interactions. Mol Ther Nucleic Acids. 2018;12:229–41.
65. Liu T, Zhang X, Gao S, Jing F, Yang Y, Du L, Zhenh G, Li P, Li C, Wang C. Exosomal long noncoding RNA CRNDE-h as a novel serum-based biomarker for diagnosis and prognosis of colorectal cancer. Oncotarget. 2016;7:85551–63.
66. Wang L, Duan W, Yan S, Xie Y, Wang C. Circulating long noncoding RNA colon cancer associated transcript 2 protected by exosome as a potential biomarker for colorectal cancer. Biomed Pharmacother. 2019;113:108758.
67. Pan B, Quin J, Liu X, He B, Wang X, et al. Identification of serum exosomal hsa-circ-0004771 as a novel diagnostic biomarker of colorectal cancer. Front Genet. 2019;10:1096.

Chapter 8
Biomarkers as Putative Therapeutic Targets in Colorectal Cancer

Sonali Pal, Manoj Garg, and Amit Kumar Pandey

Abstract Colon cancer or colorectal cancer (CRC) is a widely recognized gastrointestinal malignancy around the globe. These are a type of tumor called adenocarcinoma, which is the cancer of the cells that lines the inner tissue of the colon and rectum. CRC is highly heterogeneous and known to undergo a series of molecular alterations throughout the natural course of the disease. As our knowledge regarding the CRC carcinogenesis advances, it is indispensable to identify practical, ideal, and consistent molecular and cellular biomarkers associated with CRC. Besides, gene mutations and alteration in ncRNAs, such as lncRNA or miRNAs, have also been found to play a role in CRC tumorigenesis. A biomarker is a biological molecule that is mostly present in biological specimens such as blood, urine, tissue, and fecal matters to identify the specific pathophysiological conditions like diabetes and cancer. The introduction of such effective tools will potentially assist in early diagnosis and predict the success of the disease and its response to chemotherapy. These biomarkers are the critical part of advancing personalized therapy, and their application may restructure the course of therapy and processes in CRC. Some of the previously identified biomarkers might possess certain limitations in a clinical scenario. Thus, the identification of diagnostic, prognostic, and predictive biomarkers stays challenging. This chapter outlines the currently available and emerging biomarkers with their clinical potential and therapeutic applications. Moreover, it highlights the challenges that follow up in the path of biomarker research.

Keywords Colon cancer/colorectal cancer · Molecular characteristics · Non-coding RNAs · MicroRNAs · Long non-coding RNAs · Biomarkers · Diagnostic · Prognostic · Predictive

---

S. Pal · A. K. Pandey (✉)
Amity Institute of Biotechnology, Amity University Haryana,
Panchgaon, Manesar, Haryana, India
e-mail: akpandey1@ggn.amity.edu

M. Garg
Amity Institute of Molecular Medicine and Stem Cell Research (AIMMSCR),
Amity University, Uttar Pradesh, Noida, India

G. P. Nagaraju et al. (eds.), *Colon Cancer Diagnosis and Therapy*,
https://doi.org/10.1007/978-3-030-63369-1_8

Abbreviations

CA 19–9	Carbohydrate antigen 19–9
CEA	Carcinoembryonic antigen
CIMP	CpG island methylator phenotype
CIN	Chromosomal instability
CRC	Colorectal cancer
CSS	Cancer-specific survival
DFS	Disease-free survival
EGFR	Epidermal growth factor receptor
ENCODE	Encyclopedia of DNA Elements
EVs	Extracellular vesicles
FAP	Familial adenomatous polyposis
HNPCC	Hereditary non-polyposis colorectal cancer
IARC	International Agency for Research on Cancer
lncRNAs	long ncRNAs
LOI	Loss of imprinting
miRNAs	microRNA
MMR	Mismatch repair
MSI	Microsatellite instability
ncRNAs	non-coding RNAs
OS	Overall survival
PFS	Progression-free survival
RFS	Relapse-free survival
TBT	Telomerase biosensor technology
TCGA	Cancer Genome Atlas
TGF-β	Transforming growth factor-β

8.1 Introduction

8.1.1 Epidemiology, Etiology, and Molecular Pathway Involved in Colorectal Cancer

The revolutionary road to the global healthcare system has experienced extensive changes, developments, challenges, and improvements over the past years. This has certainly improved the diagnosis and treatment of cancer-related malignancies. CRC was uncommon in the 1950s, but lately, increasing unfavorable western dietary habits, smoking, lack of exercise, and obesity have attributed it to become the third widespread malignancy across the globe. The International Agency for Research on Cancer (IARC) in 2018 projected a rate of 1.8 million new cases and > 860,000 passing yearly worldwide [1]. New treatment options have emerged;

however, these have limited impact on both cure and survivability. Thus for early detection and treatment, the development of effective screening methods is an utmost need.

The molecular mechanism illustrating the colorectal carcinogenesis was summarized by Fearon and Vogelstein [2]. CRC is regarded as a multifactorial or polygenic disease [3, 4]. The cause of developing CRC is not exclusively dependent on genetic and epigenetic instabilities [5], but both assist in its development processes with methylation often being dominant than point mutations [6]. Mutations may arise in tumor silencer genes, oncogene, and genes involved in DNA repair mechanisms [7]. CRC is largely classified into two types based on the origin of mutation: sporadic or hereditary. The sporadic CRC encompasses 70% of all encountered cases with a seemingly genetic predisposition or no family history. The predominant factor that results in sporadic CRC is genomic instability that includes chromosomal instability (CIN), loss of heterozygosity (LOH), and aneuploidy [8]. CIN results in the majority of all sporadic CRC cases, approximately 80–85% [9]. The remaining 15% is due to the loss of DNA repair mechanism that results in a hypermutable phenotype that causes microsatellite instability (MSI) [10] and epigenetic instability that is well represented by hypermethylation of oncogene promoters that lead to low protein expression and silencing of genes [11]. These genomic aberrations also affect the principal pathways like WNT, MAPK/PI3K, and TGF-β and roles inside the cell [12, 13].

The hereditary CRC originates from inherited susceptibility working following environmental factors [14]. It has two subtypes: familial adenomatous polyposis (FAP) and hereditary non-polyposis colorectal cancer (HNPCC). The FAP develops because of germline mutations in adenomatous polyposis coli (APC) [15, 16]. The genomic location of the *APC* gene is 5q21–22; FAP accounts for approximately 0.5–1% of all CRCs [17, 18]. On the other hand, HNPCC (also named as Lynch syndrome) was described by Henry Lynch in 1966 [19]. It occurs due to the germline mutations in DNA mismatch repair (MMR) genes such as MLH1, MSH2, MSH6, and PMS2 [20] and accounts for only 1–3% of all CRCs. Some pieces of evidence suggest that in a few cases of HNPCC, mutations in the MMR system might lead to somatic APC [21]. The other alternative type of hereditary CRC includes a rare syndrome called hamartomatous polyposis syndrome which affects less than 1% of all CRCs [14].

All these pathways contribute to the development of CRC in the large intestine in normal colonic mucosa as polyps then develop into adenoma followed by carcinoma and finally metastasize. It is a multistage carcinogenic process portrayed as the adenoma-carcinoma sequence [22]. Increasing evidence suggests that various distinct molecules have been tried for their expected use in CRC screening such as DNA [23, 24], proteins [25], messenger RNA (mRNA) [26], and microRNAs (miRNAs) [27–29]. All of these molecules have demonstrated a promising role as a biomarker in preliminary studies. The non-coding RNAs (ncRNAs) including miRNAs and long non-coding RNAs (lncRNAs) have a regulatory role in CRC tumorigenesis [30]. These insights, together with others, have enhanced our knowledge of CRC. Moreover, they have paved the way for the detection of unique thera-

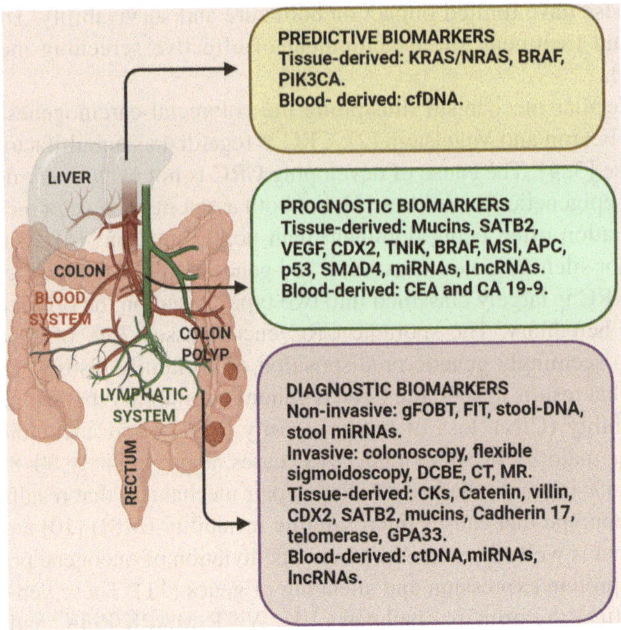

Fig. 8.1 A multistage carcinogenic process of colorectal cancer (adenoma-carcinoma sequence) with the involvement of distinct classes of biomarkers and their potential utilization at different stages (color coding used for different stages) of CRC progression

peutic targets and biomarkers. The emergence of such effective tools will improve our understanding of early diagnosis and help us predict the course of the disease and its response to other drugs (Fig. 8.1).

8.2 The Emerging Landscape of Biomarkers

The rapidly changing treatment scenario has provided wider opportunities for patients with CRC. The availability and approval of targeted therapies for metastatic CRC result in improved tumor response and overall patient survival rate, but it is still necessary to increase the efficacy of the treatment with the development of personalized therapy, curb the outcomes of each regimen, and minimize toxicity. Therefore, there is a rise in demand to classify various biomarkers that will guarantee the best possible therapeutic strategy. The amalgamation of previous knowledge and the advent of newer technologies like next-generation sequencing (NGS) and tumor panels have provided a wider platform for the discovery and validation of biomarkers [31].

In broad terms, a biomarker is a substance, structure, or process that can be can be measured to separate the typical or atypical biological state of an organism by examining the various biomolecules frequency of the outcome of disease [32–34]. An ideal CRC biomarker should fulfill the following criteria: [1] it should be

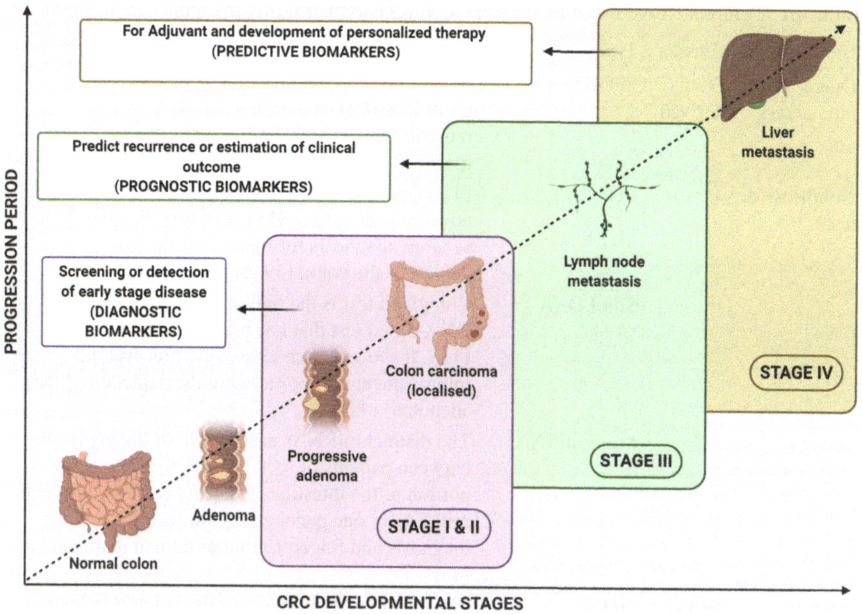

Fig. 8.2 The set of different identified diagnostic, prognostic, and predictive biomarkers in tissue, blood, and stool samples at different stages. (Color coding used for stages as above)

quantitatively measurable; [2] must be highly sensitive and specific; [3] should be reproducible and reliable; and [4] can easily distinguish affected populations [35, 36]. In terms of clinical effectiveness, cancer biomarker is of much more importance. These are capable of assessing the risk of cancer development and its progression in a specific tissue or possible response to therapy. Several subtypes of biomarkers are defined according to their function and utility in clinical applications like the diagnostic, predictive biomarkers, and prognostic biomarkers (Fig. 8.2, Table 8.1).

8.2.1 *Diagnostic Biomarkers*

These are characterized as a biological attribute that identifies the existence of a condition or detects someone with a subtype of the disease [100].

The most commonly available diagnostic screening methods for the identification of CRC in a wide range of population include the following:

8.2.1.1 Noninvasive Methods

Some of these methods are gFOBT, immunochemical testing of fecal, and DNA testing from the stool that can be used for standard screening.

Table 8.1 Comprehensive list of biomarkers according to their utility in clinical applications

Biomarker	Classes	Types	Explanation
Diagnostic biomarkers	Stool-derived	gFOBT	It recognizes blood loss from peptic ulcer and gastrointestinal cancer; it is known to deduce the mortality rate by 11–33%; it can't specify the exact location or source of bleeding in the GI tract [37, 38]
Noninvasive tests		FIT	FIT is more sensitive and specific for cancers and advanced adenomas. However, this provides a more accurate diagnosis for the lesions occurring ore in the left of the colon [39–41]
		Stool DNA	Cologuard test is the only multitarget feces DNA-based test that has been affirmed by the FDA. It shows better sensitivity; however, no improvement was observed in the detection of large adenomas [42]
		Stool miRNAs	The distinct miRNAs are capable of distinguishing between patients of rectal cancer from the other portion of the intestine. The combination of several miRNAs in one panel can be utilized for specific diagnosis and fingerprinting of human malignancies [43]
	Blood-derived	ctDNA	The integrity of ctDNA is evaluated as a ratio of longer to shorter DNA fragments during the diagnosis of CRC [44, 45]. This method has a sensitivity of 73.08% and a specificity of 97.27% [46] and a sensitivity of 90% and specificity of 85% with RT-PCR [47]
		miRNAs	These are little, endogenous, and most bountiful ncRNAs that are 20–22 nts in length and show higher stability in blood. miRNAs and their bound targets are firmly associated with CRC progression
		EV-miRNAs	EVs are a heterogeneous cluster of layer-bound particles discharged from every human cell. miRNAs are the most conspicuously considered classes of EV [48, 49]. miRNAs separated from serum exosomes are related to pathological stages and grades of the CRC patients [50]
		lncRNAs	The altered expression of several lncRNAs is observed in CRC. The first CRC-related lncRNA, the endogenous H19 gene that was found to be abundant in CRC specimens, and its overexpression played a significant role in CRC development
Invasive tests	–	Optical colonoscopy	The most primitive, standard practice of CRC evaluation. The examination is done in real time for the identification and resection/removal of precancerous polyps in the entire colon or any abnormal growths in the upper parts of the colon. It decreased the mortality rate by 60 to 70% [51]
		Flexible sigmoidoscopy DCBE	It examines only the lower portion of the colon, called the rectum and sigmoid colon. It decreases the rate by 31% and overall mortality of CRC by 38% [52, 53]

(continued)

Table 8.1 (continued)

Biomarker	Classes	Types	Explanation
		Computed tomographic colonography	It is a noninvasive, safe, and cheaper radiological technique [54]. It examines the entire colon by coating the mucosal surface with high-density barium and results in a 33% reduction in the occurrence of CRC [55]
		MRC Cytokeratin	It uses low-dose radiation CT scanning to screen for polyps in their early stages. It is a minimally invasive test and provides clearer and more detailed 2D and 3D images; it has a similar sensitivity to colonoscopy and barium enema [56, 57]
	Tissue-derived	β-Catenin Villin	It can detect precancerous lesions and can be used to assess different staging of colorectal pathology [58]. It has good reproducibility and accuracy values equal to or higher to CTC [59]
		CDX2	They function to distinguish metastatic CRC from other tumors. To differentiate, CRC samples are stained positive for CK20 and negative for CK7 [60]
		SATB2	It is a multifunctional protein that participates in cell adhesion and Wnt signaling pathway. The upregulated Wnt signaling has an important function in the progression of the CRC [61, 62]
		Mucin	It is a cytoskeleton, actin-binding protein. The immunohistochemistry analysis has proved villin to be efficient in tracking the polarity in CRCs containing a micropapillary pattern [63]
		Cadherin-17 Telomerase	It is associated with the prevention of tumor formation in the colon because of its important role in the segregation of the cells in the GI tract. CDX2 in conjunction with CK staining can distinguish adenocarcinoma of the GI tract specifically in the group of patients that are either positive for CK7+/CK20+ or negative for CK7–/CK20– Profile [64, 65]
		Glycoprotein A33 (GPA33)	The higher expression of SATB2 was noticed particularly in the glandular cells of the lower GI tract. SATB2 has a high symptomatic affectability of 97% (121 of 125 cases) in CRCs and 81% on account of CRC metastasis [66]
			These are present on the apical surfaces of normal glandular epithelial cells and luminal epithelial cells. These perform vital functions in cell adhesion, immunity, and intracellular signaling. MUC status can be used to separate typical and CRC cells [67, 68]
			Cadherins (CDH17) are transmembrane, cell-cell attachment molecules. It can separate tumors from the colorectal milieu and those from the upper GI tract. CDH17 is robustly expressed in almost all the patients with primary (96%) and metastatic CRC (100%) [69]

(continued)

Table 8.1 (continued)

Biomarker	Classes	Types	Explanation
			Telomerase, a ribonucleoprotein which is found in 85% to 90% of all malignant tumors particularly in colorectal cancer. Use of TBT showed higher specificity and sensitivity of about 95% for colorectal cancer, melanoma, and bladder cancer [70–72]
			It is highly upregulated by epithelial cells present in the colon, stomach, as well as intestine. The specificity of A33 was significantly higher compared to its sensitivity that was similar to CDX2 [73]
Prognostic biomarkers	Blood-derived	CEA	It is a180 kD membrane-associated glycoprotein and is involved in cell adhesion or signal transduction. CEA screening is recommended after surgery at particular intervals for patients with stage II or III with CRC. CEA is the main marker that has been suggested by ASCO 2006, for the administration of CRC [74, 75]
	Tissue-derived	BRAF	*BRAF*, a proto-oncogene, triggers the MAPK pathway. About 8% of patients highly developed CRC. This has been observed that 14% of stage II and III patients with CRC have to activate *BRAF* [76, 77]. *BRAF V600E* that represents over 90% of *BRAF* alterations is suggested to be assessed for its prognostic significance [78]
		MSI	It arises because of the deactivation of the MMR genes that occur in the majority of MSI CRC cases. In a few MSI CRC cases, germline mutations may occur in MMR genes [79, 80]
		APC	APC is involved in Wnt signaling. A higher APC mutation and miR-21 level in the advanced stage of CRC are associated with shorter OS [81]
		p53	*P53* mutations significantly affect the adenoma-carcinoma transition. These occur in proximal (34%) and distal (45%) colorectal tumors [82–84]
		SMAD4	SMAD4 serves as a key regulator in TGF-β signaling. The absence of SMAD4 correlates with recurrent metastasis to the lymph node, reduced differentiation, loss of immune infiltrates, and reduced response to 5-fluorouracil. It is a negative predictor of OS, cancer-specific survival (CSS), and RFS [85–87]
		miRNAs	miRNAs have prognostic value in CRC. miRNAs can be both tumor suppressors and oncomirs and may have the potential to be prognostic markers for CRC.
		lncRNAs	Some of the lncRNA has a strong association with p53 and are detectable in the circulation and could prove to be useful in the CRC prognosis

(continued)

Table 8.1 (continued)

Biomarker	Classes	Types	Explanation
Predictive biomarkers	Tissue-derived	KRAS	It is a proto-oncogene that participates in the signaling pathway from ligand-bound EGFR to the nucleus. It is altered in 50% of all the CRC cases and can be used as a predictive biomarker in response to the EGFR inhibitor [88–90]
		BRAF	It is used for discrimination between familial and sporadic CRC. *BRAF* mutation is unaffected to anti-EGFR therapy, and insufficient pieces of evidence are present to support whether *BRAF* has a significant value in anti-EGFR antibody therapy success [91–94]
	Blood-derived	PI3Ks	It has a major regulatory function in the RAS pathway and is present in 32% of all CRC cases. *PIK3CA* mutation showed contradictory results [95, 96]
		cfDNA	There was a decrease in the concentration of cfDNA after primary resection, whereas cfDNA levels radically increased upon CRC relapse, and similar results were observed in the case of chemoradiotherapy [97–99]

The Guaiac Fecal Occult Blood Test (gFOBT)
The gFOBT test evaluates blood shortage from peptic ulcer and gastrointestinal cancer. In the last 20 years of follow-up, gFOBT has deduced the mortality rate by 11–33% [37]. Yet, certain limitations curtail its validity in terms of CRC diagnosis like its inability to detect the exact location or source of bleeding in the GI tract. Moreover, gFOBTs results can be contrived by diet or drugs and are insensitive to small bleedings [38]. This results in decreased sensitivity of approximately 30–40% for cancerous and preneoplastic lesions [101].

Fecal Immunochemical Test (FIT)
The limitations exhibited by the gFOBT test resulted in the progress of FIT which identifies globins of humans using hemoglobin-specific immunoassay that provides both qualitative and quantitative results and expressed as fecal hemoglobin concentration per gram of feces. In terms of clinical applications, FIT is more sensitive and specific for cancers and advanced adenomas [39]. FIT has many advantages over gFOBT: it is cost-effective; is a user-friendly test; and thus has a higher rate of acceptance [102]. On the contrary, certain limitations do exist for FIT; it can only identify bleeding from colonic preneoplastic lesions, thus compromising the sensitivity [102]. Another very important limitation is that it can only identify lesions more in the left than the right side of the colon [40, 41].

Stool-Based Assays
These tests examine the abnormalities in the specific genes. These assays are more popular and successful for many reasons like the mucosal-cellular layer of colonic lumen consisting of debris and neoplastic cells that are shredded from

CRC polyps [103]. These molecular changes can be detected in the stool earlier than in the blood [104]. However, the survival rate of these exfoliated cells is very low if shredded in the right colon because of the dissolution of the cells [105]. Despite the lysis, most of the exfoliated cells can preserve their components such as DNA, miRNAs, and proteins, thus allowing the analysis to be conducted.

Stool DNA

The total DNA in the human stool comprises less than 0.1% human DNA, and 99.9% of it is because of the bacteria in the intestine or through food intake. Therefore, for the diagnosis of CRC, the detection of methylated or altered human DNA in the feces is critical [106]. Various methylated genes within the stool DNA have been investigated for the diagnosis of CRC. Some of the genes are *APC*, *ATM*, *CDH1*, *CDKN2A*, *KRAS*, etc. [107]. To date, the Cologuard test is the only multitarget stool DNA-based test used for screening of CRC and is permitted by the Food and Drug Administration (FDA). The test showed better sensitivity; however, it failed to detect large adenomas [42, 108]. The combined studies based on a stool DNA test and FIT showed better results in the detection of early CRC. Although many reports confirmed that the sensitivity of the combined test was higher, due to the high frequency of the false-positive results, the demand for colonoscopy was more [109, 110].

Stool miRNAs

The small single-stranded non-coding parts of the genome that are 18–25 nucleotides in length are called miRNAs. Until 1993, miRNAs were considered as "junk DNA." Their role was first functionally characterized in *Caenorhabditis elegans* acting as negative post-transcriptional regulators [111]. They can tightly control the expression of a gene at a post-transcriptional level [112, 113]. Over the last few years, miRNAs have intrigued many researchers across the globe because of its exclusive properties. This gave birth to the novel application of miRNAs to serve as a biomarker. Some of its unique properties are the stability of miRNAs in both laboratory and experimental conditions. miRNAs are resistant to degradation by RNase due to their rigid hairpin loop structure and smaller size [114]. The cell-free miRNAs are abundantly secreted and are packed in apoptotic bodies, microvesicles, large lipoproteins, and exosomes or by their binding to argonaute-2. These attributes collectively lead to improved stability [115, 116]. This makes the isolation process quite easy from different forms of clinical specimens [114]. The secretion of miRNAs is a dynamic process from the tumor cells into the digestive tract and circulatory system [117]. Hence, the circulating cell-free miRNAs and miRNAs in stool are some of the essential types of RNA that can serve as diagnostic biomarkers in the clinical settings.

The complex environment of the GI tract than that of the blood is a key hurdle in terms of the marker stability. Accumulating evidence suggests that miRNA transcripts are condition-specific, i.e., it is found to be stable at a certain condition [27, 118]. There is limiting evidence that the abundance of miRNAs in the stool is greater than that of blood. The RT-PCR and microarray analysis proved that expression of miRNAs was deregulated in the feces of patients with CRC that included a set of upregulated miR-92a, miR-106a, miR-21, miR135, miR144, and miR17–92, while few other miR-143 and miR-145, *miR-320*, *miR-126*, *miR-484-5p*, *miR-16*, and *miR-125b* were downregulated in CRC [119–121]. The distinct miRNAs, Stool miR-29 was capable of distinguishing between patients of rectal cancer from the rest part of the intestine. Thus, a defined set of miRNAs expression patterns can be helpful to develop a cancer fingerprint [43]. Despite that fact, miRNAs failed to show any diagnostic value, and further studies need to be conducted to fully exploit the clinical potential of miRNAs.

8.2.1.2 Invasive Tests

The four most common invasive tests available to date to visualize the complete colon are colonoscopy, double-contrast barium enema (DCBE), and flexible sigmoidoscopy. The newly added method in the CRC screening modalities is a computerized tomography (CT) and MR colonography [122]. The available screening tests have proved to be quite effective and efficient. These have drastically reduced the risk of CRC-associated mortality. Nevertheless, the efficacy of these methodologies is limited by properties like the quality or performance of the test, lack of ease of accessibility to CRC screening tests, and weak compliance screening.

Optical or standard colonoscopy and flexible sigmoidoscopy are the standard, nonsurgical screening tools that use a flexible, lighted tube equipped with a lens/camera for visualization. These both screening methods differ in terms of different areas of the colon they visualize. A colonoscopy uses a longer scope to visualize the entire colon which is 6 feet long, while flexible sigmoidoscopy essentially uses a shorter scope to cover only the lower part of the colon (anus, rectum, sigmoid colon, and descending colon) that is only 2 feet long.

Optical colonoscopy is the most primitive, standard practice of CRC evaluation. The examination is done in real time for the identification and resection/removal of precancerous polyps in the entire colon or any abnormal growths in the upper parts of the colon. Studies suggest that colonoscopy decreases the mortality rate by about 60–70%. Further studies are being done to assess the efficacy and effectiveness of this method [51]. The recommended duration for colonoscopy screening is every 10 years. Although colonoscopy is highly sensitive (about 95%), some of the small polyps may not be recognized. The optical colonoscopy procedure has certain disadvantages: it is a tedious and time-consuming process, it requires patients to go for a bowel cleanse preparation and dietary modification, and certain complications may arise during the process such as trouble related to the heart, bleeding in GIT, and perforation [123–125].

Flexible sigmoidoscopy is used as a diagnostic tool for examination of only the inferior portion of the colon, called the rectum and sigmoid colon. *It is a minimally invasive and cost-effective method of detection.* The recommended duration for a sigmoidoscopy is every 5 years. Flexible sigmoidoscopy reduces the incidence by 31% and overall mortality of CRC by 38% [52, 53]. Unlike colonoscopy, it is relatively easy, safe, and fairly fast to perform as no prior bowel cleanse and sedation is required, but small polyps (<5 mm) and the whole polyp may not be detected and removed due to the restriction of visualization [126, 127], but if a polyp particularly an advanced adenoma with a size ≥1 cm is found, then it must be removed via colonoscopy.

The DCBE is well-known as an air contrast barium enema; it examines the colon by coating the mucosal surface with the liquid containing barium. It is a noninvasive, safe, and cheaper radiological technique [54]. However, before examination, bowel clearance and sedation are required. A 5-year interval between DCBE examinations is recommended because DCBE is significantly less sensitive about 85% than colonoscopy in terms of examination of large size polyp [128, 129]. This method does not permit the removal of polyps or biopsy of abnormal growths; a colonoscopy must be performed. DCBE detected 48% to 53% of adenomatous polyps [130]. DCBE results in a 33% reduction in the occurrence of CRC [55].

Computerized tomography colonography (CTC) or virtual colonoscopy is a diagnostic method for screening of CRC polyps [56, 131]. This method is cost-effective and rapid. CTC uses low-dose radiation to screen early-stage polyps. The American Cancer Society (ACS) proposed that individuals should undergo CRC screening beginning at the age of 45 and should follow up once every 5 years [132]. CTC is favored in many ways over conventional colonoscopy. CTC is a minimally invasive test and provides clearer and more detailed 2D and 3D images and has a significantly lower risk of perforation, sedation not needed. Even though the method is well tolerated and more patient acceptable, some disadvantages do exist like inability to distinguish stool from artifacts and smaller polyps, flat lesions are most often missed [133], a small risk of perforation, and full bowel clearance still needed [134]. CTC overall showed similar sensitivity to colonoscopy and barium enema [56, 57].

Magnetic resonance colonography (MRC) examination detects precancerous lesions and can also be used to assess different staging of colorectal pathology [58]. MRC is a valuable alternative for CRC evaluation, but the method is not well established. In terms of the diagnostic performance, MRC can detect all lesions more than 10 mm in size [135], yet lesions less than 5 mm remained undetected [136]. The key elements required for sufficient visualization via MRC rely upon adequate colonic distension and bowel preparation that are done with the help of bowel cleansing or fecal tagging [137, 138]. MRC offers considerable advantages over CTC like no usage of ionizing radiation and the use of dark or bright lumen strategies to achieve high soft tissue contrast [139], ability to assess extracolonic structure [140, 141], and unlimited field of view with good reproducibility and accuracy values equal or higher to CTC [59]. However, certain limitations have hampered the use of MRC like the lack of consensus concerning bowel preparation, higher costs, lengthy data acquisition, and more limited availability [137].

8.2.1.3 Tissue-Based Markers

Diagnostic tissue markers provide information that complements clinical colonoscopy findings [142]. The dual advantage of the colonoscopy is that it enables both the identification and resection of the polyp that can later be used for immunohistochemical (IHC) staining [143]. It is used for the identification of GIT neoplasm and assists in precise tumor classification. In metastatic carcinoma of unspecified origin, these help to eliminate morphologic mimickers or help in the identification of closest morphological tissue or organ of origin, thus confirming the diagnosis. Additionally, it assesses the visualization and even predicts reaction to given chemotherapy [144, 145].

Cytokeratins (CKs)

These proteins are made of keratin and are found in the cytoplasm of the epithelial tissue and belong to the family of intermediate filaments. CKs primary role is to distinguish metastatic CRC from other tumors; here CRC samples are stained positive for CK20 and negative for CK7 [60]. CK20 resides in the glandular cells and Merkel cells of colonic mucosa while hardly expressed in the urothelium or other mucosas [146, 147]. Conversely, CK7 is absent in the colonic mucosa, while it is usually expressed in the epithelial and mesothelium layer of the female urinary tract and lungs while rarely observed in GIT glands [147, 148]. The CK7/CK20 staining pattern is the most useful routine procedure for the identification of the original site of metastatic lesions [149]. The majority of CRC cases of non-neoplastic colonic mucosa shows a $CK7^{-}/CK20^{+}$ phenotype [150]. The addition of CK17 that is only expressed in 10% of all CRC to the diagnostic panel resulted in improved test efficacy. Moreover, it was reported that $CK20^{+}/CK7^{+}$ phenotype is observed in highly developed cases of CRCs, whereas $CK20^{+}/CK7^{-}$ phenotype is found in the early stages of CRC. Therefore, for the assessment of the succession of CRC, CK7 expression could be used as a discriminating marker [151].

β-Catenin

It is a versatile protein that participates in cell adhesion and intracellular signaling particularly the Wnt signaling pathway [62]. Wnt signaling activation increases the concentration of free β-catenin resulting in the initiation of proliferation both in the nucleus and cytoplasm. The mutated APCor β-catenin activates the normal Wnt pathway in the majority of CRCs. Thus, the overexpression of the Wnt pathway significantly affects the onset of CRC [61]. In CRC, the expression of β-catenin is infrequent in the nucleus, but still, it can be identified immunohistochemically and has become a significant part of the diagnostic panel [152].

Villin

It is a member of the microfilament family. It is a cytoskeleton, actin-binding protein. It is constitutively present in cells that have specialized, brush border-type microvilli, for example, enterocytes [153]. Villin has an important role in altering the tissue morphology by removing the polarity of the epithelium [154]. The immunohistochemistry analysis has proved villin to be efficient in tracking the polarity in CRCs containing a micropapillary pattern [63]. However, villin is not considered to be a specific biomarker, and its application for intestinal origin is limited [155].

Caudal-Type Homeobox 2 (CDX2)

The homeobox represents a large group of genes, among which CDX2 belongs to the caudal subgroup and is transcribed by the *CDX2* gene. The primary role of CDX2 is the preservation of the cellular intestinal phenotype in in utero and ex utero

[156], which regulates the differentiation of cells of the GI tract and acts as a tumor suppressor in the colon [65]. The majority of CDX2 is present in the epithelial layer of the small intestine, colon, and rectum [64]. The absence of CDX2 expression possibly leads to CRC in humans [65]. According to the study reported in the nude mice, the upregulated CDX2 resulted in reduced age as well as motility and invasiveness of LoVo cells. Furthermore, under hypoxic culture conditions, it favors the arrest of the cell cycle while inducing apoptosis in vitro [157]. The sensitivity and specificity of CDX2 expression in CRC were reported to be greater than 90%. Nevertheless, the sole expression of CDX2 is unable to differentiate between the adenomas of the GI tract. Therefore, if conjugated with CK staining, especially $CK7^{+}/CK20^{+}$ or $CK7^{-}/CK20^{-}$ profile, it will provide valuable results [64].

Special AT-Rich Sequence Binding Protein 2 (SATB2)

SATB2 is present in the nucleus and belongs to the family of matrix-associated transcription factors; SATB2 is involved in various biological functions such as the regulation of gene expression at the epigenetic level [158]; however, its exact role in the GI tract is still unexplored. The higher expression of SATB2 is observed in the glandular portion of the inferior GI tract. SATB2 has a higher diagnostic sensitivity in CRC metastasis [66]. To further validate the sensitivity, SATB2 was added to CK7, CK20, and CDX2; however, there was no improvement in the diagnosis of CRC, and neither sensitivity nor specificity enhancement was observed. Conversely, few reports suggest that to differentiate metastatic CRC from primary ovarian carcinomas, SATB2 may be utilized as a specific marker [159, 160]. For the diagnosis of pulmonary enteric adenocarcinoma, CDH17 linked to SATB2 was used as an optimal marker for the differential diagnosis [161].

Mucins

These are large epithelial glycoproteins with highly clustered oligosaccharides linked to tandem repeat peptides rich in amino acids such as threonine, serine, and proline [162, 163]. These are present on the upper surfaces of both glandular and luminal epithelial cells. These perform vital functions in immunity, cell adhesion, and intracellular signaling [67]. MUC can be categorized based on structure and function in two groups, secreting gel-type mucin and transmembrane mucin [164]. They participate in the process of tumorigenesis and metastasis, and abnormal expression of mucin may be a predictive biomarker of CRC [165]. The varying expression of MUC is capable of separating CRC cells from the normal cells [68]. MUC is involved in proliferation, survival, metastasis, epithelial-mesenchymal transition, and anti-apoptosis in tumors [67, 166–168]. Elevated expression of MUC1 and MUC2 was associated with CRC. In the rectum, an upregulated MUC1 expression is related to invasion, metastasis to the lymph node, advanced tumor stage, and poor survival in CRC. Moreover, MUC1 is known to participate in the process of the establishment of secondary tumors [166]. In the colon, higher expression of MUC2 results in superficial lesions, negative metastasis to the lymph node, an early stage of the tumor, and increase tumor size. Downregulation of MUC2 results in inflammatory bowel disease [169]. MUC5AC is commonly expressed in colon cancer. However, it is functionally unexplored [170]. Recently, MUC21 is known to be expressed in CRCs [171]. Thus, understanding the alliance between MUC expression levels may help to clarify the associated risk of metastasis especially in asymptomatic patients, and clinically the detection of MUC is convenient to implement.

Cadherin-17 (CDH17)

Adherence is a significant property of a cell through which cells adhere themselves to one another. CDH17 are transmembrane, Ca^{2+}-dependent cell-cell adhesion molecules conserved among metazoans. These participate in tissue morphogenesis and homeostasis and in cell-cell contact formation and stability [172]. The abnormality in cadherin expression leads to various human diseases like carcinomas [173]. CDH17 was first identified in the liver and intestine of rat thus is also named as liver-intestinal cadherin or human peptide transporter 1 [174]. The specific distribution of CDH17 in normal tissues proposed that it may be a potential tool for immunohistochemical diagnosis [175, 176]. CDH17 is expressed in primary and metastatic CRC [69]. Different approaches were used to distinguish tumors from the CRC region and those derived from the upper GI tract. First, the expression of CDH17 is usually focal or scattered in adenocarcinoma of the stomach, pancreas, and bile duct, whereas in colorectal adenocarcinoma, it is usually diffuse and strong and is infrequent in tumors at different sites. The second approach is the immunostaining of cytokeratin 7. However, immunoreactivity was observed in the case of adenocarcinoma from most body sites, thus limiting the clinical applicability. The study profile using a combination of CDH17 and cytokeratin 7 significantly narrowed the candidate primary site [69, 177]. CDH17 has higher sensitivity and specificity than its transcriptional regulator CDX2 for the detection of CRC [178].

Telomerase

It is a ribonucleoprotein that is fundamental for the maintenance of chromosome stability and genetic integrity. A stretched sequence of telomere DNA consisting of variable numbers of the nucleotide sequence TTAGGG helps to prevent the sticking of chromosome ends [179]. Telomerase accounts for 85% to 90% of all malignancies, particularly in CRC [70, 71]. Recently studies revealed that longer telomere length is related to an increased prevalence of colorectal adenomas [180, 181]. The ability of telomerase to serve as a biomarker was exploited with the development of two critically important assays, the telomeric repeat amplification protocol (TRAP) that can detect telomerase activity in a few human cancer cells. However, this assay is still undergoing validation and standardization studies. Lately, studies reported another approach that is under preclinical testing, the telomerase biosensor technology (TBT) developed by Sienna Cancer Diagnostics, Melbourne, Australia. This assay has a higher specificity and sensitivity of about 95% for colorectal cancer, melanoma, and bladder cancer [72].

Glycoprotein A33 (GPA33)

It is located on human chromosome 1q24 [182], and immunohistochemical analysis revealed that A33 is expressed in the epithelial cells of the stomach, small intestine, colon, and rectum. This indicates that A33 may be a beneficial target in CRC treatment as it is expressed in 95% of human CRC patients, particularly in well-defined tumors [183]. The specificity of A33 was significantly higher compared to its sensitivity that was similar to CDX2 [73].

8.2.1.4 Blood-Derived Biomarkers

In the last few years, the focus of research has shifted on components that are derived from the bloodstream of cancer patients. The isolation of these components and their assessment has opened up a new field of the diagnostic approach called "liquid biopsy." It is minimally invasive, easily accessible, and highly specific. To date, there are no known liquid biopsy biomarkers that can be used for the diagnosis of CRC, but their development may potentially improve CRC-related mortality. The analytes used for liquid biopsy consist of circulating cell-free tumor DNA (ctDNA), proteins, exosomes, circulating tumor cells (CTCs), mRNA, and miRNAs. For instance, ctDNA and exosomes are discharged from apoptotic or necrotic cancer cells, and CTCs are exfoliated products released into the bloodstream from primary and metastatic tumor sites. Each analyte has a few limitations that must be considered while choosing a marker to answer a particular clinical question [184–186].

Circulating Cell-Free Tumor DNA (ctDNA)
The last few decades have reported the incidence of ctDNA both in serum and plasma and are released from apoptosis or necrosis tumor cells. In comparison with healthy individuals, CRC patients have a fivefold higher level of serum ctDNA and more than 25-fold higher levels of plasma ctDNA [187]. The analysis of circulating ctDNA is done via measuring the difference in the lengths of the ctDNA fragment produced by the normal and tumor cells. In a normal individual, ctDNA is about 180 bp long, whereas fragments of ctDNA released from tumor cells are much larger via necrosis that ranges from 185 to 200 bp long. Therefore, the ratio of longer to shorter DNA fragments is measured for the diagnosis of CRC [44, 45]. This method has a sensitivity of 73.08% and a specificity of 97.27% [46], and the RT-PCR method showed a sensitivity (90%) and specificity (85%) [47]. Only 15% of CRC cases have MSI with defects in DNA MMR genes. MSI markers are detected in 35% of patients with CRC [188, 189]. To date, the hypermethylated *SEPT9* gene found in the plasma of CRC patients encodes a guanosine triphosphate enzyme that has an altered methylation pattern in both diagnostic and prognostic applications [190]. Validation studies revealed that SEPT9 methylation biomarker has a sensitivity (90%) and specificity (88%) [191], whereas for advanced adenomas and precancerous lesions, the blend of SEPT9 with ALX4 attained 71% sensitivity and 95% specificity [192]. In parallel to this, apart from *SEPT9*, several other genes have been studied such as *NEUROG1*, *RUNX3*, etc. [193]. At present, three SEPT9 methylation-based commercial tests are accessible: Epi proColon 2.0 (Epigenomics), ColoVantage™ (Quest Diagnostic), and RealTime ms9 (Abbott) [191, 194].

Circulating RNA-Derived Biomarkers

Various fluids inside the human body like serum/plasma, saliva, cerebrospinal fluid, synovial fluid, amniotic fluid, and urine have cell-free RNAs [195]. Likewise, in blood, mRNA and ncRNAs can be detected (Fig. 8.3).

There are a total of 25,000 protein-coding genes that represent 1.5% of the total genomic sequence as determined by the Encyclopedia of DNA Elements (ENCODE) project. The 60–70% portion is non-protein-coding sequences like ncRNAs, regulatory sequences, and introns [196]. ncRNAs were once considered as "junk" in the genome, and the transcription associated with it was regarded as transcriptional "noise" lacking biological meaning. Later on, it was accepted that ncRNAs are a functional class of RNA molecules transcribed from non-coding regions of the genome but not translated into proteins. ncRNAs can regulate gene expression at both the transcriptional and post-transcriptional levels. In general, ncRNAs fall under two broad categories, according to the size of the transcript: small ncRNAs (18–200 nts) that comprise of miRNAs, small interfering RNAs (siRNAs), and piwi-interacting RNAs (piRNAs) and a large proportion of lncRNAs (200 nts to >100 kb). Both of these classes have a significant role in

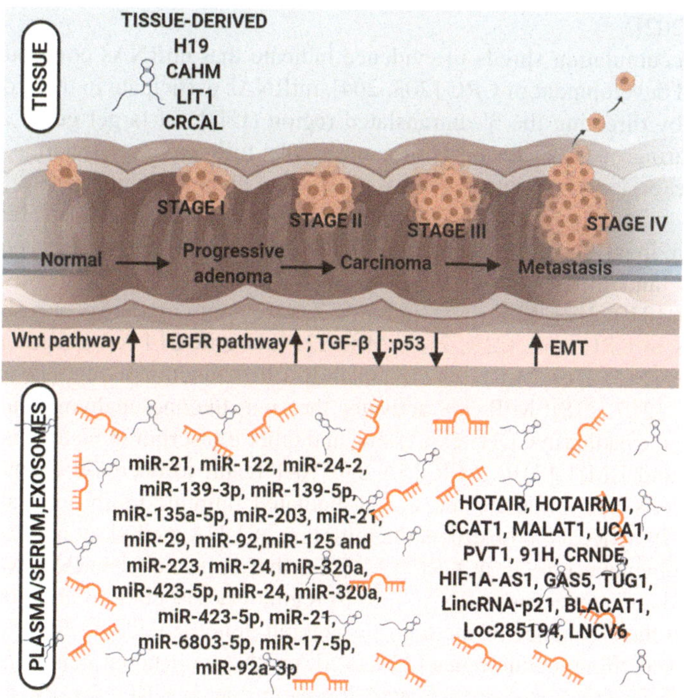

Fig. 8.3 Representation of the progression of CRC and signaling associated at each stage. Several specific miRNAs and lncRNA identified in both tissue and blood (plasma/serum, exosomes) have a potential significance to be utilized as biomarkers for the diagnosis, prognosis, and prediction of CRC

heterochromatin formation, histone modification, gene silencing, DNA methylation, and epigenetic regulation [197]. In this context, the advent of high-throughput genome sequencing tools has made it easy to summarize the role of different ncRNAs and their association with CRC, in particular. Emerging pieces of evidence suggest that miRNAs may have significant value as diagnostic and prognostic biomarkers for CRC.

miRNAs

miRNAs are the subgroup of tiny endogenous ncRNAs that are 20–22 nucleotides long and are the most abundant among other ncRNAs. In 1993, lin-4 was the first reported miRNA in *Caenorhabditis elegans* and later let-7. To date, around 10,000 miRNAs are found, among which 2500 types of encoded miRNAs have been determined in humans [198]. miRNAs regulate approximately 30% of the protein-coding genes that are involved in multiple biological processes [199]. The synthesis of miRNAs occurs intricately with the initiation in the nucleus and eventually post-transcriptional modifications in the cytoplasm [200, 201]. The miRNAs are highly stable in circulation because they are linked to carrier molecules like argonaute-2, lipoprotein complexes, and EVs that prevent their degradation from endogenous RNase and to extreme pH changes compared to mRNA [202].

The accumulating shreds of evidence indicate that miRNAs contribute to the onset and development of CRC [203, 204]. miRNAs participate in the progression of CRC by directing the 3′ untranslated region (UTR) of target genes and have some bearing on several aspects of cancer cells; miRNAs may function as either oncogene or tumor suppressor by regulating a diverse number of targets. For example, miR-18a, miR-155, and miR-205-5p are involved in the inhibition of migration, invasion, and proliferation of CRC cells [205–209], whereas miR-494, miR-598, and miR-17-3p result to promote cell multiplication, invasion, and migration [210–212]. MiR-106a and miR-7 correlate to apoptosis or resistance to apoptosis in CRC cells [213, 214]. MiR-221 and miR-214 repress autophagy in CRC cells [215, 216]. MiR-192/215 and miR-19b-1 function to regulate metabolic pathways [217, 218]. MiR-508 activates the stem-like/mesenchymal subtype by changing the cadherin CDH1 expression and other transcription factors like ZEB1, SALL4, and BMI1 [219]. MiR-15A and 16-1 result to decrease chemotaxis of IgA^+ B cells and stimulate the B-cell-mediated immune inhibition pathway in CRC [220]. MiR-21-5p obstructs the initiation of DNA methylation, thus exhibiting its epigenetic effects in CRC [221]. Furthermore, novel miRNA signatures [222, 223] and numerous miRNAs-mRNA regulatory associations are brought into light with the assistance of the high-throughput genome-wide profiling and wide range of screening technologies [224, 225]. miRNA-dependent genes and signaling pathways have been investigated for their role in CRC. NF-κB influences immune and inflammation responses and in connection with various miRNAs like miR-150-5p, miR-195-5p, and miR-203a functions to regulate the process of carcinogenesis [226, 227]. These investigations will be useful for the detection of miRNA-based biomarkers for CRC [228] (Table 8.2).

Table 8.2 Simplified list of miRNAs and their clinical potential in CRC

miRNAs	Source	Sensitivity and specificity	Clinical significance
miR-21	Plasma	82% and 90%, 65% and 85%	Diagnostic and prognostic [117, 229]
miR-122	Plasma	N/A	Prognosis [230]
miR-24-2	Serum	N/A	Diagnosis [231]
miR-139-3p, miR-139-5p, miR-135a-5p	Serum	96% and 97%, 64% and 80%	Diagnosis and prognosis [232–234]
miR-203	Serum	N/A	Prognosis and metastatic prediction [235]
miR-21, miR-29, miR-92, miR-125, and miR-223	Serum	84% and 98%	Diagnosis [236]
miR-24	Serum	78% and 83%	Early detection [237]
miR-320a	Serum	92% and 73%	Diagnosis [237]
miR-423-5p	Serum	91% and 70%	Diagnosis [237]
miR-24, miR-320a, miR-423-5p	Serum	92% and 70%	Diagnosis [237]
miR-21	Plasma exosomes	N/A	Prediction of CRC recurrence and poor prognosis [238]
miR-6803-5p	Plasma exosomes	N/A	Diagnosis and prognosis [239]
miR-17-5p	Plasma exosomes	N/A	Prognosis [50]
miR-92a-3p	Plasma exosomes	N/A	Prognosis [50]
miR-21	Saliva	97% and 91%	Diagnosis [229]
miR-4478	Fecal	N/A	Diagnosis [240]
miR-1295b-3p	Fecal	N/A	Diagnosis [240]

The increasing knowledge of miRNAs resulted in the development of expression profile for each tumor type involving conventional detection methodologies like microarray, QRT-PCR, and next-generation sequencing; however, none of them proved to be useful in clinical settings [241]. Methods like isothermal amplification techniques and near-infrared technology are developed to meet clinical requirements. A bunch of deregulation miRNAs is involved in CRC [242, 243]. In a miRNAs profile study that included miR-18a, miR-20a, miR-21, miR-29a, miR-92a, miR-106b, miR-133a, miR-143, and miR-145, it was observed that the expression levels were notably different in patients with CRC compared to healthy individuals. This suggests that these miRNAs have the potential to be used as a biomarker for CRC diagnosis [244]. Some miRNAs have relatively higher or lower expression in CRC patients like the higher miR-129 expression in plasma and a low level of miR-24-2 within CRC serum [231, 245]. A set of five miRNAs in the serum of patients with CRC and healthy controls had a different expression, including miR-31, miR-141, miR-224-3p, miR-576-5p, and miR-4669, representing a panel of miRNAs for the diagnosis of CRC. Several miRNAs are detectable in the feces such asmiR-4478, miR-1295b-3p [240], and miR-29a, miR-223, miR-224, miR-106a, and miR-135b. These could be candidates for screening and diagnosis of CRC [43, 246–249]. Evaluation of diagnostic efficiency demonstrated that a combination of five miRNAs present in the serum of CRC patients such as miR-2, miR-29, miR-92, miR-125, and miR-223 showed improved sensitivity (84.7%) and specificity (98.7%) [236]. A study anticipated some of the miRNAs as diagnostic biomarkers like miR-106a, miR-30a-3p, miR-139, miR-145, miR-125a, miR-133a, miR-145, miR-21, miR-320, miR-126, miR-484-5p, miR-143, miR-145, miR-16, miR-125b, miR-106, and miR-143 [120, 232–234, 250]. In a study conducted on miR-21, reports found that it showed specificity and sensitivity of 90% for the detection of CRC [251, 252]; for further validation of the study, a large number of samples and additional meta-analyses are required for improved determination of CRC-related diagnostic markers. To monitor the diagnostic ability of a panel of miRNAs, a combination of miR-24-2, miR-320a, and miR-423-5p showed better results with a sensitivity (92.8%) and specificity (70.8%) for detecting CRC [237]. Moreover, in comparison with available standard clinical cancer markers (CEA and CA19-9), the study report suggests that a panel of six serum-based miRNAs, miR-21, let-7 g, miR-31, miR-92a, miR-181b, and miR203, has a sensitivity of 93% and specificity of 91% for detecting CRC [253]. The global microarray expression study revealed 141 upregulated and 61 downregulated miRNAs. Furthermore, results signified 12 upregulated miRNAs whose expression increased with advancing TNM stages in CRC, *miR-7, miR-17, miR-20a, miR-21, miR-92a, miR-96, miR-106a, miR-134, miR-183, miR-196a, miR-199a-3p,* and *miR-214*. Similarly, the study pointed out eight downregulated miRNAs, *miR-9, miR-29b, miR-127-5p, miR-138, miR-143, miR146a, miR-222*, and *miR-938*, whose expression decreased with the progression of TNM stage. Therefore, this piece of evidence illustrates that the development of a chip could be a promising tool for the molecular screening of colon cancer [254, 255].

Circulating Exosome miRNAs

Circulating microRNA enclosed in extracellular vesicles (EVs) has lately emerged as a novel diagnostic marker for cancer [256, 257]. EVs are a diverse group of membrane-bound particles discharged from all human cells [48]. In the last few years, researchers have focused on EVs as these are largely secreted from tumor cells containing protected tumor-specific cargo [258, 259]. These can act in both a paracrine and endocrine manner [260, 261]. EVs are associated to promote tumor invasiveness, growth activation of stromal accessory cells to tumor-supporting phenotypes, and arrangement of pre-metastatic niches in distant organs [262, 263]. Based on the biogenesis, EVs are classified into three classes: exosomes (~40–100 nm) are formed from multivesicular bodies inside the cell endosomal compartment; microvesicles or ectosomes/microparticles (100 nm–1 μm) are derived from outer budding of the cellular membrane; and apoptotic bodies (1–5 μm) develop from fading cells undergoing apoptosis [264–268]. EVs include an assortment of cargo that reveals the origin of the parent cell, including RNA, DNA, protein, and lipids [260, 269]. To date, miRNAs are the most prominently studied classes of EV [49], and recent reports suggest that miRNA levels are higher in cancer EVs and these can process pre-miRNAs to mature miRNA [270]. In addition to tumor cells, other derivatives of circulating EVs include platelets, red blood cells, and immune cells. Pieces of evidence report that in CRC, EVs are released in abundance in in vitro conditions [271, 272]. Circulating exosomal miRNAs are considered as novel diagnostic and prognostic biomarkers for CRC [256, 273]. For instance, various specific miRNAs act as diagnostic markers, including miR-21, miR-23a, miR-1246, and miR-92a. miRNAs isolated from serum exosomes like miR-17-5p and miR-92a-3p correlate to chronic stages and grades of CRC patients [50]. In CRC patients, serum exosomes miR-6803-5p level was significantly higher and correlated with poor overall survival (OS) [239]. Another exosomal miR-4772-3p present in the serum is involved in the recurrence of tumor at stages II and III of CRC and may be an effective prognostic biomarker [240, 274]. Besides, serum exosomal miR-21could be a useful prognostic biomarker for the prediction of CRC reappearance and poor prognosis with progressive tumor stages [238].

Long Non-coding RNAs

These are a division of RNA transcripts that are 200 nucleotides in length and do not code for proteins or peptides. One of the exclusive features of lncRNAs is the presence of its secondary and three-dimensional structures that allow it to have both RNA and protein-like properties [275]. It is estimated that more than 60,000 lncRNA transcripts are found in humans and the number seems to be increasing with advancing research [276, 277]. It is noted that most of the mammalian lncRNAs have some common structural, functional, or mechanistic distinctiveness among them, and similar to mRNAs, lncRNAs often have a poly-A tail [278–280]. A large number of lncRNAs are restricted in the nucleus; however, few of them are present in the cytoplasm [281, 282]. lncRNAs have a key role in controlling the expression of a gene at various levels like epigenetic, transcriptional, and post-transcriptional for a wide range of biological and cellular processes [283].

In the last few years, only a very few numbers of lncRNAs have been functionally characterized, and there are mounting pieces of evidence that indicate that lncRNAs are concerned with a series of regulatory functions. In recent times, various methodologies have been developed like online prediction tools for the prediction of lncRNAs [284–286]. To further explore the function, expression, and distribution of lncRNAs, some of the commonly available methodologies are RNA sequencing (RNA-seq), RNA microarray, reverse transcription-polymerase chain reaction (RT-PCR), fluorescence in situ hybridization (FISH), and RNA blot analysis [287]. For the study of the lncRNA-protein interactions, some of the highly developed approaches are RNA interference (RNAi), RNA pull-down, RNA-binding protein immunoprecipitation (RIP), chromatin isolation by RNA purification (ChIRP), ChIP-sequencing (ChIP-seq), cross-linking immunoprecipitation (CLIP), and CLIP-sequencing (CLIP-seq) [288, 289]. Moreover, the development of various computational and bioinformatics approaches has enabled the researchers to further characterize and highlight other aspects of lncRNAs [290].

lncRNAs are classified based on the relative location to protein-encoding genes in the genome such as sense lncRNA, antisense lncRNA, bidirectional lncRNA, intronic lncRNA, intergenic lncRNA, and enhancer lncRNA [291]. Sense transcribed in the similar direction as the protein-coding genes with at least one exon overlapped; antisense overlaps one or more exons of another transcript on the similar or opposite strand and overlaps with sense mRNAs at the 5′ or 3′-ends; Bidirectional these are found near to the promoter or enhancer section in opposite direction. These can generate enhancer-associated RNAs (eRNAs) [292], intronic when the complete sequence of lncRNA fits into the introns of a protein-coding gene and intergenic when an lncRNA sequence belongs to two genes as a distinct unit [293–295]. To better understand the molecular mechanisms, lncRNAs can be further reclassified into (1) signaling molecules that are transcribed in a particular manner in effect to different stimuli, for example, Xist, lincRNA-p21, COLDAIR, and HOTAIR; (2) molecular decoys bind to transcription factors, miRNAs, or other targets of chromatin and competitively inhibit them, for example, MALAT1, PTENP1, IPS1, or PANDA; (3) molecular guides these binds chromatin-modifying enzymes to a particular sequence, either as cis or Trans, for example, Xist, COLD AIR, lincRNA-p21, or HOTAIR; and (4) molecular scaffolds work as a central platform to gather all the proteins to form a ribonucleoprotein complex, for example, TERC, HOTAIR, and ANRIL [296]. Altered levels of lncRNAs in tissue, plasma/serum, and exosomes can function as promising markers for CRC detection (Table 8.3).

The research conducted by Hibi and colleagues in 1996 reported the first CRC-related lncRNA, the endogenous H19 gene that was found to be abundant in CRC specimens, and its overexpression played a significant role in the development of CRC [332]. H19 is a positive moderator of EMT progression in CRC [298]. Multiple studies using a range of tools have elucidated some of the consistent and aberrant CRC-associated lncRNAs both in vivo and in vitro that could be a beneficial tool for CRC screening, diagnosis, prognosis, and therapeutic outcomes [289].

Deregulated lncRNAs are engaged at all stages of CRC and act as master gene regulators via multiple mechanisms. Some of the lncRNAs in CRC are the well-known tumor-specific growth arrest-specific 5 (*GAS5*), HOX transcript antisense intergenic RNA (HOTAIR) [299, 333], and few others like metastasis-associated lung adenocarcinoma transcript 1 (MALAT1) [301, 334] and H19 [297, 335]; colon cancer-associated transcript 1 (CCAT1); colorectal neoplasia differentially expressed (CRNDE); colorectal cancer-associated lncRNA (CRCAL) 1, colorectal cancer-associated lncRNA 2, colorectal cancer-associated lncRNA 3, and colorectal cancer-associated lncRNA 4; and urothelial carcinoma-associated 1 (UCA1) expressed in precancerous adenomas [289, 303, 317, 336, 337]. The analysis of altered levels of lncRNA patterns either in circulation, in tissues, or in exosomes can serve as a prospective marker for CRC detection, diagnosis, and treatment in the clinical scenario. Nevertheless, identification of the intricate regulatory network of lncRNAs and specific mechanisms involved will greatly add to the knowledge and will possibly decrease the number of unnecessary colonoscopies and other follow-up procedures [338].

Table 8.3 Simplified list of different lncRNAs involved with their clinical potential in CRC

lncRNAs	Cytoband	Expression	Source	Mode of action	Clinical significance
H19	11p15.5	Upregulated/ LOI	Tissue	Positive moderator of EMT progression	Prognostic [297, 298]
HOTAIR	12q13.13	Upregulated	Tissue, plasma/ serum	Associated with invasion, metastasis, and differentiation; participates in EMT	Prognosis [299, 300],
MALAT1	11q13.1	Upregulated	Tissue, plasma/ serum	Promote EMT and activates Wnt signaling	Diagnosis and prognosis [301]
CCAT1	8q24.21	Upregulated	Tissue, plasma/ serum	N/A	Screening, diagnosis, and prognosis [302, 303]
CRCAL	N/A	Upregulated	Tissue	Involved in cell cycle regulation	Prognosis [304]
UCA1	19p13.12	Upregulated	Tissue, plasma/ serum, exosomes	Associated with large tumor size, increased invasion, and less differentiated histology	Prognosis [305, 306]
HOTAIRM1	N/A	Downregulated	Tissue, plasma/ serum	Inhibit cell division; acts as tumor suppressor	Prognosis [307]
PVT-1	8q24	Upregulated	Tissue, plasma/ serum	Anti-apoptotic activity via TGF-β signaling	Prognosis [308, 309]
MEG3	14q32.2	Downregulated	Tissue, plasma/ serum	Stimulate TP53 by downregulating MDM2	Diagnostic and prognosis [304, 308, 310]
91H	N/A	Downregulated	Tissue, plasma/ serum, exosomes	Promotes tumor-cell migration and invasion via HNRNPK expression	Diagnostic and prognosis [308, 311, 312]
LIT1	11p15.5	LOI	Tissue	Associated with epigenetic status at the KvDMR1	Diagnosis [313, 314]
CAHM	6q26	Downregulated	Tissue	N/A	Screening and diagnosis [315]
CRNDE	16q12.2	Upregulated	Tissue, plasma/ serum, exosomes	Involved in developing pathological stages and increased tumor sizes. Suppress proliferation and promotes apoptosis	Diagnostic and prognosis [316–319]

(continued)

Table 8.3 (continued)

lncRNAs	Cytoband	Expression	Source	Mode of action	Clinical significance
HIF1A-AS1	N/A	Upregulated	Tissue, plasma/serum	N/A	Prognosis [320]
TUG1	N/A	Upregulated	Tissue, plasma/serum, exosomes	Promotes metastasis; participates in EMT	Prognosis [321–323]
lincRNA-p21	6p21.2	Downregulated	Tissue, plasma/serum	Functions with hnRNP-K as a transcriptional coactivator of p53	Prognosis [324, 325]
Loc285194	3q13.31	Downregulated	Tissue, plasma/serum	Activated via p53; suppresses tumor cell growth	Prognosis [326, 327]
BLACAT1	N/A	Upregulated	Tissue, plasma/serum	N/A	Prognosis [328, 329]
LNCV6	N/A	Upregulated	Exosomes	N/A	Diagnostic [330]
GAS5	1q25	Downregulated	Tissue, plasma/serum, exosomes	Acts as tumor suppressor; promotes metastasis	Prognosis [331]

HOTAIR is relatively well-studied and aberrantly expressed lncRNAs in colorectal cancer. The HOTAIR gene is present in the HoxC gene cluster from 12q13.13 on chromosome 12, specifically between HoxC11 and HoxC12 [339]. An upregulated expression of HOTAIR in the initial tumors and blood of CRC patients is associated with invasion, metastasis, and differentiation. This suggests that HOTAIR may be a valuable biomarker in sporadic CRC. The peripheral blood mononuclear cells (PBMC) of CRC blood donors also reported elevated expression of HOTAIR compared to controls. It is quite intriguing to note that levels of HOTAIR were less in patients with right-sided CRC [300]. In contrast, in a study performed using nested TaqMan RT-PCR method, results indicate that HOX antisense intergenic RNA myeloid 1 (HOTAIRM1) expression was significantly low in tumor tissue and plasma of CRC patients. It has been observed that HOTAIRM1 function as a tumor suppressor and, as a result, inhibit cell multiplication [307].

GAS5 lncRNA transcript is about 630 nts in length and is widely expressed in CRC. The *GAS5* gene is located on chromosome 1q25. In serum, GAS5 had diminished expression and is related to developing TNM stages and increased tumor size and acts as a tumor suppressor [340]. Conversely, another study revealed that overexpression of GAS5 in tissues, plasma, and exosomes of CRC patients was related to TNM and Dukes stage, metastasis to the lymph node, local distant metastasis, and recurrence [331].

In a study performed using microarray analysis, three lncRNAs were selected, namely, antisense H19 (91H), plasmacytoma variant translocation 1 (PVT1), and maternally expressed gene 3 (MEG3), and an elevated level was reported in the CRC patient's plasma compared to non-cancerous controls [308]. Exosomes lncRNA 91H expression was drastically amplified in CRC serum samples that were usually found in vesicles than in exosomes-free sera. However, elevated expression was decreased after surgery [311].

Another potentially reported lncRNA transcript called LIT1 (long QT intronic transcript 1) was identified within the KvLQT1 locus on chromosome 11. In CRC tissues, LIT1/KCNQ1OT1 was significantly higher and resulted in the loss of imprinting (LOI), while it was absent in peritumoral samples. Therefore, LIT1 may be a significant target for the diagnosis of CRC [313, 314].

The deep bisulfite sequencing analysis identified another lncRNA in CRC, colorectal adenocarcinoma hypermethylated (CAHM), earlier known as LOC100526820. It is located on chromosome 6 contiguous to the gene QKI, which codes for an RNA-binding protein. Data from methylation-specific PCR (MSP) revealed that CAHM is methylated at the sites of the MSP primers in increased concentration in colorectal adenomas but not in normal colorectal tissue. Moreover, findings suggest that CAHM is hypermethylated in 81% of adenomas and 71% of CRC, but no such findings were observed for the normal tissue [315]. Future studies investigated that in the plasma, CAHM was found to be methylated for 55% of CRC compared to adenomas (4%) and patients without neoplasia (7%). Therefore, methylated CAHM DNA in parallel with the above findings is notably a capable plasma biomarker for the initial detection of CRC [315]. The potentially diagnostic lncRNA CRNDE (colorectal neoplasia differentially expressed) present on chromosome 16 is highly overexpressed in CRC. It is involved in highly developed pathological stages and increased tumor sizes in CRC. Also, it was reported that both in vitro and in vivo the knockdown of CRNDE drastically decreased cell multiplication and caused apoptosis of CRC cells. Furthermore, CRNDE promoted CRC development via epigenetically suppressing the expressions of dual-specificity phosphatase 5 (DUSP5) and CDKN1A by binding to EZH2 (the key components of polycomb repressive complex 2 (PRC2)). Thus, these findings demonstrated that CRNDE may have diagnostic potential for CRC [316]. In another study conducted on tissue and plasma, specimen's reports found that in tissue samples, the expression levels of the CRNDE transcript were elevated in 90% of the tissues isolated from colorectal adenomas and adenocarcinomas. On the contrary, it had a decreased level in normal tissues or inflammatory bowel disease (IBD) specimens. In a plasma specimen, out of 15, only 13 CRNDE transcripts were positive in CRC patients confirming the sensitivity and specificity of 87% and 93%, respectively [317]. CRNDE lncRNA, with its splice variants particularly CRDNME-b and CRNDE-h, was found to be upregulated in both benign and malignant neoplastic colorectal tissue. The diagnostic potential of CRNDE-h was supported by the evidence that Q-PCR results of circulating CRNDE-h between CRC *and* healthy controls reported 87% sensitivity and 93% specificity, and in CRC tissues, CRNDE-h levels have the potential to differentiate from adenoma and healthy tissues with 70.4% sensitivity and 70.8%

specificity [317, 318]. In an analysis conducted on 148 CRC patient exosomes, it was revealed that CRNDE-h had an increased expression compared to healthy and benign CRC samples. These results strongly correlate with metastasis to the lymph nodes and poor OS rates [319].

CCAT1 was the first marker to be identified in the plasma of a CRC patient. It has a significantly higher expression level compared to healthy controls [324]. CCAT1 is located on chromosome 8q24.2 [303, 337]. It is 2628 nucleotide in length positioned close to c-Myc and present in the blood and fecal specimen of CRC patients. Studies indicate that in peripheral blood samples, CCAT1 was upregulated in 40% of CRC but not in healthy individuals [303, 341]. To specifically identify CRC in vitro, ex vivo, and in vivo emerged the use of a CCAT1-specific peptide nucleic acid (PNA)-based molecular beacons (TO-PNA-MB) that came out as a powerful predictor of CRC [302].

The colorectal cancer-associated lncRNA (CRCAL) 1, CRCAL 2, CRCAL 3, and CRCAL 4 are highly overexpressed and may have significant importance in the early onset of CRC. CRCAL 3 and CRCAL 4 are involved in cell cycle regulation. CRCAL1 4 is a newly identified upregulated lncRNA involved in the initial identification of CRC; however, it cannot efficiently distinguish between adenoma and CRC [304, 342].

Accumulating evidence has demonstrated the role of UCA1 lncRNA in promoting tumorigenesis of CRC [306, 336, 343]. Overexpression of UCA1 was reported with large tumor size, enhanced invasion, and attenuated differentiation in the histological sections [305]. The study performed on UCA1 using real-time PCR confirmed that UCA1 was downregulated in serum exosomes of cancerous patients [306].

The hypoxia-inducible factor 1 alpha-antisense RNA 1 (HIF1A-AS1) expression was elevated and is related to a lower 5-year survival rate indicating that it may be used as a diagnostic and prognostic biomarker in CRC [320]. Recently a study constructed a panel of six plasma exosome lncRNAs including LNCV6_116109, LNCV6_98390, LNCV6_38772, LNCV_108266, LNCV6_84003, and LNCV6_98602 with elevated expression in patients compared to healthy individuals in the early success of CRC. This suggested that these lncRNAs could be used as valuable markers for premature identification of cancer [330].

A multi-marker lncRNA panel is another diagnostic approach compared to single lncRNA. The combined measurement of circulating HOTAIR as well as CCAT1 serum or plasma levels showed better sensitivity (84.3%) and specificity (80.2%), respectively [324]. Such a combination of markers can be useful for the identification of CRC at initial stages. In a study, it was revealed that UCA1 levels in the serum exosomes can be improved by combining it with TUG1 lncRNA or with circHIPK3 [306]. A panel identified three different upregulated lncRNAs including LOC152578, XLOC_000303, and XLOC_0006844 that showed an accuracy of 85%, and it proved to be suitable for detecting the occurrence of CRC [344]. A pilot study conducted for the detection of early-stage CRCs identified a plasma-derived ncRNAs panel including 91H, PVT-1, and MEG3 that can distinguish CRC samples with higher sensitivity and specificity and can be used as a potential diagnostic biomarker [308].

8.3 Prognostic Biomarkers

The diagnosis of CRC is followed with the prognosis meaning to assess the onset of cancers aggressiveness despite adjuvant therapy. The prognostic biomarker is a molecule that provides information about overall cancer outcomes in patients, independent of the therapy [254]. To date, management is done with radiation-based techniques such as CT and MRI. Another criterion is pathological like the TNM system and lymphovascular, perineural, and venous invasion. The TNM system is the most common prognostic method that analyzes tumor depth of invasion (T), nodal involvement (N), and the presence of metastasis (M). However, the prognosis varies between patients to a patient of the same stage [345, 346]. The major limitations with the prognostic tools are that none of them provides clear evidence of which CRC cases are more prone to relapse and does not provide relevant status on metastasis or chemoresistance. Besides, they are not suitable for personalized treatment. Consequently, attempts are being made to evaluate the nature and source of various other molecules and gene alterations that can be used as prognostic biomarkers and can take a step closer to a personalized treatment [347].

8.3.1 Blood Biomarkers

Carcinoembryonic Antigen (CEA) and Carbohydrate Antigen 19-9 (CA 19-9)
The most commonly available biomarkers used to monitor CRC patients are CEA and CA 19-9. The CEA is a 180 kD membrane-associated glycoprotein from a family of 32 genes that are generally expressed in different tissues. These are involved in cell adhesion or signal transduction. CEA was acknowledged as a colon cancer antigen in 1965 by Gold and Freedman, an antigen that was found in both fetal colon and colon adenocarcinoma but not present in the healthy adult colon. It is only detectable in cancer and embryonic tissue, thus named carcinoembryonic antigen or CEA [348, 349]. The increased concentrations of CEA in 35 of 36 patients with colorectal cancer confirmed its role. Thoughtfully, the extensive usage of CEA as a marker for colorectal malignancy began 30 years later after its initial detection in serum [350]. In screening for colorectal cancer, especially in early stages, the deficit of sensitivity and specificity limits the application of CEA in diagnosing colorectal cancer [351, 352]. Serial CEA measurements can detect CRC recurrence with increased sensitivity of about 80% and specificity about 70%. CEA is the most frequent indicator of early liver metastasis in patients diagnosed with CRC, and yet it is the most suitable option to be used as a prognostic marker [353]. On the other hand, the specificity and sensitivity of CA19-9 antigen are comparatively less for CRC than for CEA.

Tissue polypeptide-specific antigen (TPS) and tissue polypeptide antigen (TPA) can detect the fragments of cytokeratins 8, 18, and 19, and levels of TPA and TPS were elevated in the metastatic stage of CRC. Moreover, TPA combined with CEA has increased sensitivity and can detect recurrence of CRC [354–357].

CEA testing is very essential for the management of CRC and should be done regularly 3 months post-surgery for stage II/IIICRC patients as affirmed by the American Society of Clinical Oncology (ASCO) 2006, and reports indicate that there was a sharp decline in the mortality rates [74, 75]. According to another study, an intensive follow-up group showed a higher cumulative 5-year survival rate than the control group (72.1% vs. 63.7%) as revealed by meta-analysis [358]. Furthermore, to support the prognostic value of preoperative CEA levels, a critical large-scale study conducted on 2230 CRC patients confirmed that the CEA level was related to patient outcomes [359, 360]. In parallel to these two other case studies, it was confirmed that the preoperative CEA level correlates to CRC prognosis that metastasized to the liver [361, 362].

8.3.2 *Tissue-Derived Prognostic Biomarkers*

Molecular Prognostic Biomarkers

Some of the diagnostic tissue-derived molecular biomarkers like mucins (MUC2), SATB2 protein, CK20/CDX2, vascular endothelial growth factor (VEGF), insulin-like growth factor 2 mRNA-binding protein 3 (IMP3), and Traf2- and Nck-interacting kinase (TNIK) have the potential to serve as promising prognostic markers [363]. Studies revealed that results obtained from the MUC2 expression profile were miscellaneous. Indeed, the absence of MUC2 expression is associated with poor prognosis in both MMR-proficient and *MLH1*-negative CRC [364]. On the contrary, an upregulated SATB2 expression is quite a good indicator of prognosis in CRC and can amplify the sensitivity to chemotherapy and radiation, whereas in cases of colorectal adenocarcinomas, SATB2 was downregulated and correlated with worse prognosis, infiltration of lymph nodes, tumor invasion, and distant metastasis [365, 366]. CDX2 has a poor prognosis rate; the absence of CDX2 expression is related to the proximal origin, infiltrative characteristics with developed TNM stage, progression-free survival (PFS), and OS [367]. One of the main angiogenic factors expressed in approximately 50% of CRC is VEGF. The expression of VEGF is significantly associated with a worse prognosis [368]. Lastly, studies on TNIK have confirmed that elevated levels of TNIK protein in primary tumors may indicate distant metastasis after surgery of stage II/III of CRC [369].

8.3.3 *DNA Alterations with Prognostic Value*

B-Rapidly Accelerated Fibrosarcoma (BRAF)

It is a proto-oncogene and stimulates the mitogen-activated protein kinase (MAPK) signaling pathway leading to the expression of various proteins that function in cell proliferation, differentiation, survival, angiogenesis, and cell motility [370]. *BRAF*-activating mutations are found in 8% of highly developed CRC and 14% of stage II/III CRC cases [76, 77]. The mutation in *BRAF* correlates with tumor location in the proximal colon, poor differentiation, and tumor size [371]. Besides, it shows poor PFS and OS rates and fewer response rates to anti-epidermal growth factor receptor (EGFR) therapy [372, 373]. In 2017, ASCO recognized *BRAF V600E* which results in 90% of *BRAF* mutations and may be of potential prognostic value [78].

Microsatellite Instability (MSI)
The coding and non-coding regions of the genome have microsatellites. These are repeating DNA sequences of about one to six pairs. During the DNA replication, process errors are fixed with the help of a mismatch repair (MMR) system. MSI arises due to the silencing of MMR genes through sporadic MLH1 promoter hypermethylation or germline mutations in MMR genes such as *MLH1*, *MSH2*, *MSH6*, or *PMS* [79, 80]. The deletion of MMR may give rise to somatic mutations and activates genomic instability, eventually resulting in cancer-related alterations [374]. For instance, germline mutations in MMR genes result in Lynch syndrome, also known as hereditary non-polyposis colon cancer [375]. In sporadic MSI CRC, hypermethylation of the MLH1 promoter region initiates MLH1 silencing [376]. The significance of MMR in correlation with CRC has proved to be quiet promising for prognostic stratification [78]. The MSI marker has higher instability of more than 30–40% and helps in better prognosis compared to low MSI; for example, BAT26 and BAT25 are mononucleotide repeats and D2S123, D5S346, and D17S250 dinucleotide repeats. To further assess the prognostic ability, a study revealed that CRC patients with MSI have increased OS and disease-free survival (DFS) compared to normal microsatellite CRC patients [377].

APC
FAP and nearly all cases of sporadic CRC occur due to mutation in the *APC* gene [378]. Functionally, *APC* is involved in the Wnt pathway and functions to maintain cellular integrity, cell multiplication, movement, and apoptosis by regulating β-catenin. *APC* mutation may lead to deregulated transcription of various oncogenes by elevating the levels of β-catenin consequently increased c-Myc expression which is involved in cell proliferation [379]. *APC* mutation may be beneficial for predicting the clinical effects of CRC. For instance, high *APC* mutation and high miR-21 in advanced stage of CRC are associated with shorter OS [81].

p53
The human *TP53* gene present on chromosome 17p consists of 11 exons and 10 introns [380]. The transcription factor P53 participates in a wide range of cellular functions that occur in response to different conditions of cellular stress like the cell cycle arrest, apoptosis, or senescence in response to DNA damage, hypoxia, or oncogene activation. The *p53* mutations arise in 34% of the proximal colon tumors and 45% of the distal colorectal tumors [82–84]. Interestingly, data from various sources have confirmed that *p53* mutations have a prognostic significance in CRC patients; however, inconsistent data was obtained [381, 382]. The overexpression of *P53* resulted in decreased DFS, relapse-free survival (RFS), and rates [83, 383].

SMAD4

It is present on cytoband 18q21 and is involved in TGF-β signaling. The absence of SMAD4 alone cannot stimulate tumor formation although it can promote tumor advancement initiated by APC inactivation in CRC [384–386]. TGF-β/SMAD4 signaling processes signals from the plasma membrane to the nucleus and participates in a diverse array of functions ranging from cell proliferation, apoptosis, and migration to cancer development and progression [387, 388]. *SMAD4* mutations occur at a frequency of about 30–40% of all CRC cases [389, 390]. In CRC, the absence of SMAD4 is related to reduced differentiation, higher stage, metastasis to the lymph node, deficit immune infiltrates, and suppressed response to 5-fluorouracil [86, 87]. Meta-analyses have revealed that the loss of SMAD4 is a negative predictor of OS, cancer-specific survival (CSS), and RFS [85, 391, 392]. Therefore, the above findings have established that SMAD4 may be a reasonable prognostic marker for optimal surveillance of patients.

miRNAs

In the past few years, the role of several miRNAs has been evaluated which has greatly helped in the identification of their prognostic value in CRC. Some of the miRNAs are tumor suppressors that include miR-101, miR-142-3p, miR-133b, miR-337, miR-126, miR-944, miR-497, and miR-646 and the let7 family [393–399]. Some of them have the potential to create a favorable microenvironment for tumor cells like miR-7, miR-155, miR-20a, miR-92a, miR-21, miR-552, miR-130b, and miR-29a [238]. These miRNAs are characterized as oncomirs or oncogenic miRNAs [400–403]. A large number of miRNAs have been identified in CRC. For instance, miR-20a-5p stimulates tumor invasion and metastasis via downregulation of SMAD4 [404]; increased miR-21 expression is related to cell multiplication, invasion, metastasis to the lymph node, highly developed clinical stage, and lower OS and DFS in distinct Duke stages [405, 406]. Elevated miR-29a expression results in metastasis [407, 408]. The miR-155 expression is related to the advanced stage, metastasis, and recurrence and may serve as a significant prognostic biomarker for DFS and OS [409]. An elevated miR-411 expression resulted in direct downregulation of PIK3R3 and AKT/mTOR indirectly. Besides, the reduced miR-411expression is related to distant metastasis and metastasis to the lymph node and worse TNM stage [410].

miRNAs function as a key regulator in the epithelial-mesenchymal transition (EMT) process during carcinogenesis. Increased expression of the miR-200 family that includes *miR-200b, miR-200c, miR-141*, and *miR-429* present in the serum of stage I and IV CRC is related to metastasis; particularly higher *miR-200c* expression was found in liver metastasis compared to primary cancer. Besides, miR-200c also acts as an independent marker for metastasis to the lymph node and recurrence. Some of the other well-known miRNAs with a prognostic value as a biomarker in CRC are miR-203, miR-224, miR-122, miR-214, miR-155, miR-182, miR-30b, and miR-124 [230, 235, 411–418].

lncRNAs

The intricate lncRNA network has a strong association with p53. Quite a few lncRNAs, such as Wrap53, MEG3, p53-eRNAs, and MALAT1, function as regulators of p53, whereas lncRNAs, such as H19, Loc285184, PANDA, and lncRNA-p21, function as an effector of p53 [419]. The tumor-suppressive lncRNA and oncogenic lncRNAs both are recognized to have significant prognostic value as an effective biomarker of CRC. A tumor-suppressive lncRNA lincRNA-p21 is a direct transcriptional target of p53 present close to cyclin-dependent kinase inhibitor p21 (CDKN1A) locus [420]. In CRC tissue, lincRNA-p21 expression was low in contrast to the adjacent tumor. However, as the CRC stage progresses, the expression in tumor tissues was significantly elevated. Therefore, it is evident that any imbalance in the p53/lincRNA-p21 network will result in CRC malignancy [325]. Loc285194 (LSAMP antisense RNA 3) is another tumor-suppressive p53 effector lncRNA found in the tumor tissues of CRC patients. It is located at Cytoband 3q13.31 and is downregulated in CRC [326]. Loc285194 acts as an endogenous sponge to inhibit CRC cell development via suppression of oncogenic miR-211 and functions as a tumor suppressor [327]. The absence of Loc285194 is positively associated with increased tumor size, poor TNM stage, higher distant metastasis, and DFS. Hence, Loc285194 might have prognostic importance in CRC [326].

The Lnc2Cancer 2.0 database has identified a few lncRNAs including H19, CRNDE-h, HOTAIR, and MALAT1 that could have promising prognostic value in CRC. The elevated H19 lncRNA expression was associated with tumor multiplication and highly developed TNM stage. Also, it may act as an independent predictor for OS, DFS, and unfavorable prognosis in CRC [309, 421, 422]. The CRNDE-h has significantly high serum exosome levels that correlate with tumor size, distant, and metastasis to lymph node [318, 319]. Moreover, elevated CRNDE-h exosomal levels in CRC patients are related to a negative predictor of OS [319, 423]. Thereby, this confirmed the prognostic capability of CRNDE-h. Similarly, HOTAIR is also related to a negative prognostic factor in CRC. In primary tumor tissue of CRC patients, upregulated HOTAIR expression is associated with higher death rate, poor histology, higher tumor depth, metastasis to liver, and lower OS [299, 300, 424]. The RT-qPCR analysis indicated that high MALAT1 lncRNA expression was related to a worse prognosis in stage II/III of CRC and resulted in decrease OS and weak response to oxaliplatin-based therapy, thus implicating its role as a prognostic and therapeutic target in CRC [334, 425].

Some of the potentially identified prognostic lncRNAs including the aforementioned lncRNAs are CCAT1 [303], CCAT2 [426], GAS5 [331], BLACAT1 [329], and 91H [311] lncRNAs. These are detectable in the circulation and could prove to be useful as minimally invasive markers for CRC prognosis. The combined effect of CCAT2 and CCAT1expression is related to predict tumor recurrence and prognosis in CRC patients [426]. GAS5 expression has a prognostic value in CRC and is inversely associated with the TNM stage and Dukes stage, metastasis to the lymph node, and local recurrence, whereas it positively correlates with the degree of differentiation and a significant 3-year OS rate [331]. The upregulated BLACAT1 expression has a prognostic value; it is related to advanced stages of CRC and shorter OS [328]. An upregulated expression of exosomal 91H lncRNA is associated with CRC recurrence and metastasis and could be used as a biomarker at the initial stages of detection [311].

8.4 Predictive Biomarkers

Individuals with malignancies exhibit a varying degree of responses to a certain drug/therapies. Therefore, determination of the most suitable therapeutic regimen or prediction of the likely response to a given therapy is of paramount importance. This is the final step in the clinical management of CRC. The emergence of predictive biomarkers is an important approach for the establishment of personalized therapies. Predictive biomarkers can help in understanding the clinical outcome to a certain treatment which further guides the final process [427, 428].

8.4.1 Tissue Biomarkers

8.4.1.1 DNA Alterations

KRAS and NRAS

KRAS belongs to a family of Ras proteins that include H-, K-, and N-RAS that are present on the inner side of the cell membrane. KRAS is involved in the signaling process from ligand-bound EGFR to the nucleus [88]. The binding of the EGFR to its ligand (EGF, TGF-α, amphiregulin) activates EGFR that results in a change of GDP- to GTP-bound form of the KRAS, followed by increased BRAF level which further activates the MAPK pathway. EGFR has a key role in CRC initiation, and progression such as *KRAS* gene is altered in 50% of all the CRC cases and has predictive value as a biomarker in response to EGFR inhibitor [89, 90]. *KRAS* mutations result in resistance to therapy with EGFR receptor monoclonal antibody (mAbs) blockers such as cetuximab [429]. For instance, metastatic CRC having *KRAS* mutations present no benefit with anti-EGFR therapy; however, it exhibited better results with P.G13D *KRAS* mutation treated with cetuximab [430, 431]. A RAS mutation includes mutations in KRAS exons 2, 3, and 4 and NRAS exons 2, 3, and 4 and has the potential to discriminate between individual responses to anti-EGFR therapy [432].

BRAF

The second most common mutations found in 8–10% of all CRC are BRAF mutations, particularly BRAF *V600E*. They can differentiate between familial and sporadic CRC [91, 92]. Studies indicate that a tumor with BRAF mutation is resistant to anti-EGFR therapy and insufficient pieces of evidence are present to support whether *BRAF* is a predictive marker for anti-EGFR antibody therapy success [93, 94].

Phosphatidylinositol 3-Kinases (PI3Ks)

PI3Ks are linked to the RAS-mediated pathway [96]. The somatic-activating mutations are the most common genetic alterations in the PI3K pathway present in 32% of all CRC [95]. Studies indicate a decreased response rate and poor PFS and OS in

KRAS wild-type metastatic CRC patients with *PIK3CA* mutation [433]. On the contrary, it was reported that *PIK3CA* mutation is not related to reducing OS or PFS from cetuximab therapy in KRAS wild-type CRC patients. Therefore, inconsistent results indicate that *PIK3CA* mutation is not suitable to be used as a predictive biomarker; however, it can be used as a predictive marker for adjuvant aspirin therapy in CRC [434]. In an observational study conducted on CRC patients with PIK3CA-mutation that showed increased cancer-specific survival and OS rates compared to *PIK3CA* wild-type CRC patients [435–437].

8.4.2 Blood Biomarkers

Cell-Free DNA

The concentration of cfDNA after CRC surgery primary resection followed by CRC relapse (collectively, postoperative cfDNA measurement) is a critical factor to predict and help in the detection of recurrence. There was a decrease in the concentration of cfDNA after primary resection, whereas cfDNA levels radically increased upon CRC relapse [97–99]. In another study, similar results were observed in the case of chemoradiotherapy. Patients who responded to the therapy showed reduced cfDNA concentration, whereas increased cDNA concentration was observed for non-responders [438, 439].

8.5 Future Challenges

Over the last decade, significant progress has been made to effectively manage CRC. The development of new efficient screening modalities has improved the diagnosis at an early stage. However, there is a compelling need for the development of highly effective and sensitive biomarkers. The understanding of cancer genomics abnormality in CRC is one of the biggest challenges; therefore, exhaustive studies would give a better insight into the early onset and development of CRC. The identification of the vulnerable genes and their associated genomic irregularity with the aid of high-throughput sequencing followed with advanced DNA approaches such as next-generation sequencing (NGS) could be a potential target for CRC therapy [440]. The emergence of NGS has significantly impacted the understanding of the changing face of CRC in terms of the development of novel biomarkers based on genomic alterations; however, more efforts are required to get desired and powerful results [441]. The understanding of intricate molecular signaling pathways involved in the metastatic phenotype is vital for the development of targeted drug molecules that may either inhibit or manage the progression of the CRC. A few anecdotes on dietary and environmental factors are present, and if taken into consideration, they might prove to be useful in understanding cancer incidence. Another great challenge is the administration of the oral drug to the target site based on polysaccharides [442]. These will carry chemotherapeutic and chemopreventive agents precisely to the colon and rectum [443, 444]. Finally, to detect CRC at its early stages, molecular biomarkers have proved as an invaluable tool in cancer detection and patient prognosis. Moreover, these can be used to control tumor growth, identify different stages of the disease, and respond to a certain therapy. There is a need for novel, reliable, targeted, and sensitive biomarkers shortly. Instead of a single biomarker, a set of biomarkers would be an efficient option in the detection and diagnosis of CRC in comparison with single biomarkers as well as to conventional therapy. However, isolating both sensitive and specific single miRNAs and miRNAs panels in CRC is itself a challenging task. Currently, for diagnostic and therapy management purposes, MSI and KRAS mutation determination in tumor samples is operational. For the diagnosis of CRC at its initial stage, various tests are under evaluations that are dependent on miRNAs expression, gene microarrays, and CpG island methylation phenotype; however, studies based on large cohort still need to be conducted for further validation. Lastly, the biggest challenge is the integration of different biomarkers into the healthcare Scheme. A blood-derived biomarker will ideally outshine on all the parameters for screening compared to fecal-based assays; therefore, the use of biomarkers in the present scenario may be beneficial in clinical practice [445].

8.6 Conclusion

CRC can affect individuals of different ages with an increased incidence and mortality worldwide. The novel findings in the diagnostics and treatment methodologies include feces, blood, and tissue that have provided better and updated insights into the understanding of CRC. Recently, researchers have focused on investigating some noninvasive screening tests for the initial diagnosis of CRC based on DNA, RNA, and protein molecules in stool, blood, and other biological fluids. The development of biomarkers has great potential in the prevention, diagnosis, and treatment of the disease. To date, several genetic and epigenetic markers have been studied; however, none of them is noninvasive, specific, sensitive, and inexpensive in clinical practice. Also, insufficient studies have been done based on RNA biomarkers compared to DNA biomarkers. Recently, transcriptome studies have gained a fresh impetus particularly miRNAs expression level as one of the valuable biomarkers for the treatment of recurrent and advanced CRC. Different protein markers like CA 19-9 and CEA and their different combined variants in tissues or biological fluids present a potential tool with increased sensitivity and specificity to detect CRC at initial stages. Finally, the present research is focused on the development of less aggressive, more sensitive, specific, and cost-effective therapies that will enhance the OS and will improve the life of CRC patients.

References

1. Bray F, Ferlay J, Soerjomataram I, Siegel RL, Torre LA, Jemal A. Global cancer statistics 2018: GLOBOCAN estimates of incidence and mortality worldwide for 36 cancers in 185 countries. CA Cancer J Clin. 2018;68(6):394–424.
2. Fearon ER, Vogelstein B. A genetic model for colorectal tumorigenesis. Cell. 1990;61(5):759–67.
3. Wan ML, Wang Y, Zeng Z, Deng B, Zhu BS, Cao T, et al. Colorectal cancer (CRC) as a multifactorial disease and its causal correlations with multiple signaling pathways. Biosci Rep. 2020;40(3):BSR20200265.
4. Migliore L, Migheli F, Spisni R, Coppede F. Genetics, cytogenetics, and epigenetics of colorectal cancer. J Biomed Biotechnol. 2011;2011:792362.
5. Grady WM, Pritchard CC. Molecular alterations and biomarkers in colorectal cancer. Toxicol Pathol. 2014;42(1):124–39.
6. Lao VV, Grady WM. Epigenetics and colorectal cancer. Nat Rev Gastroenterol Hepatol. 2011;8(12):686–700.
7. Fearon ER. Molecular genetics of colorectal cancer. Annu Rev Pathol. 2011;6:479–507.
8. Pino MS, Chung DC. The chromosomal instability pathway in colon cancer. Gastroenterology. 2010;138(6):2059–72.
9. Grady WM, Carethers JM. Genomic and epigenetic instability in colorectal cancer pathogenesis. Gastroenterology. 2008;135(4):1079–99.
10. De' Angelis GL, Bottarelli L, Azzoni C, De' Angelis N, Leandro G, Di Mario F, et al. Microsatellite instability in colorectal cancer. Acta Biomed. 2018;89(9-S):97–101.
11. Puccini A, Berger MD, Naseem M, Tokunaga R, Battaglin F, Cao S, et al. Colorectal cancer: epigenetic alterations and their clinical implications. Biochim Biophys Acta Rev Cancer. 2017;1868(2):439–48.
12. Cancer Genome Atlas N. Comprehensive molecular characterization of human colon and rectal cancer. Nature. 2012;487(7407):330–7.
13. Fransen K, Klintenas M, Osterstrom A, Dimberg J, Monstein HJ, Soderkvist P. Mutation analysis of the BRAF, ARAF and RAF-1 genes in human colorectal adenocarcinomas. Carcinogenesis. 2004;25(4):527–33.
14. Burt R. Inheritance of colorectal cancer. Drug Discov Today Dis Mech. 2007;4(4):293–300.
15. Rahmani F, Avan A, Hashemy SI, Hassanian SM. Role of Wnt/beta-catenin signaling regulatory microRNAs in the pathogenesis of colorectal cancer. J Cell Physiol. 2018;233(2):811–7.
16. Aghabozorgi AS, Bahreyni A, Soleimani A, Bahrami A, Khazaei M, Ferns GA, et al. Role of adenomatous polyposis coli (APC) gene mutations in the pathogenesis of colorectal cancer; current status and perspectives. Biochimie. 2019;157:64–71.
17. Strate LL, Syngal S. Hereditary colorectal cancer syndromes. Cancer Causes Control. 2005;16(3):201–13.
18. Snyder C, Hampel H. Hereditary colorectal cancer syndromes. Semin Oncol Nurs. 2019;35(1):58–78.
19. Lynch HT, Snyder CL, Shaw TG, Heinen CD, Hitchins MP. Milestones of Lynch syndrome: 1895–2015. Nat Rev Cancer. 2015;15(3):181–94.
20. Wells K, Wise PE. Hereditary colorectal cancer syndromes. Surg Clin North Am. 2017;97(3):605–25.
21. Huang J, Zheng S, Jin SH, Zhang SZ. Somatic mutations of APC gene in carcinomas from hereditary non-polyposis colorectal cancer patients. World J Gastroenterol. 2004;10(6):834–6.
22. Cunningham D, Atkin W, Lenz HJ, Lynch HT, Minsky B, Nordlinger B, et al. Colorectal cancer. Lancet. 2010;375(9719):1030–47.
23. Shah R, Jones E, Vidart V, Kuppen PJ, Conti JA, Francis NK. Biomarkers for early detection of colorectal cancer and polyps: systematic review. Cancer Epidemiol Biomark Prev. 2014;23(9):1712–28.

24. Alix-Panabieres C, Pantel K. Clinical applications of circulating tumor cells and circulating tumor DNA as liquid biopsy. Cancer Discov. 2016;6(5):479–91.
25. Shastri YM, Loitsch S, Hoepffner N, Povse N, Hanisch E, Rosch W, et al. Comparison of an established simple office-based immunological FOBT with fecal tumor pyruvate kinase type M2 (M2-PK) for colorectal cancer screening: prospective multicenter study. Am J Gastroenterol. 2008;103(6):1496–504.
26. Takai T, Kanaoka S, Yoshida K, Hamaya Y, Ikuma M, Miura N, et al. Fecal cyclooxygenase 2 plus matrix metalloproteinase 7 mRNA assays as a marker for colorectal cancer screening. Cancer Epidemiol Biomark Prev. 2009;18(6):1888–93.
27. Huang Z, Huang D, Ni S, Peng Z, Sheng W, Du X. Plasma microRNAs are promising novel biomarkers for early detection of colorectal cancer. Int J Cancer. 2010;127(1):118–26.
28. Pan C, Yan X, Li H, Huang L, Yin M, Yang Y, et al. Systematic literature review and clinical validation of circulating microRNAs as diagnostic biomarkers for colorectal cancer. Oncotarget. 2017;8(40):68317–28.
29. Kanaan Z, Roberts H, Eichenberger MR, Billeter A, Ocheretner G, Pan J, et al. A plasma microRNA panel for detection of colorectal adenomas: a step toward more precise screening for colorectal cancer. Ann Surg. 2013;258(3):400–8.
30. Tang X, Qiao X, Chen C, Liu Y, Zhu J, Liu J. Regulation mechanism of Long noncoding RNAs in Colon cancer development and progression. Yonsei Med J. 2019;60(4):319–25.
31. Udar N, Lofton-Day C, Dong J, Vavrek D, Jung AS, Meier K, et al. Clinical validation of the next-generation sequencing-based extended RAS panel assay using metastatic colorectal cancer patient samples from the phase 3 PRIME study. J Cancer Res Clin Oncol. 2018;144(10):2001–10.
32. Micheel CM, Nass SJ, Omenn GS, editors. Evolution of translational omics: lessons learned and the path forward. Washington, DC: National Academies Press; 2012.
33. Lassere MN. The biomarker-surrogacy evaluation schema: a review of the biomarker-surrogate literature and a proposal for a criterion-based, quantitative, multidimensional hierarchical levels of evidence schema for evaluating the status of biomarkers as surrogate endpoints. Stat Methods Med Res. 2008;17(3):303–40.
34. Vainio H. Use of biomarkers in risk assessment. Int J Hyg Environ Health. 2001;204 (2–3):91–102.
35. Ahmed FE. Development of novel diagnostic and prognostic molecular markers for sporadic colon cancer. Expert Rev Mol Diagn. 2005;5(3):337–52.
36. Chand M, Keller DS, Mirnezami R, Bullock M, Bhangu A, Moran B, et al. Novel biomarkers for patient stratification in colorectal cancer: a review of definitions, emerging concepts, and data. World J Gastrointest Oncol. 2018;10(7):145–58.
37. Faivre J, Dancourt V, Lejeune C, Tazi MA, Lamour J, Gerard D, et al. Reduction in colorectal cancer mortality by fecal occult blood screening in a French controlled study. Gastroenterology. 2004;126(7):1674–80.
38. Gonzalez-Pons M, Cruz-Correa M. Colorectal cancer biomarkers: where are we now? Biomed Res Int. 2015;2015:149014.
39. Zou H, Harrington JJ, Klatt KK, Ahlquist DA. A sensitive method to quantify human long DNA in stool: relevance to colorectal cancer screening. Cancer Epidemiol Biomark Prev. 2006;15(6):1115–9.
40. Morikawa T, Kato J, Yamaji Y, Wada R, Mitsushima T, Shiratori Y. A comparison of the immunochemical fecal occult blood test and total colonoscopy in the asymptomatic population. Gastroenterology. 2005;129(2):422–8.
41. Gupta AK, Melton LJ 3rd, Petersen GM, Timmons LJ, Vege SS, Harmsen WS, et al. Changing trends in the incidence, stage, survival, and screen-detection of colorectal cancer: a population-based study. Clin Gastroenterol Hepatol. 2005;3(2):150–8.
42. Imperiale TF, Ransohoff DF, Itzkowitz SH, Turnbull BA, Ross ME, Colorectal Cancer Study G. Fecal DNA versus fecal occult blood for colorectal-cancer screening in an average-risk population. N Engl J Med. 2004;351(26):2704–14.

43. Zhu Y, Xu A, Li J, Fu J, Wang G, Yang Y, et al. Fecal miR-29a and miR-224 as the noninvasive biomarkers for colorectal cancer. Cancer Biomark. 2016;16(2):259–64.
44. Yu J, Gu G, Ju S. Recent advances in clinical applications of circulating cell-free DNA integrity. Lab Med. 2014;45(1):6–11.
45. Jahr S, Hentze H, Englisch S, Hardt D, Fackelmayer FO, Hesch RD, et al. DNA fragments in the blood plasma of cancer patients: quantitations and evidence for their origin from apoptotic and necrotic cells. Cancer Res. 2001;61(4):1659–65.
46. Hao TB, Shi W, Shen XJ, Qi J, Wu XH, Wu Y, et al. Circulating cell-free DNA in serum as a biomarker for diagnosis and prognostic prediction of colorectal cancer. Br J Cancer. 2014;111(8):1482–9.
47. Frattini M, Gallino G, Signoroni S, Balestra D, Battaglia L, Sozzi G, et al. Quantitative analysis of plasma DNA in colorectal cancer patients: a novel prognostic tool. Ann N Y Acad Sci. 2006;1075:185–90.
48. Margolis L, Sadovsky Y. The biology of extracellular vesicles: the known unknowns. PLoS Biol. 2019;17(7):e3000363.
49. Desmond BJ, Dennett ER, Danielson KM. Circulating extracellular vesicle MicroRNA as diagnostic biomarkers in early colorectal cancer-a review. Cancers. 2019;12(1):52.
50. Fu F, Jiang W, Zhou L, Chen Z. Circulating Exosomal miR-17-5p and miR-92a-3p predict pathologic stage and grade of colorectal cancer. Transl Oncol. 2018;11(2):221–32.
51. Ransohoff DF. How much does colonoscopy reduce colon cancer mortality? Ann Intern Med. 2009;150(1):50–2.
52. Segnan N, Armaroli P, Bonelli L, Risio M, Sciallero S, Zappa M, et al. Once-only sigmoidoscopy in colorectal cancer screening: follow-up findings of the Italian randomized controlled trial--SCORE. J Natl Cancer Inst. 2011;103(17):1310–22.
53. Atkin WS, Edwards R, Kralj-Hans I, Wooldrage K, Hart AR, Northover JM, et al. Once-only flexible sigmoidoscopy screening in prevention of colorectal cancer: a multicentre randomised controlled trial. Lancet. 2010;375(9726):1624–33.
54. Halligan S, Wooldrage K, Dadswell E, Kralj-Hans I, von Wagner C, Edwards R, et al. Computed tomographic colonography versus barium enema for diagnosis of colorectal cancer or large polyps in symptomatic patients (SIGGAR): a multicentre randomised trial. Lancet. 2013;381(9873):1185–93.
55. Scheitel SM, Ahlquist DA, Wollan PC, Hagen PT, Silverstein MD. Colorectal cancer screening: a community case-control study of proctosigmoidoscopy, barium enema radiography, and fecal occult blood test efficacy. Mayo Clin Proc. 1999;74(12):1207–13.
56. Cotton PB, Durkalski VL, Pineau BC, Palesch YY, Mauldin PD, Hoffman B, et al. Computed tomographic colonography (virtual colonoscopy): a multicenter comparison with standard colonoscopy for detection of colorectal neoplasia. JAMA. 2004;291(14):1713–9.
57. Rosman AS, Korsten MA. Meta-analysis comparing CT colonography, air contrast barium enema, and colonoscopy. Am J Med. 2007;120(3):203–10.e4.
58. Luboldt W, Bauerfeind P, Wildermuth S, Marincek B, Fried M, Debatin JF. Colonic masses: detection with MR colonography. Radiology. 2000;216(2):383–8.
59. Zijta FM, Bipat S, Stoker J. Magnetic resonance (MR) colonography in the detection of colorectal lesions: a systematic review of prospective studies. Eur Radiol. 2010;20(5):1031–46.
60. Bayrak R, Yenidunya S, Haltas H. Cytokeratin 7 and cytokeratin 20 expression in colorectal adenocarcinomas. Pathol Res Pract. 2011;207(3):156–60.
61. Wang JL, Qi Z, Li YH, Zhao HM, Chen YG, Fu W. TGF beta induced factor homeobox 1 promotes colorectal cancer development through activating Wnt/beta-catenin signaling. Oncotarget. 2017;8(41):70214–25.
62. Willert K, Nusse R. Beta-catenin: a key mediator of Wnt signaling. Curr Opin Genet Dev. 1998;8(1):95–102.
63. Kuroda N, Yorita K. Colon cancer with micropapillary carcinoma component: a clinopathologic study of 9 cases. Pol J Pathol. 2017;68(2):102–8.

64. Moskaluk CA, Zhang H, Powell SM, Cerilli LA, Hampton GM, Frierson HF Jr. Cdx2 protein expression in normal and malignant human tissues: an immunohistochemical survey using tissue microarrays. Mod Pathol. 2003;16(9):913–9.
65. Werling RW, Yaziji H, Bacchi CE, Gown AM. CDX2, a highly sensitive and specific marker of adenocarcinomas of intestinal origin: an immunohistochemical survey of 476 primary and metastatic carcinomas. Am J Surg Pathol. 2003;27(3):303–10.
66. Magnusson K, de Wit M, Brennan DJ, Johnson LB, McGee SF, Lundberg E, et al. SATB2 in combination with cytokeratin 20 identifies over 95% of all colorectal carcinomas. Am J Surg Pathol. 2011;35(7):937–48.
67. Hattrup CL, Gendler SJ. Structure and function of the cell surface (tethered) mucins. Annu Rev Physiol. 2008;70:431–57.
68. Li C, Zuo D, Liu T, Yin L, Li C, Wang L. Prognostic and Clinicopathological significance of MUC family members in colorectal cancer: a systematic review and meta-analysis. Gastroenterol Res Pract. 2019;2019:2391670.
69. Su MC, Yuan RH, Lin CY, Jeng YM. Cadherin-17 is a useful diagnostic marker for adenocarcinomas of the digestive system. Mod Pathol. 2008;21(11):1379–86.
70. Shay JW, Bacchetti S. A survey of telomerase activity in human cancer. Eur J Cancer. 1997;33(5):787–91.
71. Hastie ND, Dempster M, Dunlop MG, Thompson AM, Green DK, Allshire RC. Telomere reduction in human colorectal carcinoma and with ageing. Nature. 1990;346(6287):866–8.
72. Shay JW, Werbin H, Wright WE. Telomerase assays in the diagnosis and prognosis of cancer. Ciba Found Symp. 1997;211:148–55. discussion 55–9
73. Wong N, Adamczyk LA, Evans S, Cullen J, Oniscu A, Oien KA. A33 shows similar sensitivity to but is more specific than CDX2 as an immunomarker of colorectal carcinoma. Histopathology. 2017;71(1):34–41.
74. Locker GY, Hamilton S, Harris J, Jessup JM, Kemeny N, Macdonald JS, et al. ASCO 2006 update of recommendations for the use of tumor markers in gastrointestinal cancer. J Clin Oncol. 2006;24(33):5313–27.
75. Renehan AG, Egger M, Saunders MP, O'Dwyer ST. Impact on survival of intensive follow up after curative resection for colorectal cancer: systematic review and meta-analysis of randomised trials. BMJ. 2002;324(7341):813.
76. Forbes SA, Bhamra G, Bamford S, Dawson E, Kok C, Clements J, et al. The Catalogue of Somatic Mutations in Cancer (COSMIC). Curr Protoc Hum Genet. 2008;Chapter 10:Unit 10 1.
77. Yuan ZX, Wang XY, Qin QY, Chen DF, Zhong QH, Wang L, et al. The prognostic role of BRAF mutation in metastatic colorectal cancer receiving anti-EGFR monoclonal antibodies: a meta-analysis. PLoS One. 2013;8(6):e65995.
78. Sepulveda AR, Hamilton SR, Allegra CJ, Grody W, Cushman-Vokoun AM, Funkhouser WK, et al. Molecular biomarkers for the evaluation of colorectal cancer: guideline from the American Society for Clinical Pathology, College of American Pathologists, Association for Molecular Pathology, and American Society of Clinical Oncology. Arch Pathol Lab Med. 2017;141(5):625–57.
79. Tiwari AK, Roy HK, Lynch HT. Lynch syndrome in the 21st century: clinical perspectives. QJM. 2016;109(3):151–8.
80. Ward R, Meagher A, Tomlinson I, O'Connor T, Norrie M, Wu R, et al. Microsatellite instability and the clinicopathological features of sporadic colorectal cancer. Gut. 2001;48(6):821–9.
81. Chen TH, Chang SW, Huang CC, Wang KL, Yeh KT, Liu CN, et al. The prognostic significance of APC gene mutation and miR-21 expression in advanced-stage colorectal cancer. Color Dis. 2013;15(11):1367–74.
82. López I, Oliveira LP, Tucci P, Alvarez-Valín F, Coudry RA, Marín M. Different mutation profiles associated to P53 accumulation in colorectal cancer. Gene. 2012;499(1):81–7.
83. Russo A, Bazan V, Iacopetta B, Kerr D, Soussi T, Gebbia N, et al. The TP53 colorectal cancer international collaborative study on the prognostic and predictive significance of p53 mutation: influence of tumor site, type of mutation, and adjuvant treatment. J Clin Oncol. 2005;23(30):7518–28.

84. Ryan KM, Phillips AC, Vousden KH. Regulation and function of the p53 tumor suppressor protein. Curr Opin Cell Biol. 2001;13(3):332–7.
85. Du Y, Zhou X, Huang Z, Qiu T, Wang J, Zhu W, et al. Meta-analysis of the prognostic value of smad4 immunohistochemistry in various cancers. PLoS One. 2014;9(10):e110182.
86. Wasserman I, Lee LH, Ogino S, Marco MR, Wu C, Chen X, et al. SMAD4 loss in colorectal cancer patients correlates with recurrence, loss of immune infiltrate, and Chemoresistance. Clin Cancer Res. 2019;25(6):1948–56.
87. Yoo SY, Lee JA, Shin Y, Cho NY, Bae JM, Kang GH. Clinicopathological characterization and prognostic implication of SMAD4 expression in colorectal carcinoma. J Pathol Transl Med. 2019;53(5):289–97.
88. Markman B, Javier Ramos F, Capdevila J, Tabernero J. EGFR and KRAS in colorectal cancer. Adv Clin Chem. 2010;51:71–119.
89. Kiaris H, Spandidos D. Mutations of ras genes in human tumors (review). Int J Oncol. 1995;7(3):413–21.
90. Spandidos DA, Glarakis IS, Kotsinas A, Ergazaki M, Kiaris H. Ras oncogene activation in benign and malignant colorectal tumours. Tumori. 1995;81(3 Suppl):7–11.
91. Rajagopalan H, Bardelli A, Lengauer C, Kinzler KW, Vogelstein B, Velculescu VE. Tumorigenesis RAF/RAS oncogenes and mismatch-repair status. Nature. 2002;418 (6901):934.
92. Toon CW, Walsh MD, Chou A, Capper D, Clarkson A, Sioson L, et al. BRAFV600E immunohistochemistry facilitates universal screening of colorectal cancers for Lynch syndrome. Am J Surg Pathol. 2013;37(10):1592–602.
93. Rowland A, Dias MM, Wiese MD, Kichenadasse G, McKinnon RA, Karapetis CS, et al. Meta-analysis of BRAF mutation as a predictive biomarker of benefit from anti-EGFR monoclonal antibody therapy for RAS wild-type metastatic colorectal cancer. Br J Cancer. 2015;112(12):1888–94.
94. Kuan SF, Navina S, Cressman KL, Pai RK. Immunohistochemical detection of BRAF V600E mutant protein using the VE1 antibody in colorectal carcinoma is highly concordant with molecular testing but requires rigorous antibody optimization. Hum Pathol. 2014;45(3):464–72.
95. Samuels Y, Wang Z, Bardelli A, Silliman N, Ptak J, Szabo S, et al. High frequency of mutations of the PIK3CA gene in human cancers. Science. 2004;304(5670):554.
96. Michael JV, Wurtzel JG, Goldfinger LE. Regulation of H-Ras-driven MAPK signaling, transformation and tumorigenesis, but not PI3K signaling and tumor progression, by plasma membrane microdomains. Oncogenesis. 2016;5(5):e228.
97. Diehl F, Schmidt K, Choti MA, Romans K, Goodman S, Li M, et al. Circulating mutant DNA to assess tumor dynamics. Nat Med. 2008;14(9):985–90.
98. Schwarzenbach H, Stoehlmacher J, Pantel K, Goekkurt E. Detection and monitoring of cell-free DNA in blood of patients with colorectal cancer. Ann N Y Acad Sci. 2008;1137:190–6.
99. Spindler KL, Pallisgaard N, Andersen RF, Brandslund I, Jakobsen A. Circulating free DNA as biomarker and source for mutation detection in metastatic colorectal cancer. PLoS One. 2015;10(4):e0108247.
100. Califf RM. Biomarker definitions and their applications. Exp Biol Med (Maywood). 2018;243(3):213–21.
101. Valori R, Rey JF, Atkin WS, Bretthauer M, Senore C, Hoff G, et al. European guidelines for quality assurance in colorectal cancer screening and diagnosis. First Edition–Quality assurance in endoscopy in colorectal cancer screening and diagnosis. Endoscopy. 2012;44(Suppl 3):SE88–105.
102. Young GP, Symonds EL, Allison JE, Cole SR, Fraser CG, Halloran SP, et al. Advances in fecal occult blood tests: the FIT revolution. Dig Dis Sci. 2015;60(3):609–22.
103. Ahlquist DA, Harrington JJ, Burgart LJ, Roche PC. Morphometric analysis of the "mucocellular layer" overlying colorectal cancer and normal mucosa: relevance to exfoliation and stool screening. Hum Pathol. 2000;31(1):51–7.
104. Ahlquist DA. Molecular detection of colorectal neoplasia. Gastroenterology. 2010;138(6):2127–39.

105. Loktionov A, O'Neill IK, Silvester KR, Cummings JH, Middleton SJ, Miller R. Quantitation of DNA from exfoliated colonocytes isolated from human stool surface as a novel noninvasive screening test for colorectal cancer. Clin Cancer Res. 1998;4(2):337–42.
106. Diehl F, Schmidt K, Durkee KH, Moore KJ, Goodman SN, Shuber AP, et al. Analysis of mutations in DNA isolated from plasma and stool of colorectal cancer patients. Gastroenterology. 2008;135(2):489–98.
107. Itzkowitz S, Brand R, Jandorf L, Durkee K, Millholland J, Rabeneck L, et al. A simplified, noninvasive stool DNA test for colorectal cancer detection. Am J Gastroenterol. 2008;103(11):2862–70.
108. Oh HH, Joo YE. Novel biomarkers for the diagnosis and prognosis of colorectal cancer. Intest Res. 2020;18(2):168–83.
109. Sheng JQ, Li SR, Su H, Li JS, Sun ZQ, Wu ZT, et al. Fecal cytology in conjunction with immunofecal occult blood test for colorectal cancer screening. Anal Quant Cytol Histol. 2010;32(3):131–5.
110. Parente F, Marino B, Ilardo A, Fracasso P, Zullo A, Hassan C, et al. A combination of faecal tests for the detection of colon cancer: a new strategy for an appropriate selection of referrals to colonoscopy? A prospective multicentre Italian study. Eur J Gastroenterol Hepatol. 2012;24(10):1145–52.
111. Lee RC, Feinbaum RL, Ambros V. The C. elegans heterochronic gene lin-4 encodes small RNAs with antisense complementarity to lin-14. Cell. 1993;75(5):843–54.
112. He L, Hannon GJ. MicroRNAs: small RNAs with a big role in gene regulation. Nat Rev Genet. 2004;5(7):522–31.
113. Mendell JT. MicroRNAs: critical regulators of development, cellular physiology and malignancy. Cell Cycle. 2005;4(9):1179–84.
114. Creemers EE, Tijsen AJ, Pinto YM. Circulating microRNAs: novel biomarkers and extracellular communicators in cardiovascular disease? Circ Res. 2012;110(3):483–95.
115. Vickers KC, Palmisano BT, Shoucri BM, Shamburek RD, Remaley AT. MicroRNAs are transported in plasma and delivered to recipient cells by high-density lipoproteins. Nat Cell Biol. 2011;13(4):423–33.
116. Arroyo JD, Chevillet JR, Kroh EM, Ruf IK, Pritchard CC, Gibson DF, et al. Argonaute2 complexes carry a population of circulating microRNAs independent of vesicles in human plasma. Proc Natl Acad Sci U S A. 2011;108(12):5003–8.
117. Toiyama Y, Takahashi M, Hur K, Nagasaka T, Tanaka K, Inoue Y, et al. Serum miR-21 as a diagnostic and prognostic biomarker in colorectal cancer. J Natl Cancer Inst. 2013;105(12):849–59.
118. Mitchell PS, Parkin RK, Kroh EM, Fritz BR, Wyman SK, Pogosova-Agadjanyan EL, et al. Circulating microRNAs as stable blood-based markers for cancer detection. Proc Natl Acad Sci U S A. 2008;105(30):10513–8.
119. Link A, Balaguer F, Shen Y, Nagasaka T, Lozano JJ, Boland CR, et al. Fecal MicroRNAs as novel biomarkers for colon cancer screening. Cancer Epidemiol Biomark Prev. 2010;19(7):1766–74.
120. Masuda T, Hayashi N, Kuroda Y, Ito S, Eguchi H, Mimori K. MicroRNAs as biomarkers in colorectal cancer. Cancers. 2017;9(9):124.
121. Schee K, Fodstad O, Flatmark K. MicroRNAs as biomarkers in colorectal cancer. Am J Pathol. 2010;177(4):1592–9.
122. Geenen RW, Hussain SM, Cademartiri F, Poley JW, Siersema PD, Krestin GP. CT and MR colonography: scanning techniques, postprocessing, and emphasis on polyp detection. Radiographics. 2004;24(1):e18.
123. Liang PS, Dominitz JA. Colorectal cancer screening: is colonoscopy the best option? Med Clin North Am. 2019;103(1):111–23.
124. Church J. Complications of colonoscopy. Gastroenterol Clin N Am. 2013;42(3):639–57.
125. Alves Martins BA, de Bulhoes GF, Cavalcanti IN, Martins MM, de Oliveira PG, Martins AMA. Biomarkers in colorectal cancer: the role of translational proteomics research. Front Oncol. 2019;9:1284.

126. Schoen RE, Machicado JD. Detection of advanced neoplasia with FIT versus flexible sigmoidoscopy versus colonoscopy: more is more. Dig Dis Sci. 2015;60(5):1123–5.
127. Scholefield JH. ABC of colorectal cancer: screening. BMJ. 2000;321(7267):1004–6.
128. Winawer SJ, Stewart ET, Zauber AG, Bond JH, Ansel H, Waye JD, et al. A comparison of colonoscopy and double-contrast barium enema for surveillance after polypectomy. National Polyp Study Work Group. N Engl J Med. 2000;342(24):1766–72.
129. Rockey DC, Paulson E, Niedzwiecki D, Davis W, Bosworth HB, Sanders L, et al. Analysis of air contrast barium enema, computed tomographic colonography, and colonoscopy: prospective comparison. Lancet. 2005;365(9456):305–11.
130. Rex DK, Rahmani EY, Haseman JH, Lemmel GT, Kaster S, Buckley JS. Relative sensitivity of colonoscopy and barium enema for detection of colorectal cancer in clinical practice. Gastroenterology. 1997;112(1):17–23.
131. Chaparro M, Gisbert JP, Del Campo L, Cantero J, Mate J. Accuracy of computed tomographic colonography for the detection of polyps and colorectal tumors: a systematic review and meta-analysis. Digestion. 2009;80(1):1–17.
132. Scalise P, Mantarro A, Pancrazi F, Neri E. Computed tomography colonography for the practicing radiologist: a review of current recommendations on methodology and clinical indications. World J Radiol. 2016;8(5):472–83.
133. Galdino GM, Yee J. Carpet lesion on CT colonography: a potential pitfall. AJR Am J Roentgenol. 2003;180(5):1332–4.
134. Pickhardt PJ, Hassan C, Halligan S, Marmo R. Colorectal cancer: CT colonography and colonoscopy for detection–systematic review and meta-analysis. Radiology. 2011;259(2):393–405.
135. Pappalardo G, Polettini E, Frattaroli FM, Casciani E, D'Orta C, D'Amato M, et al. Magnetic resonance colonography versus conventional colonoscopy for the detection of colonic endoluminal lesions. Gastroenterology. 2000;119(2):300–4.
136. Angtuaco TL, Banaad-Omiotek GD, Howden CW. Differing attitudes toward virtual and conventional colonoscopy for colorectal cancer screening: surveys among primary care physicians and potential patients. Am J Gastroenterol. 2001;96(3):887–93.
137. Lauenstein T, Holtmann G, Schoenfelder D, Bosk S, Ruehm SG, Debatin JF. MR colonography without colonic cleansing: a new strategy to improve patient acceptance. AJR Am J Roentgenol. 2001;177(4):823–7.
138. Florie J, Birnie E, van Gelder RE, Jensch S, Haberkorn B, Bartelsman JF, et al. MR colonography with limited bowel preparation: patient acceptance compared with that of full-preparation colonoscopy. Radiology. 2007;245(1):150–9.
139. Debatin JF, Lauenstein TC. Virtual magnetic resonance colonography. Gut. 2003;52(Suppl 4):iv17–22.
140. Zalis ME, Barish MA, Choi JR, Dachman AH, Fenlon HM, Ferrucci JT, et al. CT colonography reporting and data system: a consensus proposal. Radiology. 2005;236(1):3–9.
141. Yusuf E, Florie J, Nio CY, Jensch S, Nievelstein RA, Baak L, et al. Incidental extracolonic findings on bright lumen MR colonography in a population at increased risk for colorectal carcinoma. Eur J Radiol. 2011;78(1):135–41.
142. Kuipers EJ, Rosch T, Bretthauer M. Colorectal cancer screening–optimizing current strategies and new directions. Nat Rev Clin Oncol. 2013;10(3):130–42.
143. Taliano RJ, LeGolvan M, Resnick MB. Immunohistochemistry of colorectal carcinoma: current practice and evolving applications. Hum Pathol. 2013;44(2):151–63.
144. Sharma MR, Schilsky RL. GI cancers in 2010: new standards and a predictive biomarker for adjuvant therapy. Nat Rev Clin Oncol. 2011;8(2):70–2.
145. Anderson GG, Weiss LM. Determining tissue of origin for metastatic cancers: meta-analysis and literature review of immunohistochemistry performance. Appl Immunohistochem Mol Morphol. 2010;18(1):3–8.
146. Stenling R, Lindberg J, Rutegard J, Palmqvist R. Altered expression of CK7 and CK20 in preneoplastic and neoplastic lesions in ulcerative colitis. APMIS. 2007;115(11):1219–26.
147. Righi A, Betts CM, Marchetti C, Marucci G, Montebugnoli L, Prati C, et al. Merkel cells in the oral mucosa. Int J Surg Pathol. 2006;14(3):206–11.

148. Radovic S, Selak I, Babic M, Vukobrat-Bijedic Z, Knezevic Z. Anti-cytokeratin 7: a positive marker for epithelial dysplasia in flat bowel mucosa. Bosn J Basic Med Sci. 2004;4(3):24–30.
149. Gurzu S, Jung I. Aberrant pattern of the cytokeratin 7/cytokeratin 20 immunophenotype in colorectal adenocarcinomas with BRAF mutations. Pathol Res Pract. 2012;208(3):163–6.
150. Chu P, Wu E, Weiss LM. Cytokeratin 7 and cytokeratin 20 expression in epithelial neoplasms: a survey of 435 cases. Mod Pathol. 2000;13(9):962–72.
151. Hernandez BY, Frierson HF, Moskaluk CA, Li YJ, Clegg L, Cote TR, et al. CK20 and CK7 protein expression in colorectal cancer: demonstration of the utility of a population-based tissue microarray. Hum Pathol. 2005;36(3):275–81.
152. Clevers H. Wnt/beta-catenin signaling in development and disease. Cell. 2006;127(3):469–80.
153. Bretscher A, Weber K. Villin: the major microfilament-associated protein of the intestinal microvillus. Proc Natl Acad Sci U S A. 1979;76(5):2321–5.
154. Patnaik S, George SP, Pham E, Roy S, Singh K, Mariadason JM, et al. By moonlighting in the nucleus, villin regulates epithelial plasticity. Mol Biol Cell. 2016;27(3):535–48.
155. Bacchi CE, Gown AM. Distribution and pattern of expression of villin, a gastrointestinal-associated cytoskeletal protein, in human carcinomas: a study employing paraffin-embedded tissue. Lab Investig. 1991;64(3):418–24.
156. Silberg DG, Swain GP, Suh ER, Traber PG. Cdx1 and cdx2 expression during intestinal development. Gastroenterology. 2000;119(4):961–71.
157. Zheng J, He S, Qi J, Wang X, Yu J, Wu Y, et al. Targeted CDX2 expression inhibits aggressive phenotypes of colon cancer cells in vitro and in vivo. Int J Oncol. 2017;51(2):478–88.
158. Dobreva G, Dambacher J, Grosschedl R. SUMO modification of a novel MAR-binding protein, SATB2, modulates immunoglobulin mu gene expression. Genes Dev. 2003;17(24):3048–61.
159. Perez Montiel D, Arispe Angulo K, Cantu-de Leon D, Bornstein Quevedo L, Chanona Vilchis J, Herrera Montalvo L. The value of SATB2 in the differential diagnosis of intestinal-type mucinous tumors of the ovary: primary vs metastatic. Ann Diagn Pathol. 2015;19(4):249–52.
160. Moh M, Krings G, Ates D, Aysal A, Kim GE, Rabban JT. SATB2 expression distinguishes ovarian metastases of colorectal and appendiceal origin from primary ovarian tumors of mucinous or endometrioid type. Am J Surg Pathol. 2016;40(3):419–32.
161. Bian T, Zhao J, Feng J, Zhang Q, Qian L, Liu J, et al. Combination of cadherin-17 and SATB homeobox 2 serves as potential optimal makers for the differential diagnosis of pulmonary enteric adenocarcinoma and metastatic colorectal adenocarcinoma. Oncotarget. 2017;8(38):63442–52.
162. Andrianifahanana M, Moniaux N, Batra SK. Regulation of mucin expression: mechanistic aspects and implications for cancer and inflammatory diseases. Biochim Biophys Acta. 2006;1765(2):189–222.
163. Hollingsworth MA, Swanson BJ. Mucins in cancer: protection and control of the cell surface. Nat Rev Cancer. 2004;4(1):45–60.
164. Itoh Y, Kamata-Sakurai M, Denda-Nagai K, Nagai S, Tsuiji M, Ishii-Schrade K, et al. Identification and expression of human epiglycanin/MUC21: a novel transmembrane mucin. Glycobiology. 2008;18(1):74–83.
165. Krishn SR, Kaur S, Smith LM, Johansson SL, Jain M, Patel A, et al. Mucins and associated glycan signatures in colon adenoma-carcinoma sequence: prospective pathological implication(s) for early diagnosis of colon cancer. Cancer Lett. 2016;374(2):304–14.
166. Hayashi T, Takahashi T, Motoya S, Ishida T, Itoh F, Adachi M, et al. MUC1 mucin core protein binds to the domain 1 of ICAM-1. Digestion. 2001;63(Suppl 1):87–92.
167. Mohr AM, Bailey JM, Lewallen ME, Liu X, Radhakrishnan P, Yu F, et al. MUC1 regulates expression of multiple microRNAs involved in pancreatic tumor progression, including the miR-200c/141 cluster. PLoS One. 2013;8(10):e73306.
168. Roy LD, Sahraei M, Subramani DB, Besmer D, Nath S, Tinder TL, et al. MUC1 enhances invasiveness of pancreatic cancer cells by inducing epithelial to mesenchymal transition. Oncogene. 2011;30(12):1449–59.
169. Hansson GC, Johansson ME. The inner of the two Muc2 mucin-dependent mucus layers in colon is devoid of bacteria. Gut Microbes. 2010;1(1):51–4.

170. Hoshi H, Sawada T, Uchida M, Saito H, Iijima H, Toda-Agetsuma M, et al. Tumor-associated MUC5AC stimulates in vivo tumorigenicity of human pancreatic cancer. Int J Oncol. 2011;38(3):619–27.
171. King RJ, Yu F, Singh PK. Genomic alterations in mucins across cancers. Oncotarget. 2017;8(40):67152–68.
172. Maitre JL, Heisenberg CP. Three functions of cadherins in cell adhesion. Curr Biol. 2013;23(14):R626–33.
173. Makrilia N, Kollias A, Manolopoulos L, Syrigos K. Cell adhesion molecules: role and clinical significance in cancer. Cancer Investig. 2009;27(10):1023–37.
174. Dantzig AH, Hoskins JA, Tabas LB, Bright S, Shepard RL, Jenkins IL, et al. Association of intestinal peptide transport with a protein related to the cadherin superfamily. Science. 1994;264(5157):430–3.
175. Gessner R, Tauber R. Intestinal cell adhesion molecules. Liver-intestine cadherin. Ann N Y Acad Sci. 2000;915:136–43.
176. Takamura M, Ichida T, Matsuda Y, Kobayashi M, Yamagiwa S, Genda T, et al. Reduced expression of liver-intestine cadherin is associated with progression and lymph node metastasis of human colorectal carcinoma. Cancer Lett. 2004;212(2):253–9.
177. Dennis JL, Hvidsten TR, Wit EC, Komorowski J, Bell AK, Downie I, et al. Markers of adenocarcinoma characteristic of the site of origin: development of a diagnostic algorithm. Clin Cancer Res. 2005;11(10):3766–72.
178. Panarelli NC, Yantiss RK, Yeh MM, Liu Y, Chen YT. Tissue-specific cadherin CDH17 is a useful marker of gastrointestinal adenocarcinomas with higher sensitivity than CDX2. Am J Clin Pathol. 2012;138(2):211–22.
179. Murnane JP. Telomere dysfunction and chromosome instability. Mutat Res. 2012;730(1–2):28–36.
180. Fernandez-Rozadilla C, Kartsonaki C, Woolley C, McClellan M, Whittington D, Horgan G, et al. Telomere length and genetics are independent colorectal tumour risk factors in an evaluation of biomarkers in normal bowel. Br J Cancer. 2018;118(5):727–32.
181. Peacock SD, Massey TE, Vanner SJ, King WD. Telomere length in the colon is related to colorectal adenoma prevalence. PLoS One. 2018;13(10):e0205697.
182. Heath JK, White SJ, Johnstone CN, Catimel B, Simpson RJ, Moritz RL, et al. The human A33 antigen is a transmembrane glycoprotein and a novel member of the immunoglobulin superfamily. Proc Natl Acad Sci U S A. 1997;94(2):469–74.
183. Pereira-Fantini PM, Judd LM, Kalantzis A, Peterson A, Ernst M, Heath JK, et al. A33 antigen-deficient mice have defective colonic mucosal repair. Inflamm Bowel Dis. 2010; 16(4):604–12.
184. Heitzer E, Perakis S, Geigl JB, Speicher MR. The potential of liquid biopsies for the early detection of cancer. NPJ Precis Oncol. 2017;1(1):36.
185. Buder A, Tomuta C, Filipits M. The potential of liquid biopsies. Curr Opin Oncol. 2016;28(2):130–4.
186. Perakis S, Speicher MR. Emerging concepts in liquid biopsies. BMC Med. 2017;15(1):75.
187. El-Gayar D, El-Abd N, Hassan N, Ali R. Increased free circulating DNA integrity index as a serum biomarker in patients with colorectal carcinoma. Asian Pac J Cancer Prev. 2016;17(3):939–44.
188. Taback B, Saha S, Hoon DS. Comparative analysis of mesenteric and peripheral blood circulating tumor DNA in colorectal cancer patients. Ann N Y Acad Sci. 2006;1075:197–203.
189. Lazarev I, Leibovitch L, Czeiger D, Sion-Vardi N, Geffen DB, Douvdevani A, et al. Cell-free DNA blood levels in colorectal cancer patients do not correlate with mismatch repair-proficiency. In Vivo. 2014;28(3):349–54.
190. Hauptman N, Glavac D. Colorectal cancer blood-based biomarkers. Gastroenterol Res Pract. 2017;2017:2195361.
191. Warren JD, Xiong W, Bunker AM, Vaughn CP, Furtado LV, Roberts WL, et al. Septin 9 methylated DNA is a sensitive and specific blood test for colorectal cancer. BMC Med. 2011;9:133.

192. Tanzer M, Balluff B, Distler J, Hale K, Leodolter A, Rocken C, et al. Performance of epigenetic markers SEPT9 and ALX4 in plasma for detection of colorectal precancerous lesions. PLoS One. 2010;5(2):e9061.
193. Danese E, Montagnana M. Epigenetics of colorectal cancer: emerging circulating diagnostic and prognostic biomarkers. Ann Transl Med. 2017;5(13):279.
194. Church TR, Wandell M, Lofton-Day C, Mongin SJ, Burger M, Payne SR, et al. Prospective evaluation of methylated SEPT9 in plasma for detection of asymptomatic colorectal cancer. Gut. 2014;63(2):317–25.
195. Weber JA, Baxter DH, Zhang S, Huang DY, Huang KH, Lee MJ, et al. The microRNA spectrum in 12 body fluids. Clin Chem. 2010;56(11):1733–41.
196. Pennisi E. Genomics ENCODE project writes eulogy for junk DNA. Science. 2012;337(6099):1159. 61
197. Mattick JS, Makunin IV. Non-coding RNA. Human Mol Genet. 2006;15 Spec No 1:R17–29.
198. Harfe BD. MicroRNAs in vertebrate development. Curr Opin Genet Dev. 2005;15(4):410–5.
199. Chen B, Li H, Zeng X, Yang P, Liu X, Zhao X, et al. Roles of microRNA on cancer cell metabolism. J Transl Med. 2012;10:228.
200. Vannini I, Fanini F, Fabbri M. Emerging roles of microRNAs in cancer. Curr Opin Genet Dev. 2018;48:128–33.
201. Wahid F, Shehzad A, Khan T, Kim YY. MicroRNAs: synthesis, mechanism, function, and recent clinical trials. Biochim Biophys Acta. 2010;1803(11):1231–43.
202. Berger F, Reiser MF. Micro-RNAs as potential new molecular biomarkers in oncology: have they reached relevance for the clinical imaging sciences? Theranostics. 2013;3(12):943–52.
203. Chen B, Liu Y, Jin X, Lu W, Liu J, Xia Z, et al. MicroRNA-26a regulates glucose metabolism by direct targeting PDHX in colorectal cancer cells. BMC Cancer. 2014;14:443.
204. Wei WT, Nian XX, Wang SY, Jiao HL, Wang YX, Xiao ZY, et al. miR-422a inhibits cell proliferation in colorectal cancer by targeting AKT1 and MAPK1. Cancer Cell Int. 2017;17:91.
205. Humphreys KJ, McKinnon RA, Michael MZ. miR-18a inhibits CDC42 and plays a tumour suppressor role in colorectal cancer cells. PLoS One. 2014;9(11):e112288.
206. Liu J, Chen Z, Xiang J, Gu X. MicroRNA-155 acts as a tumor suppressor in colorectal cancer by targeting CTHRC1 in vitro. Oncol Lett. 2018;15(4):5561–8.
207. Chen S, Wang Y, Su Y, Zhang L, Zhang M, Li X, et al. miR2055p/PTK7 axis is involved in the proliferation, migration and invasion of colorectal cancer cells. Mol Med Rep. 2018;17(5):6253–60.
208. Gulei D, Magdo L, Jurj A, Raduly L, Cojocneanu-Petric R, Moldovan A, et al. The silent healer: miR-205-5p up-regulation inhibits epithelial to mesenchymal transition in colon cancer cells by indirectly up-regulating E-cadherin expression. Cell Death Dis. 2018;9(2):66.
209. Liu N, Jiang F, Han XY, Li M, Chen WJ, Liu QC, et al. MiRNA-155 promotes the invasion of colorectal cancer SW-480 cells through regulating the Wnt/beta-catenin. Eur Rev Med Pharmacol Sci. 2018;22(1):101–9.
210. Lu D, Tang L, Zhuang Y, Zhao P. miR-17-3P regulates the proliferation and survival of colon cancer cells by targeting Par4. Mol Med Rep. 2018;17(1):618–23.
211. Li KP, Fang YP, Liao JQ, Duan JD, Feng LG, Luo XZ, et al. Upregulation of miR598 promotes cell proliferation and cell cycle progression in human colorectal carcinoma by suppressing INPP5E expression. Mol Med Rep. 2018;17(2):2991–7.
212. Zhang Y, Guo L, Li Y, Feng GH, Teng F, Li W, et al. MicroRNA-494 promotes cancer progression and targets adenomatous polyposis coli in colorectal cancer. Mol Cancer. 2018;17(1):1.
213. Pothoulakis C, Torre-Rojas M, Duran-Padilla MA, Gevorkian J, Zoras O, Chrysos E, et al. CRHR2/Ucn2 signaling is a novel regulator of miR-7/YY1/Fas circuitry contributing to reversal of colorectal cancer cell resistance to Fas-mediated apoptosis. Int J Cancer. 2018;142(2):334–46.
214. Qin Y, Huo Z, Song X, Chen X, Tian X. Wang X. mir-106a regulates cell proliferation and apoptosis of colon cancer cells through targeting the PTEN/PI3K/AKT signaling pathway. Oncol Lett. 2018;15(3):3197–201.

215. Hu JL, He GY, Lan XL, Zeng ZC, Guan J, Ding Y, et al. Inhibition of ATG12-mediated autophagy by miR-214 enhances radiosensitivity in colorectal cancer. Oncogenesis. 2018;7(2):16.
216. Liao D, Li T, Ye C, Zeng L, Li H, Pu X, et al. miR-221 inhibits autophagy and targets TP53INP1 in colorectal cancer cells. Exp Ther Med. 2018;15(2):1712–7.
217. Cruz-Gil S, Sanchez-Martinez R, Gomez de Cedron M, Martin-Hernandez R, Vargas T, Molina S, et al. Targeting the lipid metabolic axis ACSL/SCD in colorectal cancer progression by therapeutic miRNAs: miR-19b-1 role. J Lipid Res. 2018;59(1):14–24.
218. Zhao J, Xu J, Zhang R. SRPX2 regulates colon cancer cell metabolism by miR-192/215 via PI3K-Akt. Am J Transl Res. 2018;10(2):483–90.
219. Yan TT, Ren LL, Shen CQ, Wang ZH, Yu YN, Liang Q, et al. miR-508 defines the stem-like/mesenchymal subtype in colorectal cancer. Cancer Res. 2018;78(7):1751–65.
220. Liu R, Lu Z, Gu J, Liu J, Huang E, Liu X, et al. MicroRNAs 15A and 16-1 activate signaling pathways that mediate chemotaxis of immune regulatory B cells to colorectal tumors. Gastroenterology. 2018;154(3):637–51.e7.
221. Cheng YW, Chou CJ, Yang PM. Ten-eleven translocation 1 (TET1) gene is a potential target of miR-21-5p in human colorectal cancer. Surg Oncol. 2018;27(1):76–81.
222. Du B, Wu D, Yang X, Wang T, Shi X, Lv Y, et al. The expression and significance of microRNA in different stages of colorectal cancer. Medicine (Baltimore). 2018;97(5):e9635.
223. Kandimalla R, Gao F, Matsuyama T, Ishikawa T, Uetake H, Takahashi N, et al. Genome-wide discovery and identification of a novel miRNA signature for recurrence prediction in stage II and III colorectal cancer. Clin Cancer Res. 2018;24(16):3867–77.
224. Xu P, Wang J, Sun B, Xiao Z. Integrated analysis of miRNA and mRNA expression data identifies multiple miRNAs regulatory networks for the tumorigenesis of colorectal cancer. Gene. 2018;659:44–51.
225. Vishnubalaji R, Hamam R, Abdulla MH, Mohammed MA, Kassem M, Al-Obeed O, et al. Genome-wide mRNA and miRNA expression profiling reveal multiple regulatory networks in colorectal cancer. Cell Death Dis. 2015;6:e1614.
226. Slattery ML, Mullany LE, Sakoda L, Samowitz WS, Wolff RK, Stevens JR, et al. The NF-kappaB signalling pathway in colorectal cancer: associations between dysregulated gene and miRNA expression. J Cancer Res Clin Oncol. 2018;144(2):269–83.
227. Chen B, Xia Z, Deng YN, Yang Y, Zhang P, Zhu H, et al. Emerging microRNA biomarkers for colorectal cancer diagnosis and prognosis. Open Biol. 2019;9(1):180212.
228. Tanaka T, Tanaka M, Tanaka T, Ishigamori R. Biomarkers for colorectal cancer. Int J Mol Sci. 2010;11(9):3209–25.
229. Sazanov AA, Kiselyova EV, Zakharenko AA, Romanov MN, Zaraysky MI. Plasma and saliva miR-21 expression in colorectal cancer patients. J Appl Genet. 2017;58(2):231–7.
230. Maierthaler M, Benner A, Hoffmeister M, Surowy H, Jansen L, Knebel P, et al. Plasma miR-122 and miR-200 family are prognostic markers in colorectal cancer. Int J Cancer. 2017;140(1):176–87.
231. He HW, Wang NN, Yi XM, Tang CP, Wang D. Low-level serum miR-24-2 is associated with the progression of colorectal cancer. Cancer Biomark. 2018;21(2):261–7.
232. Wang Q, Zhang H, Shen X, Ju S. Serum microRNA-135a-5p as an auxiliary diagnostic biomarker for colorectal cancer. Ann Clin Biochem. 2017;54(1):76–85.
233. Miyoshi J, Toden S, Yoshida K, Toiyama Y, Alberts SR, Kusunoki M, et al. MiR-139-5p as a novel serum biomarker for recurrence and metastasis in colorectal cancer. Sci Rep. 2017;7:43393.
234. Ng L, Wan TM, Man JH, Chow AK, Iyer D, Chen G, et al. Identification of serum miR-139-3p as a non-invasive biomarker for colorectal cancer. Oncotarget. 2017;8(16):27393–400.
235. Hur K, Toiyama Y, Okugawa Y, Ide S, Imaoka H, Boland CR, et al. Circulating microRNA-203 predicts prognosis and metastasis in human colorectal cancer. Gut. 2017;66(4):654–65.
236. Liu HN, Liu TT, Wu H, Chen YJ, Tseng YJ, Yao C, et al. Serum microRNA signatures and metabolomics have high diagnostic value in colorectal cancer using two novel methods. Cancer Sci. 2018;109(4):1185–94.

237. Fang Z, Tang J, Bai Y, Lin H, You H, Jin H, et al. Plasma levels of microRNA-24, microRNA-320a, and microRNA-423-5p are potential biomarkers for colorectal carcinoma. J Exp Clin Cancer Res. 2015;34:86.
238. Tsukamoto M, Iinuma H, Yagi T, Matsuda K, Hashiguchi Y. Circulating Exosomal MicroRNA-21 as a biomarker in each tumor stage of colorectal cancer. Oncology. 2017;92(6):360–70.
239. Yan S, Jiang Y, Liang C, Cheng M, Jin C, Duan Q, et al. Exosomal miR-6803-5p as potential diagnostic and prognostic marker in colorectal cancer. J Cell Biochem. 2018;119(5):4113–9.
240. Ghanbari R, Mosakhani N, Asadi J, Nouraee N, Mowla SJ, Poustchi H, et al. Decreased expression of fecal miR-4478 and miR-1295b-3p in early-stage colorectal cancer. Cancer Biomark. 2015;15(2):189–95.
241. Berindan-Neagoe I, Monroig Pdel C, Pasculli B, Calin GA. MicroRNAome genome: a treasure for cancer diagnosis and therapy. CA Cancer J Clin. 2014;64(5):311–36.
242. Wu WK, Law PT, Lee CW, Cho CH, Fan D, Wu K, et al. MicroRNA in colorectal cancer: from benchtop to bedside. Carcinogenesis. 2011;32(3):247–53.
243. Dong Y, Wu WK, Wu CW, Sung JJ, Yu J, Ng SS. MicroRNA dysregulation in colorectal cancer: a clinical perspective. Br J Cancer. 2011;104(6):893–8.
244. Giraldez MD, Lozano JJ, Ramirez G, Hijona E, Bujanda L, Castells A, et al. Circulating microRNAs as biomarkers of colorectal cancer: results from a genome-wide profiling and validation study. Clin Gastroenterol Hepatol. 2013;11(6):681–8.e3.
245. Ya G, Wang H, Ma Y, Hu A, Ma Y, Hu J, et al. Serum miR-129 functions as a biomarker for colorectal cancer by targeting estrogen receptor (ER) beta. Pharmazie. 2017;72(2):107–12.
246. Wu CW, Ng SC, Dong Y, Tian L, Ng SS, Leung WW, et al. Identification of microRNA-135b in stool as a potential noninvasive biomarker for colorectal cancer and adenoma. Clin Cancer Res. 2014;20(11):2994–3002.
247. Koga Y, Yamazaki N, Yamamoto Y, Yamamoto S, Saito N, Kakugawa Y, et al. Fecal miR-106a is a useful marker for colorectal cancer patients with false-negative results in immunochemical fecal occult blood test. Cancer Epidemiol Biomark Prev. 2013;22(10):1844–52.
248. Chang PY, Chen CC, Chang YS, Tsai WS, You JF, Lin GP, et al. MicroRNA-223 and microRNA-92a in stool and plasma samples act as complementary biomarkers to increase colorectal cancer detection. Oncotarget. 2016;7(9):10663–75.
249. Wang YN, Chen ZH, Chen WC. Novel circulating microRNAs expression profile in colon cancer: a pilot study. Eur J Med Res. 2017;22(1):51.
250. Ma Y, Zhang P, Yang J, Liu Z, Yang Z, Qin H. Candidate microRNA biomarkers in human colorectal cancer: systematic review profiling studies and experimental validation. Int J Cancer. 2012;130(9):2077–87.
251. Ahmed FE, Amed NC, Vos PW, Bonnerup C, Atkins JN, Casey M, et al. Diagnostic microRNA markers to screen for sporadic human colon cancer in blood. Cancer Genomics Proteomics. 2012;9(4):179–92.
252. Kanaan Z, Rai SN, Eichenberger MR, Roberts H, Keskey B, Pan J, et al. Plasma miR-21: a potential diagnostic marker of colorectal cancer. Ann Surg. 2012;256(3):544–51.
253. Wang J, Huang SK, Zhao M, Yang M, Zhong JL, Gu YY, et al. Identification of a circulating microRNA signature for colorectal cancer detection. PLoS One. 2014;9(4):e87451.
254. Ahmed FE, Ahmed NC, Vos PW, Bonnerup C, Atkins JN, Casey M, et al. Diagnostic microRNA markers to screen for sporadic human colon cancer in stool: I. Proof of principle. Cancer Genomics Proteomics. 2013;10(3):93–113.
255. Yiu AJ, Yiu CY. Biomarkers in colorectal cancer. Anticancer Res. 2016;36(3):1093–102.
256. Ogata-Kawata H, Izumiya M, Kurioka D, Honma Y, Yamada Y, Furuta K, et al. Circulating exosomal microRNAs as biomarkers of colon cancer. PLoS One. 2014;9(4):e92921.
257. Uratani R, Toiyama Y, Kitajima T, Kawamura M, Hiro J, Kobayashi M, et al. Diagnostic potential of cell-free and Exosomal MicroRNAs in the identification of patients with high-risk colorectal adenomas. PLoS One. 2016;11(10):e0160722.
258. Kalluri R. The biology and function of exosomes in cancer. J Clin Invest. 2016;126(4):1208–15.

259. Szajnik M, Derbis M, Lach M, Patalas P, Michalak M, Drzewiecka H, et al. Exosomes in plasma of patients with ovarian carcinoma: potential biomarkers of tumor progression and response to therapy. Gynecol Obstet (Sunnyvale). 2013;Suppl 4:3.
260. Valadi H, Ekstrom K, Bossios A, Sjostrand M, Lee JJ, Lotvall JO. Exosome-mediated transfer of mRNAs and microRNAs is a novel mechanism of genetic exchange between cells. Nat Cell Biol. 2007;9(6):654–9.
261. Lotvall J, Valadi H. Cell to cell signalling via exosomes through esRNA. Cell Adhes Migr. 2007;1(3):156–8.
262. Lucchetti D, Calapa F, Palmieri V, Fanali C, Carbone F, Papa A, et al. Differentiation affects the release of exosomes from colon cancer cells and their ability to modulate the behavior of recipient cells. Am J Pathol. 2017;187(7):1633–47.
263. Rai A, Greening DW, Chen M, Xu R, Ji H, Simpson RJ. Exosomes derived from human primary and metastatic colorectal cancer cells contribute to functional heterogeneity of activated fibroblasts by reprogramming their proteome. Proteomics. 2019;19(8):e1800148.
264. Zaborowski MP, Balaj L, Breakefield XO, Lai CP. Extracellular vesicles: composition, biological relevance, and methods of study. Bioscience. 2015;65(8):783–97.
265. Andaloussi SEL, Mäger I, Breakefield XO, Wood MJA. Extracellular vesicles: biology and emerging therapeutic opportunities. Nat Rev Drug Discov. 2013;12(5):347–57.
266. Thery C, Boussac M, Veron P, Ricciardi-Castagnoli P, Raposo G, Garin J, et al. Proteomic analysis of dendritic cell-derived exosomes: a secreted subcellular compartment distinct from apoptotic vesicles. J Immunol. 2001;166(12):7309–18.
267. Gasser O, Hess C, Miot S, Deon C, Sanchez JC, Schifferli JA. Characterisation and properties of ectosomes released by human polymorphonuclear neutrophils. Exp Cell Res. 2003;285(2):243–57.
268. Heijnen HF, Schiel AE, Fijnheer R, Geuze HJ, Sixma JJ. Activated platelets release two types of membrane vesicles: microvesicles by surface shedding and exosomes derived from exocytosis of multivesicular bodies and alpha-granules. Blood. 1999;94(11):3791–9.
269. Simpson RJ, Lim JW, Moritz RL, Mathivanan S. Exosomes: proteomic insights and diagnostic potential. Expert Rev Proteomics. 2009;6(3):267–83.
270. Melo SA, Sugimoto H, O'Connell JT, Kato N, Villanueva A, Vidal A, et al. Cancer exosomes perform cell-independent microRNA biogenesis and promote tumorigenesis. Cancer Cell. 2014;26(5):707–21.
271. Popena I, Abols A, Saulite L, Pleiko K, Zandberga E, Jekabsons K, et al. Effect of colorectal cancer-derived extracellular vesicles on the immunophenotype and cytokine secretion profile of monocytes and macrophages. Cell Commun Signal. 2018;16(1):17.
272. Manning S, Danielson KM. The immunomodulatory role of tumor-derived extracellular vesicles in colorectal cancer. Immunol Cell Biol. 2018; https://doi.org/10.1111/imcb.12038.
273. Matsumura T, Sugimachi K, Iinuma H, Takahashi Y, Kurashige J, Sawada G, et al. Exosomal microRNA in serum is a novel biomarker of recurrence in human colorectal cancer. Br J Cancer. 2015;113(2):275–81.
274. Liu C, Eng C, Shen J, Lu Y, Takata Y, Mehdizadeh A, et al. Serum exosomal miR-4772-3p is a predictor of tumor recurrence in stage II and III colon cancer. Oncotarget. 2016;7(46):76250–60.
275. Novikova IV, Hennelly SP, Sanbonmatsu KY. Tackling structures of long noncoding RNAs. Int J Mol Sci. 2013;14(12):23672–84.
276. Iyer MK, Niknafs YS, Malik R, Singhal U, Sahu A, Hosono Y, et al. The landscape of long noncoding RNAs in the human transcriptome. Nat Genet. 2015;47(3):199–208.
277. Uszczynska-Ratajczak B, Lagarde J, Frankish A, Guigo R, Johnson R. Towards a complete map of the human long non-coding RNA transcriptome. Nat Rev Genet. 2018;19(9):535–48.
278. Kashi K, Henderson L, Bonetti A, Carninci P. Discovery and functional analysis of lncRNAs: methodologies to investigate an uncharacterized transcriptome. Biochim Biophys Acta. 2016;1859(1):3–15.
279. Jia H, Osak M, Bogu GK, Stanton LW, Johnson R, Lipovich L. Genome-wide computational identification and manual annotation of human long noncoding RNA genes. RNA. 2010;16(8):1478–87.

280. Hombach S, Kretz M. Non-coding RNAs: classification, biology and functioning. Adv Exp Med Biol. 2016;937:3–17.
281. Derrien T, Johnson R, Bussotti G, Tanzer A, Djebali S, Tilgner H, et al. The GENCODE v7 catalog of human long noncoding RNAs: analysis of their gene structure, evolution, and expression. Genome Res. 2012;22(9):1775–89.
282. Cabili MN, Dunagin MC, McClanahan PD, Biaesch A, Padovan-Merhar O, Regev A, et al. Localization and abundance analysis of human lncRNAs at single-cell and single-molecule resolution. Genome Biol. 2015;16:20.
283. Hung T, Chang HY. Long noncoding RNA in genome regulation: prospects and mechanisms. RNA Biol. 2010;7(5):582–5.
284. Zeng P, Chen J, Meng Y, Zhou Y, Yang J, Cui Q. Defining essentiality score of protein-coding genes and long noncoding RNAs. Front Genet. 2018;9:380.
285. Antonov IV, Mazurov E, Borodovsky M, Medvedeva YA. Prediction of lncRNAs and their interactions with nucleic acids: benchmarking bioinformatics tools. Brief Bioinform. 2019;20(2):551–64.
286. Kang YJ, Yang DC, Kong L, Hou M, Meng YQ, Wei L, et al. CPC2: a fast and accurate coding potential calculator based on sequence intrinsic features. Nucleic Acids Res. 2017;45(W1):W12–W6.
287. Xu MD, Qi P, Du X. Long non-coding RNAs in colorectal cancer: implications for pathogenesis and clinical application. Mod Pathol. 2014;27(10):1310–20.
288. Rowley MJ, Bohmdorfer G, Wierzbicki AT. Analysis of long non-coding RNAs produced by a specialized RNA polymerase in Arabidopsis thaliana. Methods. 2013;63(2):160–9.
289. Yang Y, Junjie P, Sanjun C, Ma Y. Long non-coding RNAs in colorectal cancer: progression and future directions. J Cancer. 2017;8(16):3212–25.
290. Da Sacco L, Baldassarre A, Masotti A. Bioinformatics tools and novel challenges in long non-coding RNAs (lncRNAs) functional analysis. Int J Mol Sci. 2012;13(1):97–114.
291. Hu G, Niu F, Humburg BA, Liao K, Bendi S, Callen S, et al. Molecular mechanisms of long noncoding RNAs and their role in disease pathogenesis. Oncotarget. 2018;9(26): 18648–63.
292. Chi Y, Wang D, Wang J, Yu W, Yang J. Long non-coding RNA in the pathogenesis of cancers. Cell. 2019;8(9):1015.
293. Rinn JL, Chang HY. Genome regulation by long noncoding RNAs. Annu Rev Biochem. 2012;81:145–66.
294. Moran VA, Perera RJ, Khalil AM. Emerging functional and mechanistic paradigms of mammalian long non-coding RNAs. Nucleic Acids Res. 2012;40(14):6391–400.
295. Spurlock CF 3rd, Crooke PS 3rd, Aune TM. Biogenesis and transcriptional regulation of long noncoding RNAs in the human immune system. J Immunol. 2016;197(12):4509–17.
296. Wang KC, Chang HY. Molecular mechanisms of long noncoding RNAs. Mol Cell. 2011;43(6):904–14.
297. Tsang WP, Ng EK, Ng SS, Jin H, Yu J, Sung JJ, et al. Oncofetal H19-derived miR-675 regulates tumor suppressor RB in human colorectal cancer. Carcinogenesis. 2010;31(3):350–8.
298. Liang WC, Fu WM, Wong CW, Wang Y, Wang WM, Hu GX, et al. The lncRNA H19 promotes epithelial to mesenchymal transition by functioning as miRNA sponges in colorectal cancer. Oncotarget. 2015;6(26):22513–25.
299. Kogo R, Shimamura T, Mimori K, Kawahara K, Imoto S, Sudo T, et al. Long noncoding RNA HOTAIR regulates polycomb-dependent chromatin modification and is associated with poor prognosis in colorectal cancers. Cancer Res. 2011;71(20):6320–6.
300. Svoboda M, Slyskova J, Schneiderova M, Makovicky P, Bielik L, Levy M, et al. HOTAIR long non-coding RNA is a negative prognostic factor not only in primary tumors, but also in the blood of colorectal cancer patients. Carcinogenesis. 2014;35(7):1510–5.
301. Xu C, Yang M, Tian J, Wang X, Li Z. MALAT-1: a long non-coding RNA and its important 3′ end functional motif in colorectal cancer metastasis. Int J Oncol. 2011;39(1):169–75.
302. Kam Y, Rubinstein A, Naik S, Djavsarov I, Halle D, Ariel I, et al. Detection of a long non-coding RNA (CCAT1) in living cells and human adenocarcinoma of colon tissues using FIT-PNA molecular beacons. Cancer Lett. 2014;352(1):90–6.

303. Nissan A, Stojadinovic A, Mitrani-Rosenbaum S, Halle D, Grinbaum R, Roistacher M, et al. Colon cancer associated transcript-1: a novel RNA expressed in malignant and pre-malignant human tissues. Int J Cancer. 2012;130(7):1598–606.
304. Yamada A, Yu P, Lin W, Okugawa Y, Boland CR, Goel A. A RNA-sequencing approach for the identification of novel long non-coding RNA biomarkers in colorectal cancer. Sci Rep. 2018;8(1):575.
305. Han Y, Yang YN, Yuan HH, Zhang TT, Sui H, Wei XL, et al. UCA1, a long non-coding RNA up-regulated in colorectal cancer influences cell proliferation, apoptosis and cell cycle distribution. Pathology. 2014;46(5):396–401.
306. Barbagallo C, Brex D, Caponnetto A, Cirnigliaro M, Scalia M, Magnano A, et al. LncRNA UCA1, upregulated in CRC biopsies and downregulated in serum exosomes, controls mRNA expression by RNA-RNA interactions. Mol Ther Nucleic Acids. 2018;12:229–41.
307. Wan L, Kong J, Tang J, Wu Y, Xu E, Lai M, et al. HOTAIRM1 as a potential biomarker for diagnosis of colorectal cancer functions the role in the tumour suppressor. J Cell Mol Med. 2016;20(11):2036–44.
308. Liu H, Ye D, Chen A, Tan D, Zhang W, Jiang W, et al. A pilot study of new promising non-coding RNA diagnostic biomarkers for early-stage colorectal cancers. Clin Chem Lab Med. 2019;57(7):1073–83.
309. Li Q, Dai Y, Wang F, Hou S. Differentially expressed long non-coding RNAs and the prognostic potential in colorectal cancer. Neoplasma. 2016;63(6):977–83.
310. Li L, Shang J, Zhang Y, Liu S, Peng Y, Zhou Z, et al. MEG3 is a prognostic factor for CRC and promotes chemosensitivity by enhancing oxaliplatin-induced cell apoptosis. Oncol Rep. 2017;38(3):1383–92.
311. Gao T, Liu X, He B, Nie Z, Zhu C, Zhang P, et al. Exosomal lncRNA 91H is associated with poor development in colorectal cancer by modifying HNRNPK expression. Cancer Cell Int. 2018;18:11.
312. Deng Q, He B, Gao T, Pan Y, Sun H, Xu Y, et al. Up-regulation of 91H promotes tumor metastasis and predicts poor prognosis for patients with colorectal cancer. PLoS One. 2014;9(7):e103022.
313. Nakano S, Murakami K, Meguro M, Soejima H, Higashimoto K, Urano T, et al. Expression profile of LIT1/KCNQ1OT1 and epigenetic status at the KvDMR1 in colorectal cancers. Cancer Sci. 2006;97(11):1147–54.
314. Tanaka K, Shiota G, Meguro M, Mitsuya K, Oshimura M, Kawasaki H. Loss of imprinting of long QT intronic transcript 1 in colorectal cancer. Oncology. 2001;60(3):268–73.
315. Pedersen SK, Mitchell SM, Graham LD, McEvoy A, Thomas ML, Baker RT, et al. CAHM, a long non-coding RNA gene hypermethylated in colorectal neoplasia. Epigenetics. 2014;9(8):1071–82.
316. Ding J, Li J, Wang H, Tian Y, Xie M, He X, et al. Long noncoding RNA CRNDE promotes colorectal cancer cell proliferation via epigenetically silencing DUSP5/CDKN1A expression. Cell Death Dis. 2017;8(8):e2997.
317. Graham LD, Pedersen SK, Brown GS, Ho T, Kassir Z, Moynihan AT, et al. Colorectal neoplasia differentially expressed (CRNDE), a novel gene with elevated expression in colorectal adenomas and adenocarcinomas. Genes Cancer. 2011;2(8):829–40.
318. Liu T, Zhang X, Yang YM, Du LT, Wang CX. Increased expression of the long noncoding RNA CRNDE-h indicates a poor prognosis in colorectal cancer, and is positively correlated with IRX5 mRNA expression. Onco Targets Ther. 2016;9:1437–48.
319. Liu T, Zhang X, Gao S, Jing F, Yang Y, Du L, et al. Exosomal long noncoding RNA CRNDE-h as a novel serum-based biomarker for diagnosis and prognosis of colorectal cancer. Oncotarget. 2016;7(51):85551–63.
320. Gong W, Tian M, Qiu H, Yang Z. Elevated serum level of lncRNA-HIF1A-AS1 as a novel diagnostic predictor for worse prognosis in colorectal carcinoma. Cancer Biomark. 2017;20(4):417–24.
321. Sun J, Ding C, Yang Z, Liu T, Zhang X, Zhao C, et al. The long non-coding RNA TUG1 indicates a poor prognosis for colorectal cancer and promotes metastasis by affecting epithelial-mesenchymal transition. J Transl Med. 2016;14:42.

322. Wang L, Zhao Z, Feng W, Ye Z, Dai W, Zhang C, et al. Long non-coding RNA TUG1 promotes colorectal cancer metastasis via EMT pathway. Oncotarget. 2016;7(32):51713–9.
323. Zhai HY, Sui MH, Yu X, Qu Z, Hu JC, Sun HQ, et al. Overexpression of long non-coding RNA TUG1 promotes colon cancer progression. Med Sci Monit. 2016;22:3281–7.
324. Zhao W, Song M, Zhang J, Kuerban M, Wang H. Combined identification of long non-coding RNA CCAT1 and HOTAIR in serum as an effective screening for colorectal carcinoma. Int J Clin Exp Pathol. 2015;8(11):14131–40.
325. Zhai H, Fesler A, Schee K, Fodstad O, Flatmark K, Ju J. Clinical significance of long intergenic noncoding RNA-p21 in colorectal cancer. Clin Colorectal Cancer. 2013;12(4):261–6.
326. Qi P, Xu MD, Ni SJ, Huang D, Wei P, Tan C, et al. Low expression of LOC285194 is associated with poor prognosis in colorectal cancer. J Transl Med. 2013;11:122.
327. Liu Q, Huang J, Zhou N, Zhang Z, Zhang A, Lu Z, et al. LncRNA loc285194 is a p53-regulated tumor suppressor. Nucleic Acids Res. 2013;41(9):4976–87.
328. Su J, Zhang E, Han L, Yin D, Liu Z, He X, et al. Long noncoding RNA BLACAT1 indicates a poor prognosis of colorectal cancer and affects cell proliferation by epigenetically silencing of p15. Cell Death Dis. 2017;8(3):e2665.
329. Dai M, Chen X, Mo S, Li J, Huang Z, Huang S, et al. Meta-signature LncRNAs serve as novel biomarkers for colorectal cancer: integrated bioinformatics analysis, experimental validation and diagnostic evaluation. Sci Rep. 2017;7:46572.
330. Hu D, Zhan Y, Zhu K, Bai M, Han J, Si Y, et al. Plasma Exosomal long non-coding RNAs serve as biomarkers for early detection of colorectal cancer. Cell Physiol Biochem. 2018;51(6):2704–15.
331. Liu L, Meng T, Yang XH, Sayim P, Lei C, Jin B, et al. Prognostic and predictive value of long non-coding RNA GAS5 and mircoRNA-221 in colorectal cancer and their effects on colorectal cancer cell proliferation, migration and invasion. Cancer Biomark. 2018;22(2):283–99.
332. Hibi K, Nakamura H, Hirai A, Fujikake Y, Kasai Y, Akiyama S, et al. Loss of H19 imprinting in esophageal cancer. Cancer Res. 1996;56(3):480–2.
333. Gupta RA, Shah N, Wang KC, Kim J, Horlings HM, Wong DJ, et al. Long non-coding RNA HOTAIR reprograms chromatin state to promote cancer metastasis. Nature. 2010;464(7291):1071–6.
334. Zheng HT, Shi DB, Wang YW, Li XX, Xu Y, Tripathi P, et al. High expression of lncRNA MALAT1 suggests a biomarker of poor prognosis in colorectal cancer. Int J Clin Exp Pathol. 2014;7(6):3174–81.
335. Yang W, Ning N, Jin X. The lncRNA H19 promotes cell proliferation by competitively binding to miR-200a and Derepressing beta-catenin expression in colorectal cancer. Biomed Res Int. 2017;2017:2767484.
336. Kalmar A, Nagy ZB, Galamb O, Csabai I, Bodor A, Wichmann B, et al. Genome-wide expression profiling in colorectal cancer focusing on lncRNAs in the adenoma-carcinoma transition. BMC Cancer. 2019;19(1):1059.
337. Alaiyan B, Ilyayev N, Stojadinovic A, Izadjoo M, Roistacher M, Pavlov V, et al. Differential expression of colon cancer associated transcript1 (CCAT1) along the colonic adenoma-carcinoma sequence. BMC Cancer. 2013;13:196.
338. Qi P, Du X. The long non-coding RNAs, a new cancer diagnostic and therapeutic gold mine. Mod Pathol. 2013;26(2):155–65.
339. Woo CJ, Kingston RE. HOTAIR lifts noncoding RNAs to new levels. Cell. 2007;129(7):1257–9.
340. Li Y, Li Y, Huang S, He K, Zhao M, Lin H, et al. Long non-coding RNA growth arrest specific transcript 5 acts as a tumour suppressor in colorectal cancer by inhibiting interleukin-10 and vascular endothelial growth factor expression. Oncotarget. 2017;8(8):13690–702.
341. Cheng J, Kapranov P, Drenkow J, Dike S, Brubaker S, Patel S, et al. Transcriptional maps of 10 human chromosomes at 5-nucleotide resolution. Science. 2005;308(5725):1149–54.
342. Galamb O, Bartak BK, Kalmar A, Nagy ZB, Szigeti KA, Tulassay Z, et al. Diagnostic and prognostic potential of tissue and circulating long non-coding RNAs in colorectal tumors. World J Gastroenterol. 2019;25(34):5026–48.

343. Tao K, Yang J, Hu Y, Sun Y, Tan Z, Duan J, et al. Clinical significance of urothelial carcinoma associated 1 in colon cancer. Int J Clin Exp Med. 2015;8(11):21854–60.
344. Shi J, Li X, Zhang F, Zhang C, Guan Q, Cao X, et al. Circulating lncRNAs associated with occurrence of colorectal cancer progression. Am J Cancer Res. 2015;5(7):2258–65.
345. Edge SB, Compton CC. The American Joint Committee on Cancer: the 7th edition of the AJCC cancer staging manual and the future of TNM. Ann Surg Oncol. 2010;17(6): 1471–4.
346. Oldenhuis CN, Oosting SF, Gietema JA, de Vries EG. Prognostic versus predictive value of biomarkers in oncology. Eur J Cancer. 2008;44(7):946–53.
347. Weiser MR. AJCC 8th Edition: colorectal cancer. Ann Surg Oncol. 2018;25(6):1454–5.
348. Gold P, Freedman SO. Specific carcinoembryonic antigens of the human digestive system. J Exp Med. 1965;122(3):467–81.
349. Gold P, Freedman SO. Demonstration of tumor-specific antigens in human colonic Carcinomata by immunological tolerance and absorption techniques. J Exp Med. 1965;121:439–62.
350. Thomson DM, Krupey J, Freedman SO, Gold P. The radioimmunoassay of circulating carcinoembryonic antigen of the human digestive system. Proc Natl Acad Sci U S A. 1969;64(1):161–7.
351. Sheahan K, O'Brien MJ, Burke B, Dervan PA, O'Keane JC, Gottlieb LS, et al. Differential reactivities of carcinoembryonic antigen (CEA) and CEA-related monoclonal and polyclonal antibodies in common epithelial malignancies. Am J Clin Pathol. 1990;94(2):157–64.
352. Tan E, Gouvas N, Nicholls RJ, Ziprin P, Xynos E, Tekkis PP. Diagnostic precision of carcinoembryonic antigen in the detection of recurrence of colorectal cancer. Surg Oncol. 2009;18(1):15–24.
353. Duffy MJ. Carcinoembryonic antigen as a marker for colorectal cancer: is it clinically useful? Clin Chem. 2001;47(4):624–30.
354. Holdenrieder S, Stieber P, Liska V, Treska V, Topolcan O, Dreslerova J, et al. Cytokeratin serum biomarkers in patients with colorectal cancer. Anticancer Res. 2012;32(5):1971–6.
355. Bystrom P, Berglund A, Nygren P, Wernroth L, Johansson B, Larsson A, et al. Evaluation of predictive markers for patients with advanced colorectal cancer. Acta Oncol. 2012;51(7): 849–59.
356. Levy M, Visokai V, Lipska L, Topolcan O. Tumor markers in staging and prognosis of colorectal carcinoma. Neoplasma. 2008;55(2):138–42.
357. Nicolini A, Ferrari P, Duffy MJ, Antonelli A, Rossi G, Metelli MR, et al. Intensive risk-adjusted follow-up with the CEA, TPA, CA19.9, and CA72.4 tumor marker panel and abdominal ultrasonography to diagnose operable colorectal cancer recurrences: effect on survival. Arch Surg. 2010;145(12):1177–83.
358. Rosen M, Chan L, Beart RW Jr, Vukasin P, Anthone G. Follow-up of colorectal cancer: a meta-analysis. Dis Colon Rectum. 1998;41(9):1116–26.
359. Li Destri G, Rubino AS, Latino R, Giannone F, Lanteri R, Scilletta B, et al. Preoperative carcinoembryonic antigen and prognosis of colorectal cancer. An independent prognostic factor still reliable. Int Surg. 2015;100(4):617–25.
360. Park YJ, Park KJ, Park JG, Lee KU, Choe KJ, Kim JP. Prognostic factors in 2230 Korean colorectal cancer patients: analysis of consecutively operated cases. World J Surg. 1999;23(7):721–6.
361. Fong Y, Fortner J, Sun RL, Brennan MF, Blumgart LH. Clinical score for predicting recurrence after hepatic resection for metastatic colorectal cancer: analysis of 1001 consecutive cases. Ann Surg. 1999;230(3):309–18. discussion 18–21
362. Nordlinger B, Guiguet M, Vaillant JC, Balladur P, Boudjema K, Bachellier P, et al. Surgical resection of colorectal carcinoma metastases to the liver. A prognostic scoring system to improve case selection, based on 1568 patients. Association Francaise de Chirurgie. Cancer. 1996;77(7):1254–62.
363. Nikolouzakis TK, Vassilopoulou L, Fragkiadaki P, Mariolis Sapsakos T, Papadakis GZ, Spandidos DA, et al. Improving diagnosis, prognosis and prediction by using biomarkers in CRC patients (review). Oncol Rep. 2018;39(6):2455–72.

364. Perez RO, Bresciani BH, Bresciani C, Proscurshim I, Kiss D, Gama-Rodrigues J, et al. Mucinous colorectal adenocarcinoma: influence of mucin expression (Muc1, 2 and 5) on clinico-pathological features and prognosis. Int J Color Dis. 2008;23(8):757–65.
365. Eberhard J, Gaber A, Wangefjord S, Nodin B, Uhlen M, Ericson Lindquist K, et al. A cohort study of the prognostic and treatment predictive value of SATB2 expression in colorectal cancer. Br J Cancer. 2012;106(5):931–8.
366. Wang S, Zhou J, Wang XY, Hao JM, Chen JZ, Zhang XM, et al. Down-regulated expression of SATB2 is associated with metastasis and poor prognosis in colorectal cancer. J Pathol. 2009;219(1):114–22.
367. Bae JM, Lee TH, Cho NY, Kim TY, Kang GH. Loss of CDX2 expression is associated with poor prognosis in colorectal cancer patients. World J Gastroenterol. 2015;21(5):1457–67.
368. Falchook GS, Kurzrock R. VEGF and dual-EGFR inhibition in colorectal cancer. Cell Cycle. 2015;14(8):1129–30.
369. Takahashi H, Ishikawa T, Ishiguro M, Okazaki S, Mogushi K, Kobayashi H, et al. Prognostic significance of Traf2- and Nck-interacting kinase (TNIK) in colorectal cancer. BMC Cancer. 2015;15:794.
370. Ascierto PA, Kirkwood JM, Grob JJ, Simeone E, Grimaldi AM, Maio M, et al. The role of BRAF V600 mutation in melanoma. J Transl Med. 2012;10:85.
371. Li Y, Li W. BRAF mutation is associated with poor clinicopathological outcomes in colorectal cancer: a meta-analysis. Saudi J Gastroenterol. 2017;23(3):144–9.
372. Lochhead P, Kuchiba A, Imamura Y, Liao X, Yamauchi M, Nishihara R, et al. Microsatellite instability and BRAF mutation testing in colorectal cancer prognostication. J Natl Cancer Inst. 2013;105(15):1151–6.
373. Gavin PG, Colangelo LH, Fumagalli D, Tanaka N, Remillard MY, Yothers G, et al. Mutation profiling and microsatellite instability in stage II and III colon cancer: an assessment of their prognostic and oxaliplatin predictive value. Clin Cancer Res. 2012;18(23):6531–41.
374. Graham DM, Coyle VM, Kennedy RD, Wilson RH. Molecular subtypes and personalized therapy in metastatic colorectal cancer. Curr Colorectal Cancer Rep. 2016;12:141–50.
375. Lynch HT, de la Chapelle A. Hereditary colorectal cancer. N Engl J Med. 2003;348(10):919–32.
376. Deng G, Peng E, Gum J, Terdiman J, Sleisenger M, Kim YS. Methylation of hMLH1 promoter correlates with the gene silencing with a region-specific manner in colorectal cancer. Br J Cancer. 2002;86(4):574–9.
377. Guastadisegni C, Colafranceschi M, Ottini L, Dogliotti E. Microsatellite instability as a marker of prognosis and response to therapy: a meta-analysis of colorectal cancer survival data. Eur J Cancer. 2010;46(15):2788–98.
378. Carethers JM, Jung BH. Genetics and genetic Biomarkers in sporadic colorectal cancer. Gastroenterology. 2015;149(5):1177–90.e3.
379. Narayan S, Roy D. Role of APC and DNA mismatch repair genes in the development of colorectal cancers. Mol Cancer. 2003;2:41.
380. Saha MN, Qiu L, Chang H. Targeting p53 by small molecules in hematological malignancies. J Hematol Oncol. 2013;6:23.
381. Popat S, Chen Z, Zhao D, Pan H, Hearle N, Chandler I, et al. A prospective, blinded analysis of thymidylate synthase and p53 expression as prognostic markers in the adjuvant treatment of colorectal cancer. Ann Oncol. 2006;17(12):1810–7.
382. Petersen S, Thames HD, Nieder C, Petersen C, Baumann M. The results of colorectal cancer treatment by p53 status: treatment-specific overview. Dis Colon Rectum. 2001;44(3):322–33. discussion 33–4
383. Westra JL, Schaapveld M, Hollema H, de Boer JP, Kraak MM, de Jong D, et al. Determination of TP53 mutation is more relevant than microsatellite instability status for the prediction of disease-free survival in adjuvant-treated stage III colon cancer patients. J Clin Oncol. 2005;23(24):5635–43.
384. Mamot C, Mild G, Reuter J, Laffer U, Metzger U, Terracciano L, et al. Infrequent mutation of the tumour-suppressor gene Smad4 in early-stage colorectal cancer. Br J Cancer. 2003;88(3):420–3.

385. Xu Y, Pasche B. TGF-beta signaling alterations and susceptibility to colorectal cancer. Human Mol Genet. 2007;16 Spec No 1:R14–20.
386. Attisano L, Wrana JL. Signal transduction by the TGF-beta superfamily. Science. 2002;296(5573):1646–7.
387. Shi Y, Massague J. Mechanisms of TGF-beta signaling from cell membrane to the nucleus. Cell. 2003;113(6):685–700.
388. Nikolic A, Kojic S, Knezevic S, Krivokapic Z, Ristanovic M, Radojkovic D. Structural and functional analysis of SMAD4 gene promoter in malignant pancreatic and colorectal tissues: detection of two novel polymorphic nucleotide repeats. Cancer Epidemiol. 2011;35(3):265–71.
389. Riggins GJ, Kinzler KW, Vogelstein B, Thiagalingam S. Frequency of Smad gene mutations in human cancers. Cancer Res. 1997;57(13):2578–80.
390. Salovaara R, Roth S, Loukola A, Launonen V, Sistonen P, Avizienyte E, et al. Frequent loss of SMAD4/DPC4 protein in colorectal cancers. Gut. 2002;51(1):56–9.
391. Alazzouzi H, Alhopuro P, Salovaara R, Sammalkorpi H, Jarvinen H, Mecklin JP, et al. SMAD4 as a prognostic marker in colorectal cancer. Clin Cancer Res. 2005;11(7):2606–11.
392. Voorneveld PW, Jacobs RJ, De Miranda NF, Morreau H, van Noesel CJ, Offerhaus GJ, et al. Evaluation of the prognostic value of pSMAD immunohistochemistry in colorectal cancer. Eur J Cancer Prev. 2013;22(5):420–4.
393. Wang P, Meng X, Huang Y, Lv Z, Liu J, Wang G, et al. MicroRNA-497 inhibits thyroid cancer tumor growth and invasion by suppressing BDNF. Oncotarget. 2017;8(2):2825–34.
394. Dai H, Hou K, Cai Z, Zhou Q, Zhu S. Low-level miR-646 in colorectal cancer inhibits cell proliferation and migration by targeting NOB1 expression. Oncol Lett. 2017;14(6):6708–14.
395. Wen L, Li Y, Jiang Z, Zhang Y, Yang B, Han F. miR-944 inhibits cell migration and invasion by targeting MACC1 in colorectal cancer. Oncol Rep. 2017;37(6):3415–22.
396. Liu X, Wang Y, Zhao J. MicroRNA337 inhibits colorectal cancer progression by directly targeting KRAS and suppressing the AKT and ERK pathways. Oncol Rep. 2017;38(5):3187–96.
397. Shen WW, Zeng Z, Zhu WX, Fu GH. MiR-142-3p functions as a tumor suppressor by targeting CD133, ABCG2, and Lgr5 in colon cancer cells. J Mol Med (Berl). 2013;91(8):989–1000.
398. Xuan Y, Yang H, Zhao L, Lau WB, Lau B, Ren N, et al. MicroRNAs in colorectal cancer: small molecules with big functions. Cancer Lett. 2015;360(2):89–105.
399. Schee K, Boye K, Abrahamsen TW, Fodstad O, Flatmark K. Clinical relevance of microRNA miR-21, miR-31, miR-92a, miR-101, miR-106a and miR-145 in colorectal cancer. BMC Cancer. 2012;12:505.
400. Cao J, Yan XR, Liu T, Han XB, Yu JJ, Liu SH, et al. MicroRNA-552 promotes tumor cell proliferation and migration by directly targeting DACH1 via the Wnt/beta-catenin signaling pathway in colorectal cancer. Oncol Lett. 2017;14(3):3795–802.
401. Peng Q, Zhang X, Min M, Zou L, Shen P, Zhu Y. The clinical role of microRNA-21 as a promising biomarker in the diagnosis and prognosis of colorectal cancer: a systematic review and meta-analysis. Oncotarget. 2017;8(27):44893–909.
402. Bovell LC, Shanmugam C, Putcha BD, Katkoori VR, Zhang B, Bae S, et al. The prognostic value of microRNAs varies with patient race/ethnicity and stage of colorectal cancer. Clin Cancer Res. 2013;19(14):3955–65.
403. Yang IP, Tsai HL, Miao ZF, Huang CW, Kuo CH, Wu JY, et al. Development of a deregulating microRNA panel for the detection of early relapse in postoperative colorectal cancer patients. J Transl Med. 2016;14(1):108.
404. Cheng D, Zhao S, Tang H, Zhang D, Sun H, Yu F, et al. MicroRNA-20a-5p promotes colorectal cancer invasion and metastasis by downregulating Smad4. Oncotarget. 2016;7(29):45199–213.
405. Shibuya H, Iinuma H, Shimada R, Horiuchi A, Watanabe T. Clinicopathological and prognostic value of microRNA-21 and microRNA-155 in colorectal cancer. Oncology. 2010;79(3–4):313–20.

406. Fukushima Y, Iinuma H, Tsukamoto M, Matsuda K, Hashiguchi Y. Clinical significance of microRNA-21 as a biomarker in each Dukes' stage of colorectal cancer. Oncol Rep. 2015;33(2):573–82.
407. He PY, Yip WK, Chai BL, Chai BY, Jabar MF, Dusa N, et al. Inhibition of cell migration and invasion by miR29a3p in a colorectal cancer cell line through suppression of CDC42BPA mRNA expression. Oncol Rep. 2017;38(6):3554–66.
408. Wang LG, Gu J. Serum microRNA-29a is a promising novel marker for early detection of colorectal liver metastasis. Cancer Epidemiol. 2012;36(1):e61–7.
409. Lv ZC, Fan YS, Chen HB, Zhao DW. Investigation of microRNA-155 as a serum diagnostic and prognostic biomarker for colorectal cancer. Tumour Biol. 2015;36(3):1619–25.
410. Zhao J, Xu J, Zhang R. MicroRNA-411 inhibits malignant biological behaviours of colorectal cancer cells by directly targeting PIK3R3. Oncol Rep. 2018;39(2):633–42.
411. Ling H, Pickard K, Ivan C, Isella C, Ikuo M, Mitter R, et al. The clinical and biological significance of MIR-224 expression in colorectal cancer metastasis. Gut. 2016;65(6):977–89.
412. Lou X, Qi X, Zhang Y, Long H, Yang J. Decreased expression of microRNA-625 is associated with tumor metastasis and poor prognosis in patients with colorectal cancer. J Surg Oncol. 2013;108(4):230–5.
413. Liao WT, Ye YP, Zhang NJ, Li TT, Wang SY, Cui YM, et al. MicroRNA-30b functions as a tumour suppressor in human colorectal cancer by targeting KRAS, PIK3CD and BCL2. J Pathol. 2014;232(4):415–27.
414. Wang MJ, Li Y, Wang R, Wang C, Yu YY, Yang L, et al. Downregulation of microRNA-124 is an independent prognostic factor in patients with colorectal cancer. Int J Color Dis. 2013;28(2):183–9.
415. Liu H, Du L, Wen Z, Yang Y, Li J, Wang L, et al. Up-regulation of miR-182 expression in colorectal cancer tissues and its prognostic value. Int J Color Dis. 2013;28(5):697–703.
416. Chen DL, Wang ZQ, Zeng ZL, Wu WJ, Zhang DS, Luo HY, et al. Identification of microRNA-214 as a negative regulator of colorectal cancer liver metastasis by way of regulation of fibroblast growth factor receptor 1 expression. Hepatology. 2014;60(2):598–609.
417. Lee BH. Commentary on: "comprehensive molecular characterization of papillary renal-cell carcinoma." Cancer Genome Atlas Research Network.: N Engl J Med. 2016 Jan 14;374(2):135–45. Urol Oncol. 2017;35(9):578–9.
418. Toiyama Y, Hur K, Tanaka K, Inoue Y, Kusunoki M, Boland CR, et al. Serum miR-200c is a novel prognostic and metastasis-predictive biomarker in patients with colorectal cancer. Ann Surg. 2014;259(4):735–43.
419. Pal S, Garg M, Pandey AK. Deciphering the mounting complexity of the p53 regulatory network in correlation to long non-coding RNAs (lncRNAs) in ovarian cancer. Cells. 2020;9(3):527.
420. Riley T, Sontag E, Chen P, Levine A. Transcriptional control of human p53-regulated genes. Nat Rev Mol Cell Biol. 2008;9(5):402–12.
421. Han D, Gao X, Wang M, Qiao Y, Xu Y, Yang J, et al. Long noncoding RNA H19 indicates a poor prognosis of colorectal cancer and promotes tumor growth by recruiting and binding to eIF4A3. Oncotarget. 2016;7(16):22159–73.
422. Ohtsuka M, Ling H, Ivan C, Pichler M, Matsushita D, Goblirsch M, et al. H19 noncoding RNA, an independent prognostic factor, regulates essential Rb-E2F and CDK8-beta-catenin signaling in colorectal cancer. EBioMedicine. 2016;13:113–24.
423. Yu B, Du Q, Li H, Liu HY, Ye X, Zhu B, et al. Diagnostic potential of serum exosomal colorectal neoplasia differentially expressed long non-coding RNA (CRNDE-p) and microRNA-217 expression in colorectal carcinoma. Oncotarget. 2017;8(48):83745–53.
424. Xiao Z, Qu Z, Chen Z, Fang Z, Zhou K, Huang Z, et al. LncRNA HOTAIR is a prognostic biomarker for the proliferation and Chemoresistance of colorectal cancer via MiR-203a-3p-mediated Wnt/ss-catenin signaling pathway. Cell Physiol Biochem. 2018;46(3):1275–85.
425. Li P, Zhang X, Wang H, Wang L, Liu T, Du L, et al. MALAT1 is associated with poor response to Oxaliplatin-based chemotherapy in colorectal cancer patients and promotes Chemoresistance through EZH2. Mol Cancer Ther. 2017;16(4):739–51.

426. Ozawa T, Matsuyama T, Toiyama Y, Takahashi N, Ishikawa T, Uetake H, et al. CCAT1 and CCAT2 long noncoding RNAs, located within the 8q.24.21 'gene desert', serve as important prognostic biomarkers in colorectal cancer. Ann Oncol. 2017;28(8):1882–8.
427. Chauvin A, Boisvert FM. Clinical proteomics in colorectal cancer, a promising tool for improving personalised medicine. Proteomes. 2018;6(4):49.
428. Alnabulsi A, Murray GI. Integrative analysis of the colorectal cancer proteome: potential clinical impact. Expert Rev Proteomics. 2016;13(10):917–27.
429. Dinu D, Dobre M, Panaitescu E, Birla R, Iosif C, Hoara P, et al. Prognostic significance of KRAS gene mutations in colorectal cancer–preliminary study. J Med Life. 2014;7(4):581–7.
430. Peeters M, Douillard JY, Van Cutsem E, Siena S, Zhang K, Williams R, et al. Mutant KRAS codon 12 and 13 alleles in patients with metastatic colorectal cancer: assessment as prognostic and predictive biomarkers of response to panitumumab. J Clin Oncol. 2013;31(6):759–65.
431. De Roock W, Jonker DJ, Di Nicolantonio F, Sartore-Bianchi A, Tu D, Siena S, et al. Association of KRAS p.G13D mutation with outcome in patients with chemotherapy-refractory metastatic colorectal cancer treated with cetuximab. JAMA. 2010;304(16):1812–20.
432. Hecht JR, Douillard JY, Schwartzberg L, Grothey A, Kopetz S, Rong A, et al. Extended RAS analysis for anti-epidermal growth factor therapy in patients with metastatic colorectal cancer. Cancer Treat Rev. 2015;41(8):653–9.
433. Huang L, Liu Z, Deng D, Tan A, Liao M, Mo Z, et al. Anti-epidermal growth factor receptor monoclonal antibody-based therapy for metastatic colorectal cancer: a meta-analysis of the effect of PIK3CA mutations in KRAS wild-type patients. Arch Med Sci. 2014;10(1):1–9.
434. Karapetis CS, Jonker D, Daneshmand M, Hanson JE, O'Callaghan CJ, Marginean C, et al. PIK3CA, BRAF, and PTEN status and benefit from cetuximab in the treatment of advanced colorectal cancer–results from NCIC CTG/AGITG CO.17. Clin Cancer Res. 2014;20(3):744–53.
435. Liao X, Lochhead P, Nishihara R, Morikawa T, Kuchiba A, Yamauchi M, et al. Aspirin use, tumor PIK3CA mutation, and colorectal-cancer survival. N Engl J Med. 2012;367(17):1596–606.
436. Din FV, Theodoratou E, Farrington SM, Tenesa A, Barnetson RA, Cetnarskyj R, et al. Effect of aspirin and NSAIDs on risk and survival from colorectal cancer. Gut. 2010;59(12):1670–9.
437. Algra AM, Rothwell PM. Effects of regular aspirin on long-term cancer incidence and metastasis: a systematic comparison of evidence from observational studies versus randomised trials. Lancet Oncol. 2012;13(5):518–27.
438. Agostini M, Pucciarelli S, Enzo MV, Del Bianco P, Briarava M, Bedin C, et al. Circulating cell-free DNA: a promising marker of pathologic tumor response in rectal cancer patients receiving preoperative chemoradiotherapy. Ann Surg Oncol. 2011;18(9):2461–8.
439. Zitt M, Muller HM, Rochel M, Schwendinger V, Zitt M, Goebel G, et al. Circulating cell-free DNA in plasma of locally advanced rectal cancer patients undergoing preoperative chemoradiation: a potential diagnostic tool for therapy monitoring. Dis Markers. 2008;25(3):159–65.
440. Yamagishi H, Kuroda H, Imai Y, Hiraishi H. Molecular pathogenesis of sporadic colorectal cancers. Chin J Cancer. 2016;35:4.
441. Kim TM, Lee SH, Chung YJ. Clinical applications of next-generation sequencing in colorectal cancers. World J Gastroenterol. 2013;19(40):6784–93.
442. Das V, Kalita J, Pal M. Predictive and prognostic biomarkers in colorectal cancer: a systematic review of recent advances and challenges. Biomed Pharmacother. 2017;87:8–19.
443. Henaine AM, Chahine G, Salameh P, Elias E, Massoud M, Hartmann D, et al. Management of metastatic colorectal cancer: current treatments and new therapies. J Med Liban. 2015;63(4):218–27.
444. Gulbake A, Jain A, Jain A, Jain A, Jain SK. Insight to drug delivery aspects for colorectal cancer. World J Gastroenterol. 2016;22(2):582–99.
445. Gangadhar T, Schilsky RL. Molecular markers to individualize adjuvant therapy for colon cancer. Nat Rev Clin Oncol. 2010;7(6):318–25.

Chapter 9
Proteins Involved in Colorectal Cancer: Identification Strategies and Possible Roles

Sudhir Kumar, Divya Goel, Neeraj, and Vineet Kumar Maurya

Abstract Colorectal cancer is one of the five types of commonly occurring cancer in the world. Like other cancers, it is also a result of uncontrolled cell divisions. Each disease bears clear proteomic signatures, which if identified properly would assist in its early diagnosis and timely treatment. Comparative proteomics and microarray technologies enable the study of differential proteomics signatures of a disease. Using these two technologies, some proteins like beta-subunit of 14-3-3 proteins (14-3-3β) and aldehyde dehydrogenase 1 (ALDH1), etc. have been identified as possible biomarkers for detection of colorectal cancer (CRC). Proteomics signature not only provides clue about biomarkers for colon cancer but also indicates drug targets that can be utilized for treatment of cancer. Most common drug targets for cancer are expected to be the proteins involved in cell cycle, protein synthesis, signaling and transport, etc. Tumor antigen p53 (p53), E2F transcription factor 1 (E2F1), ribosomal protein L15 (RPL15), vascular endothelial growth factor (VEGF), G protein-coupled receptor 35 (GPR35), nucleoside diphosphate kinases (NM23), erythroblastic oncogene-B (c-erbB-2), and urokinase-type plasminogen activator (uPA) are some of the proteins which have been explored for their possible roles in colorectal cancer. These proteins along with other crucial proteins are described in the present chapter for their role either as biomarker or drug target for colorectal cancer. Besides "omics," "data mining technology"-based studies were also explored for their possible role in proteomic profiling of colorectal cancer.

Keywords p53 · GPR35 · E2F1 · RPL-15 · CD44 · ATM/ATR · JAK/STAT · Microarray · Data mining

---

S. Kumar · D. Goel
Department of Biotechnology, H.N.B. Garhwal University (A Central University), Srinagar (Garhwal), Uttarakhand, India

Neeraj
Department of Computer Science and Engineering, H. N. B. Garhwal University (A Central University), Srinagar (Garhwal), Uttarakhand, India

V. K. Maurya (✉)
Department of Botany and Microbiology, H.N.B. Garhwal University (A Central University), Srinagar (Garhwal), Uttarakhand, India

G. P. Nagaraju et al. (eds.), *Colon Cancer Diagnosis and Therapy*,
https://doi.org/10.1007/978-3-030-63369-1_9

Abbreviations

AKT	RAC-alpha serine/threonine-specific protein kinase
ALDH1	Aldehyde dehydrogenase 1
APC	Adenomatous polyposis coli protein
AREG	Amphiregulin
ATM	Ataxia telangiectasia mutated
ATR	Ataxia telangiectasia and Rad3-related
BAG4	Bcl-2-associated athanogene co-chaperone 4
BMP	Bone morphogenetic protein
BRCA1	Breast cancer type 1 susceptibility protein homolog
BTC	Betacellulin
CD	Cluster of differentiation
CHK1	Checkpoint kinase 1
CHK2	Checkpoint kinase 2
CNTF	Ciliary neurotrophic factor
CoA	Coenzyme A
CRC	Colorectal cancer
CXCL17	Chemokine (C-X-C motif) ligand 17
DIGE	Difference gel electrophoresis
E2F1	E2F transcription factor 1
ECM	Extracellular matrix
EF-G	Elongation factor G
EGFR	Epidermal growth factor receptor
ENO1	Enolase 1
EPGN	Epithelial mitogen
ErbB2	Epidermal growth factor receptor-related protein B2
EREG	Epiregulin
FAP	Familial adenomatous polyposis
GAPDH	Glyceraldehyde 3-phosphate dehydrogenase
GPR35	G protein-coupled receptor 35
HNPCC	Hereditary non-polyposis colorectal cancer
IDH1	Isocitrate dehydrogenase 1
IL6	Interleukin-6
IL6ST	Interleukin-6 signal transducer
JAKs	Janus kinases
JNK	c-Jun N-terminal kinase
KLF14	Kruppel-like Transcription Factor 14
KRAS	Kirsten rat sarcoma viral oncogenic protein
LDHB	Lactate dehydrogenase beta-subunit
LIF	Leukemia inhibitory factor
MAPK	Mitogen-activated protein kinase
mTOR	Mechanistic/mammalian target of rapamycin
NAD	Nicotinamide adenine dinucleotide

NADP	Nicotinamide adenine dinucleotide phosphate
NDP	Nucleoside diphosphates
NM23	Nucleoside diphosphate kinases
NTP	Nucleoside triphosphates
OSM	Oncostatin M
p53	Tumor antigen or tumor protein p53
PCR	Polymerase chain reaction
Raf	RAF proto-oncogene serine/threonine-protein kinase
RAPD	Randomly amplified polymorphic DNA
Ras	GTPaseHRas
RB	Retinoblastoma
RFLP	Restriction fragment length polymorphism
RPL15	Ribosomal protein L15
STAT3	Signal transducer and activator of transcription 3
TGF-α	Tumor growth factor-alpha
TGF-β	Tumor growth factor-beta
TNFRSF1A	Tumor necrosis factor receptor superfamily member 1A
uPA	Urokinase-type plasminogen activator
VEGF	Vascular endothelial growth factor
VWF	von Willebrand factor
WNT	Wingless-related integration site

9.1 Introduction

Colorectal cancer (CRC) is the fourth most commonly diagnosed cancer and the third leading cause of cancer-related deaths worldwide. CRC emerges from the glandular epithelial cells of inner intestinal lining. Colon stem cells are pluripotent cells which are situated at the bottom of intestinal crypts and differentiated into Paneth, goblet, enteroendocrine, and enterocytes. Under normal conditions, these stem cells differentiate, migrate out of the crypt, and shift gradually up to the villus. Once at the top of the villus, these cells undergo apoptosis after 14 days. This process is under strict regulation of various signaling proteins including Wingless-related integration site (Wnt) protein, bone morphogenetic protein (BMP), and tumor growth factor-beta (TGF-β). Mutations leading to disturbance of signaling process, cell cycle, or apoptosis lead to CRC.

Usually CRC begins as non-cancerous growth arising from inner epithelial surface of the intestine called polyp (adenoma), which grows slowly for 10–20 years before converting into CRC. Both genetic and environmental factors are responsible for CRC, and it was also estimated that 25–30% cases of CRC have a family history. Inherited syndromes include "Lynch syndrome," also known as "hereditary non-polyposis colorectal cancer" (HNPCC), and familial adenomatous polyposis (FAP). FAP is characterized by development of hundreds of polyps at the age of 10–12, which may develop CRC after the age of 40. HNPCC account for 2–4% cases of

CRCs, while FAP account for <1% case of CRCs. Among the CRC patients with familial history of CRC, only 5% are due to mutations, and the risk of developing CRC is increased if their first-degree relatives were diagnosed with CRC. This reveals an interesting fact that since only 5% cases of CRC are genetic, the other 95% may be related to lifestyle and diet. Since family members normally follow similar lifestyles and dietary patterns, there is a high probability of other family members developing CRC after the age of 50, if a first-degree relative (parents) has developed CRC.

Environmental factors include exposure to carcinogens; heavy alcohol consumption; red meat; low-fiber, high-fat diets; sedentary working style; smoking; and abstaining from physical workouts. Patients with inflammatory bowel disease have increased risk of CRC because inflammation is one of the risk factors for cancer [56].

Chemotherapy, radiation therapy, targeted therapy, and tumor resection are the available treatment options for CRC, but chemo-/radiation therapy has proved to be less effective compared to tumor resection, especially when tumor has metastasized. Patient survival after treatment depends upon the stage at which cancer was diagnosed and treated. 90% patients survive for approximately 5 years if colon cancer is detected at early non-metastasized stage and treated simultaneously. With late diagnosis, i.e., after the start of metastasis, survival rate drops to 12% [45]. The colon can be divided into two parts: proximal colon (consists of ascending colon and transverse colon) and distal colon (consists of descending colon and sigmoid colon). Survival of patients after colon cancer also depends upon location of tumor. Tumors of the proximal colon are much more common in older than in younger patients and in women than in men; these patients have lower survival rates than patients with tumors in the distal colon or rectum. An adenomatous polyp is common in the colon along with non-adenomatous polyps. There are three types of adenomatous polyps: tubular (65–80%), villous (5–10%), and tubulovillous (10–25%), depending upon their shape. The villous types of polyps have highest risk of transforming into a carcinoma, followed by tubulovillous and tubular types of polyps [52].

Complete understanding of CRC development patterns, environmental and genetic risk factors, and molecular mechanism of disease progression is required for effective prevention and treatment of CRC. As mentioned earlier, the early diagnosis of CRC is helpful in providing proper treatment of CRCs. Available visual examination and molecular examination methods are effective in diagnosis of CRCs. Although tumor formation is a definite indicator of cancer, it is a late-stage indicator. A biomarker-based CRC detection method that could diagnose CRC and its development stages is the need of the hour. A biomarker is a protein, enzyme, or metabolite whose expression level is the direct indication of the disease and its severity. The role of biomarkers in diagnosis and management of diseases is well-known. According to "Human Genome Project," there are 20,000–25,000 protein-coding genes in human genome. Among these proteins, the ones identified as potential biomarker for CRCs and probable drug targets by various research groups are briefly described in this chapter. Besides that, the involvement of "omics" and "data mining" approaches in detection of biomarkers and drug targets for CRC is also described.

9.2 Biomarker

A biomarker is any visual/anatomical/physiological or biochemical indicator that is directly correlated to disease or developmental stage of any organism. Proteins, genes, enzymes, and metabolites are the molecular biomarkers whose level can be detected in the blood easily, while tumor is an example of anatomical biomarker. Tumor formation occurs at late stage of cancer, the stage having high probability of treatment failures or metastasis. Hence, blood-based biomarkers which can detect CRC at early stages and clearly indicate the developmental stages of CRC are urgently required. Various proteins have been identified as probable biomarkers by various research groups which are mentioned below.

9.2.1 Proteins Involved in Bioenergetics Pathways as Biomarkers

9.2.1.1 Enolase-1 (ENO1)

ENO1 is an important enzyme of glycolytic pathway. Glycolysis is a basic metabolic process used in aerobic respiration. Overexpression of ENO1 has been observed in many types of cancer like lung, liver, thyroid, prostrate, and pancreas [54]; hence it can be used as a potential CRC biomarker [11]. Since it degrades extracellular matrix and helps in tumor metastasis, it could be a drug target for cancer [23].

9.2.1.2 Glyceraldehyde 3-Phosphate Dehydrogenase (GAPDH)

It is also an enzyme of glycolysis pathway, which is involved in energy generation. Besides glycolysis, GAPDH also participates in apoptosis initiation and transcription activation. Its overexpression has been reported in many types of human cancers [43, 63]. GAPDH is also upregulated in CRC samples and can be used as a biomarker for CRC [5, 20].

9.2.1.3 Isocitrate Dehydrogenase 1 (IDH1)

It is also a protein involved in energy metabolism in Krebs cycle. Mutations in IDH1 are found responsible for many types of cancer including CRCs [12, 59, 74]. IDH1 becomes hyperacetylated during an early stage of CRC development, and any deacetylating agents like sirtuin 2 can inhibit CRC by deacetylating IDH1 [67].

9.2.1.4 Aldehyde Dehydrogenase 1 (ALDH1)

It is a stem cell marker and potential marker for cancer stem cells [35, 57]. ALDH1 is a nicotinamide adenine dinucleotide phosphate (NADP)-dependent enzyme, which oxidizes endogenous and exogenous aldehydes to carboxylic acid or coenzyme A (CoA) esters, thus protecting the cell from oxidative stress. It is also used for the synthesis of molecules that regulate cellular homeostasis, such as retinoic acid, γ-aminobutyric acid, and betaine [57]. Protein microarray-based studies showed upregulation of ALDH1 in CRC tissues; hence, it can be used as a CRC biomarker [36].

9.2.1.5 Lactate Dehydrogenase Beta-Subunit (LDHB)

This protein is also linked to bioenergetics pathways which catalyze the interconversion of pyruvate by oxidation of reduced form of nicotinamide adenine dinucleotide (NADH) to NAD. LDHB upregulation in CRC increases the rate of glycolysis, which is required for meeting the increased energy demand of cancer cells. High expression of LDHB has been observed during CRC and other cancers and thus can also be used as a CRC biomarker [72].

9.2.2 Transcription Factors as Biomarkers

9.2.2.1 Kruppel-Like Transcription Factor-14 (KLF14)

It is a transcription factor which controls many metabolic processes. It controls the process of glycolysis by regulating the level of LDHB. Level of KLF14 is downregulated in CRC samples, due to which control of glycolysis is released and cancer cells meet their energy demand, required for rapid proliferation. KLF14 is a potential biomarker whose downregulation is an indicator of cancer [69].

9.2.2.2 E2F transcription factor 1

It is one of the members of E2F transcription factor family, whose activity is regulated by its binding to retinoblastoma (RB) tumor suppressor protein. Dissociation of E2F1 from retinoblastoma protein activates the downstream transcription processes, and cell enters the S stage of cell cycle. Overexpression of E2F1 along with thymidine synthase promotes growth of cancer [24]. It promotes CRC by activating small unit of ribonucleotide reductase [16, 18].

9.2.2.3 Ribosomal Protein L15 (RPL15)

The role of RPL15 as a CRC biomarker and drug target was analyzed by Dong et al. [15]. RPL15 belongs to a large subunit of ribosome and is responsible for maintenance of nucleolar structure and formation of pre-60S subunits in the nucleoli. In addition, it is also required for ribosome regeneration and cell proliferation. Overexpression of RPL15 was reported in esophageal cancer [62], gastric cancer [21], and CRC [15]. Its depletion induces anti-cancerous effect in colon cancer cell by inducing apoptosis in them. In normal cells, RPL15 depletion causes cell cycle arrest at G1 to S cell stage by causing ribosomal stress. Since its overexpression indicates cancer and depletion protects from cancer, it can be used as both cancer biomarker and drug target for CRC.

9.2.3 *Proteins Involved in Cell Cycle Regulations as Biomarkers*

9.2.3.1 "Ataxia Telangiectasia Mutated" (ATM) and "Ataxia Telangiectasia and Rad3 Related" (ATR)

These two proteins are the members of "PI3 kinase-like protein kinase" family. Both these proteins are activated by DNA damage response, and upon activation, they stop the process of cell division by phosphorylating the proteins involved in cell cycle till DNA damage is corrected. ATM activates tumor antigen p53 (p53), breast cancer type 1 susceptibility protein homolog (BRCA1), checkpoint kinase 2 (CHK2), etc., while ATR activates p53 and checkpoint kinase 1 (CHK1); thus p53 is the common point between ATR and ATM [4, 13]. Normal expression level of ATM and ATR prevents cancer, and their downregulation or any mutation affecting their function may lead to cancer; hence, these two proteins can be exploited as drug targets for cancer [68]. Their role as a CRC biomarker and drug target has also been evaluated in many studies [8, 43, 53].

9.2.3.2 Tumor Antigen p53 (p53)

It is a well-established tumor suppressor gene and is also known as the "guardian of the genome." p53 plays a critical role in cell cycle, DNA repair, and apoptosis. Normal level of p53 induces apoptosis, prevents cancer, and is an indicator of non-cancerous conditions. Downregulation, suppression, or mutation of p53 is found to be involved in various types of cancers including CRC [33, 66, 75]. Detection of p53 in blood is a clear biomarker of late stage of CRC, while adenomatous polyposis coli (APC) protein and Kirsten rat sarcoma viral oncogenic protein (KRAS) are early stage CRC biomarkers in blood [61]. p53 was also used as an early stage biomarker of CRC for screening of a large population using p53 antibody-based microarray. These studies along with one metadata study highlighted that p53 can be used as reliable biomarker for CRC and its different stages [28, 37, 64].

9.2.4 *Growth Factors as Biomarkers*

9.2.4.1 Proto-oncogene NEU (NEU)

It is also known as the cluster of differentiation 340 (CD340) and epidermal growth factor receptor-related protein (ErbB2). NEU is a transmembrane glycoprotein with intrinsic kinase activity and is proto-oncogenic in nature [31, 64]. NEU degrades extracellular matrix by promoting proteinase cascade, thus playing a key role in tumor proliferation and metastasis. Upregulation of NEU leads to metastasis of CRC and can be used as noninvasive prognosis marker [17, 38].

9.2.4.2 Vascular Endothelial Growth Factor (VEGF)

It is dimeric heparin-binding signaling protein which is found in four isoforms (VEGF121, VEGF165, VEGF189, and VEGF206). It is an essential factor for growth of vascular endothelium, and its upregulation is related with tumor growth and metastasis by angiogenesis activation [19, 32]. Overexpression of VEGF as a CRC biomarker was evaluated in platelets of CRC patients [39] to study the period of survival after their treatment [14], and a positive correlation was found in VEGF upregulation and CRC.

9.2.4.3 Epidermal Growth Factor Receptor (EGFR)

This is a cell surface receptor of tyrosine kinase receptor family. It binds with many ligands like elongation factor G (EF-G), tumor growth factor-alpha (TGF-α), amphiregulin (AREG), epithelial mitogen (EPGN), betacellulin (BTC), epiregulin (EREG), etc. Binding of ligands with epidermal growth factor receptor (EGFR) induces dimerization, phosphorylation, and activation of downstream signaling cascade like mitogen-activated protein kinase (MAPK), RAC alpha serine/threonine-specific protein kinase (AKT), and c-Jun N-terminal kinase (JNK). The downstream signaling finally leads to DNA synthesis and cell proliferation. Under CRC conditions, regulation of EGFR signaling is disturbed; hence, cell proliferation becomes uncontrolled. Upregulation of EGFR has been reported by many groups; hence, it can work as a CRC biomarker [65]. Inhibition of EGFR is effective in CRC; thus, EGFR and related downstream signaling proteins can be used as possible drug targets [10].

9.2.5 *Kinase Proteins as Biomarkers*

9.2.5.1 Urokinase-Type Plasminogen Activator (uPA)

It is also known as urokinase. uPA is a serine-type kinase which breaks inactive plasminogen into active plasmin enzyme. Plasmin activates downstream protease cascade and degrades extracellular matrix (ECM). Degradation of ECM helps in angiogenesis and cancer metastasis [7, 25]. Many studies analyzed the significance of increased uPA level in blood as biomarker for CRC [17, 41] using graphene nanosheets [47] and proteomics [1].

9.2.5.2 Nucleoside Diphosphate Kinase (NDPK/NM23)

It is a multifunctional, hexameric, ubiquitously distributed kinase enzyme, which acts as metastasis suppressor and transcription factor too. The main function of NM23 is to catalyze exchange of terminal phosphate residue between nucleoside diphosphates (NDP) and nucleoside triphosphates (NTP) to produce NTP in a reversible manner, by phosphorylation of histidine [51]. Two genes *NM23-H1* and *NM23-H2* have 88% similarity in their amino acids sequence, code for A and B subunits of NM23, respectively. NM23-H1 is a metastatic suppressor, and its down-regulation has been reported in many cancers including CRC [6, 73]. There are some contradicting reports showing positive correlation (upregulation) [3] or no correlation (no changes in expression level) [42] between expression level of NM23 and metastasis of CRC. This could be due to 88% similarity in amino acid sequence of NM23-H1 and NM23-H2, leading to nonspecific binding of antibodies to NM23-H2, whose expression level during CRC is not well documented yet. Although there are reports advocating the use of NM23 as a CRC biomarker [22], due to its contradictory status, use of NM23 as a CRC biomarker demands further investigations.

9.2.6 *Receptors and Signaling Molecules as Biomarkers*

9.2.6.1 G Protein-Coupled Receptor 35 (GPR35)

GPR35 is a member of cell surface receptor family, having five to seven transmembrane helix and cytoplasmic G protein binding sites. Initially it was considered as an orphan receptor having no known endogenous ligand. Any high-affinity ligand for GPR35 is yet unknown, although some low-affinity ligands like kynurenic acid and chemokine (C-X-C motif) ligand 17 (CXCL17) have been identified. Overexpression of GPR35 is responsible for the development of drug resistance in cancer cells. This drug resistance is caused by GPR35 in association with Akt and β-arrestin-2 signaling molecules. GPR35 expression is high in cancer cells, and it can be used a biomarker and drug target for treatment of CRC [2, 9].

9.2.6.2 Beta-Subunit of 14-3-3 Proteins (14-3-3β)

It is a serine/threonine binding membrane receptor, which transfers signals by homo- and heterodimerization. These proteins are involved in various signaling processes related to cell cycle regulation, apoptosis, metabolism, protein transport, and transcription by their autophosphorylation. In addition, they also take part in GTPaseHRas/RAF proto-oncogene serine/threonine-protein kinase (Ras/Raf) and AKT/mechanistic or mammalian target of rapamycin (mTOR) pathways which are involved in tumor formation. Two-dimensional gel electrophoresis, two-dimensional difference gel electrophoresis (DIGE), and immunohistochemistry-based studies showed that the level of 14-3-3β was upregulated in CRC samples compared to normal samples [26]. Depleted level of 14-3-3β indicates non-cancerous stage. Hence it can be used as a potential biomarker for CRC [36].

9.2.6.3 Interleukin-6 Signal Transducer (IL6ST)

It is a subunit of tyrosine kinase receptor and acts as a single transducer for many cytokines like interleukin-6 (IL6), ciliary neurotrophic factor (CNTF), leukemia inhibitory factor (LIF), and oncostatin M (OSM). IL6 is a pro-inflammatory cytokine which via IL6ST induces downstream Janus kinases (JAKs) and signal transducer and activator of transcription 3 (STAT3) [60] signaling pathways, thus inducing cell proliferation as well as inflammation. Increased level of IL6 and activation of IL6ST and STAT3 with/without IL6 lead to CRC; hence, increased level of both IL6 and IL6ST can be used as a CRC biomarker [49].

9.2.7 Glycoproteins as Biomarkers

9.2.7.1 von Willebrand Factor (VWF)

It is an adhesive and multimeric glycoprotein of plasma, which maintain primary homeostasis at the site of vascular injury. It helps in adhesion of platelets to the subendothelium of blood vessels using coagulation factor VIII. High plasma level of VWF has been reported in various cancers, e.g., larynx, cervical [40], and CRC [46, 48]. Recently, VWF has been successfully used as a marker to predict the outcome of hepatic cancer resection [50]. Significant difference in expression of VWF was not observed under different stages of CRC; hence, it can't be used as a biomarker to differentiate CRC stages.

9.2.7.2 Cluster of Differentiation (CD44) Antigen

It is a glycoprotein that acts as a cell surface receptor. CD44 is involved in cell-cell interaction, cell adhesion, lymphocyte activation, hematopoiesis, and tumor metastasis. It is an anti-apoptotic protein whose expression level was found to be upregulated in CRC samples. Xia and Xu [70] validated CD44 as a potential biomarker using bioinformatics-based data mining for CRC wherein CD4 and CD74 expressions were also found to be high during CRC. Downregulation of CD44 was reported in LSC human colon cancer cell lines via "Core 1-mediated O-glycosylation," which can be used as a possible CRC drug target [20].

9.2.8 Chaperon Regulator as a Biomarker

9.2.8.1 BAG Family Molecular Chaperone Regulator 4 (BAG4)

It is an anti-apoptotic protein and member of chaperon regulator family. It has a BAC domain at its C-terminal which binds with HSP70 and inhibits its activity. BAG4 also binds with tumor necrosis factor receptor superfamily member 1A (TNFRSF1A) and death receptors, thus inhibiting apoptosis [34, 55]. Upregulation of BAG4 was reported by Rho et al. [45] and Xiong et al. [69] using protein and mRNA microarray, respectively.

The abovementioned CRC biomarkers are not absolute. Some more proteins that require further validation as CRC biomarkers could be pyruvate kinase M2, cyclo-oxygenase-2, phosphoinositide 3-kinase, transferrin, caveolin-1, serum C-peptide, cyclin D, etc. There are approximately 25,000 proteins encoded by human genomes; limited numbers of proteins clearly indicate that there are yet many unexplored proteins that can be used as a reliable biomarker for CRC and other types of cancers.

9.3 Methods for Identification of Disease Biomarkers

9.3.1 Genomics Technologies

Genomics technologies include (i) gene sequencing and their comparison; (ii) randomly amplified polymorphic DNA (RAPD), restriction fragment length polymorphism (RFLP), etc.; (iii) polymerase chain reaction (PCR) and real-time PCR; and (iv) metagenomics. All these technologies are based on the principle that mutations cause cancer and during mutation there is change in gene sequence. These changes in gene sequence can be identified using any of the technologies mentioned above, and comparison of gene sequence from normal and CRC samples would reveal the role of that mutation in CRC.

9.3.2 *Proteomics Technologies*

All cancers are not due to changes in gene sequence; some are results of up-/down-regulation of various proteins. Up-/downregulation of proteins can be studied only by proteomics (gel-based, gel-free methods or Western blotting). Proteins from normal and disease samples are isolated and compared using either gel-based or gel-free methods. Up-/downregulated proteins between disease and normal samples are identified for further validation as biomarkers or drug targets.

9.3.3 *Microarray Technologies*

Microarray technology compares the gene expression of thousands of proteins simultaneously between two and more samples. Unlike genomics and proteomics technologies which focus exclusively and respectively on genes or proteins, the microarray can deal with both genes and proteins. Microarray can be mRNA, cDNA, or protein based and is being utilized widely for the comparison of gene expression between diseased and normal samples.

9.3.4 *In Silico Methods (Metadata Analysis and Big Data Mining)*

Research groups across the globe are producing lots of biological (genomics, proteomics, image data, etc.) data on daily basis. Usually research groups are focused on their limited objective, and the information not related to those objectives remains unprocessed. Metadata is the data in the form of millions of research papers published worldwide and available on the Internet. Analysis of this metadata provides much useful information [27, 30]. In the above description, metadata analysis identified p53 and CD44 as CRC biomarkers. Data mining is the analysis of large, multidimensional, and diverse data. Microarray data is the perfect example of such big data, using which CRC samples are compared with normal samples, and many biomarkers have been identified at theoretical level. Using feature selection algorithms and classification algorithms of data mining, microarray datasets have been analyzed by various data scientists [29, 58].

9.4 Conclusion

Colorectal cancer (CRC) is one of the most prevailing types of cancer, and millions of peoples are affected with it worldwide. Although treatment options for CRCs are available, the type of treatment and its efficiency depends upon the developmental stage of CRCs. Detection at an early stage not only helps in proper treatment but also reduces the changes of CRC re-occurrence. A blood serum-based biomarker assists in early diagnosis of CRC and identification of its developmental stage. Studies focused on CRCs have identified p53, ALDH1, 14-3-3β, EGFR, CD44, etc. as CRC biomarkers, which have been identified using genomics, proteomics, microarray, or in silico-based methods. Although a number of proteins, described above, have been identified as CRC biomarkers, the list is not exhaustive. There can be other proteins in the human body that may serve as better and reliable CRC biomarkers.

References

1. Ahn SB, Mohamedali A, et al. Proteomics reveals cell-surface urokinase plasminogen activator receptor expression impacts most hallmarks of cancer. Proteomics. 2019;19(21–22):1900026.
2. Ali H, AbdelMageed M, et al. Utility of G protein-coupled receptor 35 expression for predicting outcome in colon cancer. Tumor Biol. 2019;41(6):1010428319858885.
3. Alvarez-Chaver P, Rodriguez-Pineiro AM, et al. Selection of putative colorectal cancer markers by applying PCA on the soluble proteome of tumors: NDK a as a promising candidate. J Proteome. 2011;74(6):874–86.
4. Awasthi P, Foiani M, et al. ATM and ATR signaling at a glance. J Cell Sci. 2015;128(23):4255–62.
5. Bednarz-Misa I, Neubauer K, et al. Whole blood ACTB, B2M and GAPDH expression reflects activity of inflammatory bowel disease, advancement of colorectal cancer, and correlates with circulating inflammatory and angiogenic factors: relevance for real-time quantitative PCR. Adv Clin Exp Med. 2020;29(5):547–56.
6. Boissan M, De Wever O, et al. Implication of metastasis suppressor NM23-H1 in maintaining adherens junctions and limiting the invasive potential of human cancer cells. Cancer Res. 2010;70(19):7710–22.
7. Booyse FM, Aikens ML, et al. Endothelial cell fibrinolysis: transcriptional regulation of fibrinolytic protein gene expression (t-PA, u-PA, and PAI-1) by low alcohol. Alcohol Clin Exp Res. 1999;23(6):1119–24.
8. Bradbury A, Hall S, et al. Targeting ATR as cancer therapy: a new era for synthetic lethality and synergistic combinations? Pharmacol Ther. 2020;207:107450.
9. Chaitanya AK, Kumari S, et al. Mechanisms and pathways of metabolic reprogramming of colorectal cancer. In: Theranostics approaches to gastric and colon cancer. New York: Springer; 2020. p. 69–80.
10. Chan DLH, Segelov E, et al. Epidermal growth factor receptor (EGFR) inhibitors for metastatic colorectal cancer. Cochrane Database Syst Rev. 2017;6(6):CD007047.
11. Cheng Z, Shao X, et al. ENO1 acts as a prognostic biomarker candidate and promotes tumor growth and migration ability through the regulation of Rab1A in colorectal cancer. Cancer Manag Res. 2019;11:9969.
12. Clark O, Yen K, et al. Molecular pathways: isocitrate dehydrogenase mutations in cancer. Clin Cancer Res. 2016;22(8):1837–42.
13. Cortez D, Guntuku S, et al. ATR and ATRIP: partners in checkpoint signaling. Science. 2001;294(5547):1713–6.
14. Dinami R, Porru M, et al. TRF2 and VEGF-A: an unknown relationship with prognostic impact on survival of colorectal cancer patients. J Exp Clin Cancer Res. 2020;39(1):1–13.
15. Dong Z, Jiang H, et al. Ribosomal protein L15 is involved in colon carcinogenesis. Int J Med Sci. 2019;16(8):1132.

16. Fang Z, Gong C, et al. E2F1 promote the aggressiveness of human colorectal cancer by activating the ribonucleotide reductase small subunit M2. Biochem Biophys Res Commun. 2015;464(2):407–15.
17. Fang Z, Li C, et al. MicroRNA-193b acts as a tumor suppressor in colon cancer progression via targeting RAB22A. Exp Ther Med. 2019;17(5):3921–8.
18. Fang Z, Lin M, et al. A comprehensive review of the roles of E2F1 in colon cancer. Am J Cancer Res. 2020;10(3):757.
19. Frezzetti D, Gallo M, et al. VEGF as a potential target in lung cancer. Expert Opin Ther Targets. 2017;21(10):959–66.
20. Gao T, Wen T, et al. Disruption of Core 1-mediated O-glycosylation oppositely regulates CD44 expression in human colon cancer cells and tumor-derived exosomes. Biochem Biophys Res Commun. 2020;521(2):514–20.
21. Goudarzi KM, Lindstrom MS. Role of ribosomal protein mutations in tumor development. Int J Oncol. 2016;48(4):1313–24.
22. Han W, Ma J, et al. The role of NM23 in patients with colorectal cancer: a systematic review and meta-analysis. J Huazhong Univ Sci Technol Med Sci. 2017;37(1):1–10.
23. Hsiao K-C, Shih N-Y, et al. Surface α-enolase promotes extracellular matrix degradation and tumor metastasis and represents a new therapeutic target. PLoS One. 2013;8(7):e69354.
24. Huang C-L, Liu D, et al. E2F1 overexpression correlates with thymidylate synthase and survivin gene expressions and tumor proliferation in non small-cell lung cancer. Clin Cancer Res. 2007;13(23):6938–46.
25. Huang S-F, Chu S-C, et al. Antimetastatic effects of gossypol on colon cancer cells by targeting the u-PA and FAK pathways. Food Funct. 2019;10(12):8172–81.
26. Kirana C, Peng L, et al. Combination of laser microdissection, 2D-DIGE and MALDI-TOF MS to identify protein biomarkers to predict colorectal cancer spread. Clin Proteomics. 2019;16(1):1–13.
27. Kong JC, Guerra GR, et al. Prognostic impact of tumor-infiltrating lymphocytes in primary and metastatic colorectal cancer: a systematic review and meta-analysis. Dis Colon Rectum. 2019;62(4):498–508.
28. Liu S, Tan Q, et al. Anti-p53 autoantibody in blood as a diagnostic biomarker for colorectal cancer: a meta-analysis. Scand J Immunol. 2020;91(2):e12829.
29. Loey M, Jasim MW, et al. Breast and colon cancer classification from gene expression profiles using data mining techniques. Symmetry. 2020;12(3):408.
30. Lu X, Guo W, et al. Prognostic value of the Glasgow prognostic score in colorectal cancer: a meta-analysis of 9,839 patients. Cancer Manag Res. 2019;11:229.
31. Maguire HC Jr, Greene MI. The neu (c-erbB-2) oncogene. Semin Oncol. 1989;16(2):148–55.
32. Melincovici CS, Bosca AB, et al. Vascular endothelial growth factor (VEGF)-key factor in normal and pathological angiogenesis. Romanian J Morphol Embryol. 2018;59(2):455–67.
33. Mello SS, Attardi LD. Deciphering p53 signaling in tumor suppression. Curr Opin Cell Biol. 2018;51:65–72.
34. Miki K, Eddy EM. Tumor necrosis factor receptor 1 is an ATPase regulated by silencer of death domain. Mol Cell Biol. 2002;22(8):2536–43.
35. Nakahata K, Uehara S, et al. Aldehyde dehydrogenase 1 (ALDH1) is a potential marker for cancer stem cells in embryonal rhabdomyosarcoma. PLoS One. 2015;10(4):e0125454.
36. O'Dwyer D, Ralton LD, et al. The proteomics of colorectal cancer: identification of a protein signature associated with prognosis. PLoS One. 2011;6(11):e27718.
37. Pedersen JW, Gentry-Maharaj A, et al. Early detection of cancer in the general population: a blinded case-control study of p53 autoantibodies in colorectal cancer. Br J Cancer. 2013;108(1):107–14.
38. Pellino G, Gallo G, et al. Noninvasive biomarkers of colorectal cancer: role in diagnosis and personalised treatment perspectives. Gastroenterol Res Pract. 2018;2018:2397863.
39. Peterson JE, Zurakowski D, et al. VEGF, PF4 and PDGF are elevated in platelets of colorectal cancer patients. Angiogenesis, 2011;15(2):265-273.

40. Peyvandi F, Garagiola I, et al. Role of von Willebrand factor in the haemostasis. Blood Transfus. 2011;9(Suppl 2):s3.
41. Prasad M, Lalmbe U, et al. An insight in biomarkers for colorectal cancer. J Gastroenterol Liver Dis. 2018;3(1):1010.
42. Qian L-Y, Li P, et al. Multivariate analysis of molecular indicators for postoperative liver metastasis in colorectal cancer cases. Asian Pac J Cancer Prev. 2012;13(8):3967–71.
43. Ramos D, Pellin-Carcelen A, et al. Deregulation of glyceraldehyde-3-phosphate dehydrogenase expression during tumor progression of human cutaneous melanoma. Anticancer Res. 2015;35(1):439–44.
44. Randon G, Fucã G, et al. Prognostic impact of ATM mutations in patients with metastatic colorectal cancer. Sci Rep. 2019;9(1):1–7.
45. Rho J-H, Ladd JJ, et al. Protein and glycomic plasma markers for early detection of adenoma and colon cancer. Gut. 2016;67(3):473–84.
46. Rho J-H, Ladd JJ, et al. Protein and glycomic plasma markers for early detection of adenoma and colon cancer. Gut. 2018;67(3):473–84.
47. Roberts A, Tripathi PP, et al. Graphene nanosheets as an electric mediator for ultrafast sensing of urokinase plasminogen activator receptor-a biomarker of cancer. Biosens Bioelectron. 2019;141:111398.
48. Schellerer VS, Mueller-Bergh L, et al. The clinical value of von Willebrand factor in colorectal carcinomas. Am J Transl Res. 2011;3(5):445.
49. Schumacher N, Rose-John S. Adam17 activity and IL-6 trans-signaling in inflammation and cancer. Cancers. 2019;11(11):1736.
50. Schwarz C, Fitschek F, et al. von Willebrand factor antigen predicts outcomes in patients after liver resection of hepatocellular carcinoma. Gut Liver. 2020;14(2):218.
51. Sharma S, Sengupta A, et al. NM23/NDPK proteins in transcription regulatory functions and chromatin modulation: emerging trends. Lab Investig. 2018;98(2):175–81.
52. Shussman N, Wexner SD. Colorectal polyps and polyposis syndromes. Gastroenterol Rep. 2014;2(1):1–15.
53. Sundar R, Miranda S, et al. Ataxia telangiectasia mutated protein loss and benefit from oxaliplatin-based chemotherapy in colorectal cancer. Clin Colorectal Cancer. 2018;17(4):280–4.
54. Song Y, Luo Q, et al. Alpha-enolase as a potential cancer prognostic marker promotes cell growth, migration, and invasion in glioma. Molecular cancer, 2014;13(1):1–12.
55. Takayama S, Xie Z, et al. An evolutionarily conserved family of Hsp70/Hsc70 molecular chaperone regulators. J Biol Chem. 1999;274(2):781–6.
56. Ullman TA, Itzkowitz SH. Intestinal inflammation and cancer. Gastroenterology. 2011;140(6):1807–1816.e1.
57. Vassalli G. Aldehyde dehydrogenases: not just markers, but functional regulators of stem cells. Stem Cells Int. 2019;2019:3904645.
58. Vlachavas EI, Pilalis E, et al. Radiogenomic analysis of F-18-fluorodeoxyglucose positron emission tomography and gene expression data elucidates the epidemiological complexity of colorectal cancer landscape. Comput Struct Biotechnol J. 2019;17:177–85.
59. Waitkus MS, Diplas BH, et al. Biological role and therapeutic potential of IDH mutations in cancer. Cancer Cell. 2018;34(2):186–95.
60. Waldner MJ, Foersch S, et al. Interleukin-6-a key regulator of colorectal cancer development. Int J Biol Sci. 2012;8(9):1248.
61. Wang J-Y, Hsieh J-S, et al. Molecular detection of APC, K-ras, and p53 mutations in the serum of colorectal cancer patients as circulating biomarkers. World J Surg. 2004;28(7):721–6.
62. Wang H, Zhao L-N, et al. Overexpression of ribosomal protein L15 is associated with cell proliferation in gastric cancer. BMC Cancer. 2006;6(1):1–8.
63. Wang D, Moothart DR, et al. The expression of glyceraldehyde-3-phosphate dehydrogenase associated cell cycle (GACC) genes correlates with cancer stage and poor survival in patients with solid tumors. PLoS One. 2013;8(4):e61262.

64. Wang M-J, Ping J, et al. The prognostic factors and multiple biomarkers in young patients with colorectal cancer. Sci Rep. 2015;5:10645.
65. Wang H, Ma C, et al. The primary study of the correlation between mRNA expression and protein phosphorylation of epidermal growth factor receptor EGFR in colorectal and breast cancer cell lines. Cancer Res. 2017;77(13):4654.
66. Wang S, Zhang Y, et al. TRIM67 activates p53 to suppress colorectal cancer initiation and progression. Cancer Res. 2019;79(16):4086–98.
67. Wang B, Ye Y, et al. SIRT 2-dependent IDH 1 deacetylation inhibits colorectal cancer and liver metastases. EMBO Rep. 2020;21(4):e48183.
68. Weber AM, Ryan AJ. ATM and ATR as therapeutic targets in cancer. Pharmacol Ther. 2015;149:124–38.
69. Wu G, Yuan S, et al. The KLF14 transcription factor regulates glycolysis by downregulating LDHB in colorectal cancer. Int J Biol Sci. 2019;15(3):628.
70. Xia P, Xu X-Y. Prognostic significance of CD44 in human colon cancer and gastric cancer: evidence from bioinformatic analyses. Oncotarget. 2016;7(29):45538.
71. Xiong W, Ai Y-Q, et al. Microarray analysis of circular RNA expression profile associated with 5-fluorouracil-based chemoradiation resistance in colorectal cancer cells. Biomed Res Int. 2017;2017:8421614.
72. Yamamoto T, Kudo M, et al. Identification of aldolase A as a potential diagnostic biomarker for colorectal cancer based on proteomic analysis using formalin-fixed paraffin-embedded tissue. Tumor Biol. 2016;37(10):13595–606.
73. Yang T, Chen B-Z, et al. Reduced NM23 protein level correlates with worse clinicopathologic features in colorectal cancers: a meta-analysis of pooled data. Medicine. 2016;95(4):e2589.
74. Yen KE, Schenkein DP. Cancer-associated isocitrate dehydrogenase mutations. Oncologist. 2012;17(1):5.
75. Zhang X, Zhao Y, et al. Expression of circZNF609 is down-regulated in colorectal cancer tissue and promotes apoptosis in colorectal cancer cells by upregulating p53. Med Sci Monit. 2019;25:5977–85.

Chapter 10
Short-Chain Fatty Acids as Therapeutic Agents in Colon Malignancies

Arundhati Mehta, Vivek Kumar Soni, Yashwant Kumar Ratre, Rajat Pratap Singh, Dhananjay Shukla, Naveen Kumar Vishvakarma, Rakesh Kumar Rai, and Navaneet Chaturvedi

Abstract Colon cancer has taken a large number of lives worldwide and stands among the few topmost killer malignancies. Although several approaches to combat the detrimental effects of neoplastic cells have been implemented in preclinical and clinical settings, these transformed cells display aggressive and recalcitrant behaviour during progression as well as treatment. Natural metabolites of microbial origin have recently attracted the biomedical investigators to owing to vast diversity and bioactivity. Short-chain fatty acids (SCFA) are products of fermentative metabolism of the microbiota of the gut. They contain fewer than six carbons and include butyrate, propionate, acetate, and lactate. SCFA are known for their ability to hinder the process of oncogenesis at the earliest and can serve as therapeutic agents. Apart from their metabolite nature, SCFA butyrate and propionate can stimulate cell surface receptors and alter the phenotypic behaviour of affected cells. Dedicated but ambiguous transporters for these SCFAs are known, and their cellular presence has a distinct consequence on metabolic modulation of normal as well as transformed cells. Further, SCFA can modulate the key enzymes governing the epigenetic state of cells. Targeted members of epigenetic machinery include, but not limited to,

Arundhati Mehta and Vivek Kumar Soni contributed equally as first author, with all other contributors.

A. Mehta · V. K. Soni · Y. K. Ratre · R. P. Singh · D. Shukla · N. K. Vishvakarma (✉)
Department of Biotechnology, Guru Ghasidas Vishwavidyalaya, Bilaspur, Chhattisgarh, India

R. K. Rai (✉)
Uttar Pradesh-State AIDS Control Society (UPSACS), National AIDS Control Organization-Public Health foundation of India-Technical Support Unit (NACO-PHFI-TSU), Lucknow, Uttar Pradesh, India

N. Chaturvedi (✉)
Department of Molecular and Cell Biology, Henry Welcome Building, University of Leicester, Leicester, UK

School of Biochemical Engineering, Indian Institute of Technology-Banaras Hindu University (IIT-BHU), Varanasi, Uttar Pradesh, India

G. P. Nagaraju et al. (eds.), *Colon Cancer Diagnosis and Therapy*,
https://doi.org/10.1007/978-3-030-63369-1_10

HDACs and HAT. SCFA has shown potential in the management of cancers of various etiological origins. Moreover, SCFA can potentiate the ability of standard anti-cancer drugs through modulation of chemo-resistant conduct of transformed cells. This book chapter discusses the potential of SCFAs in colon cancer treatment with their possible mechanisms. Understanding the impending role of SCFA as therapeutic moieties will assist in designing therapeutic strategies using SCFA.

Keywords Colorectal cancer · Short-chain fatty acids · Gut microbiota · Micro-metabolites

Abbreviations

AML	Acute myeloid leukaemia
AT	Acetate
BT	Butyrate
CDK	Cyclin-dependent kinase
CKIs	Cyclin-dependent kinase inhibitors
CRC	Colorectal cancer
DCA	Dichloroacetate
DF	Dietary fibres
EMP	Embden-Meyerhof-Parnas pathway
FFAR	Free fatty acid receptor
GI tract	Gastrointestinal tract
GPCR/GPR	G protein-coupled receptor
HAT	Histone acetyltransferase
HDAC	Histone deacetylase
HDACi	HDAC inhibitors
IL	Interleukin
IMC	Intramucosal carcinoma
LPS	Lipopolysaccharide
MAPK or MAP kinase	Mitogen-activated protein kinase
MCA	Multiple colorectal adenomas
MCP-1	Monocyte chemoattractant protein-*1*
NaBT	Sodium butyrate
NF-kβ	Nuclear factor-kappa β
NOS	Nitric oxide synthase
PDK-2	Pyruvate dehydrogenase kinase isoform *2*
PEP	Phosphoenolpyruvate
PGC	Peroxisome proliferator-activated receptor-gamma coactivator
PKS	Polyketide synthase
PPARs	Peroxisome proliferator-activated receptors
PT	Propionate

RS	Resistant starch
SCFAs	Short-chain fatty acids
TNFα	Tumour necrosis factor α
TSGs	Tumour suppressor genes

10.1 Introduction

Divergent strategies to combat neoplastic disorders are currently underway in clinical settings as well as being tested for their efficacy in preclinical/laboratory investigations. However, many laboratories optimized strategies do meet unfavourable outcomes when they come to the battleground. Further, conventional therapeutic approaches against malignant disorders also have a variety of unwanted provokes including non-specific toxicity and onset of chemoresistance as few major ill effects. The ranges of malignancies including those of colorectal aetiology are not the exception of this. The colorectal cancers (CRCs) currently are being treated with interventional measures including surgical removal of cancer tissues, implementation of chemo–/radiotherapy, and their combinations. However, the detrimental and undesirable consequences associated with these therapeutic interventions encompass therapy insensitivity, immune derailment, infections, and multiple organ damages [7, 51]. The recent development of metabolomics and epigenetic acquaintance, along with inter–/transdisciplinary approaches to solving tribulations, has given new insight into this health deteriorating group of diseases [79, 92].

Microbial association with cancer development and progression has been sought in the earliest development of the subject, however, initially rejected in the absence of any firm evidence. Later on, an association has been proven in the case of gastric cancer with *Helicobacter pylori* [101]. On the other hand, the microbial world has also offered many molecules to fight various medical conditions. These microbes have also served as manufacturing machinery for the molecular farming of therapeutic entities. The range of molecules of microbial origins, especially those bacterial and fungal sources, has demonstrated gracious success in the management of malignancies, at least in laboratory settings. Even the association of human and normal flora of the human body has been explored for their role in the maintenance of health. These microbes of residing on or in human bodies have been linked with a diverse role in physiology and well-being [64].

The most abundant site for the microbial population in the human body is the gut, inhabited by trillions of microbes of diverse forms. Collectively known as ‘gut microbiota’, it is majorly populated by bacterial variety [50]. They have been helping us, humans, in digestion as well as maintaining colonic health. They have a unique repertoire of metabolic tackle and generate a variety of molecular products. Short-chain fatty acids are also one of these gut microbe-produced chemicals, having several benefits for human health. Similar biochemical has been suggested as a supplement to improve the efficacy of human bodies. Moreover, these SCFAs have demonstrated significant promise in the treatment of gastrointestinal malignancies including CRC [15, 35, 42]. As these SCFA and their derivatives are part of supplements, retrospective studies also suggest their efficacy in the prevention of CRC. In vitro investigations and animal studies have also suggested their potential in the treatment of colon malignancies. Diverse mechanistic targets have been associated with beneficial outcomes of SCFA in cancer. Therefore, its critical comprehension is presented here to assess the known specifics in its implementation in therapeutic settings for humans. The range of discussion is also warranted to evaluate its pledge in clinical investigations.

10.2 An Athletic Tale of Gut Microbiome

The intestinal consortium of microorganisms also known as 'gut microbiota' is a cosmic and an assorted group of microbes that reside in the gastrointestinal (GI) tract. They constitute a large population, approximately 100 trillion microorganisms of diverse taxa (including bacteria, eukaryotes, viruses, and even archaeon) encompassed in the human GI tract, which is about ten times of the number of cells found in a human body [50]. Among all the taxa residing in the gut, the chief and fundamental proportion is occupied by bacteria. Out of about half of a thousand divergent species inhabitant in the colonic space, researchers assessed the bacterial cell density to be 10^{11} to 10^{12} per millilitre, involving ~50 different phyla. Moreover, among these unicellular entities, the overriding group comprises of *Bacteroidetes* and *Firmicutes* [19, 64]. For instance, taking into account of gut microflora attributes like a wide variety, stability, and durability, the host-microbe symbiotic relationship could be recognized as 'a superorganism', executing metabolic and immunological roles [64].

Numerous experiments have shown that diet and medications greatly affect the number and composition of intestinal microbiota and therefore influence the structure of gut microbiota and their metabolic outcome. In the meantime, several metabolites are co-produced by intestinal microbiota and host, which function as a shuttle between human cells and gut microbiota and can, therefore, produce a significant share of favourable or pernicious effects of food and remedial products on the human body [18]. The GI tract's digestion is primarily synchronized by gut bacteria where they play a crucial part in the biophysiological function of various nutrient and metabolites, together with lipids, amino acids, short-chain fatty acids (SCFAs), bile acids, vitamins, indole derivatives, organic acids, and polyamines [19, 50]. Among all these biomolecules, the most copious are the bacteria-derived short-chain fatty acids (SCFAs), mainly acetate, propionate, and butyrate, which exist in the lumen of the human intestine in a ratio of around 3:1:1; correspondingly, yet, this proportion is, at least in part, reliant on both microbial composition and diet [50]. In addition to these (acetate, butyrate, and propionate), other SCFAs constitute about 5% part includes caproate, valerate, formate, etc. [15].

10.3 Short-Chain Fatty Acids (SCFAs) Production and Metabolism

Short-chain fatty acids (SCFAs) are free saturated aliphatic fatty acid moieties generated by gut microbiota by saccharolytic fermentative metabolism of dietary fibres (DF) [38, 53]. When the amount consumed surpasses the digestion rate or resists preliminary digestion, the prime macronutrients (carbohydrates, proteins, and fats) escape and enter the colon due to their innate structural intricacies [55]. Resistant starch (RS), inulin, oat bran, wheat bran, cellulose, guar gum, and pectin are the key substrates among the non-digestible DF for bacterial fermentation and SCFA generation. Especially, RS is a significant source for the production of butyrate. The synthesis of butyrate (BT) and propionate (PT) primarily comes from glycolysis (carbohydrate metabolism) but also added through the metabolism of organic acids and amino acids. Moreover, the acetate in the bowel, generated by glycolysis, is the most abundant SCFA and can also be converted into butyrate by the enzyme butyryl-CoA and acetyl-CoA transferases [56]. Structures of few SCFA compounds are given in Fig. 10.1.

In the intestinal microbiota, foremost metabolic pathways are employed in the development of SCFAs from non-comestible saccharides, initially through the development of pyruvates by glycolysis in the Embden-Meyerhof-Parnas (EMP) pathway or via pentose phosphate shunt (PPS) utilizing phosphoenolpyruvate (PEP). This transitional biomolecule is being used to generate specific SCFA utilizing certain bacterial synthesis pathways. With the concomitant production of H_2 and CO_2, much of the pyruvate is transformed into acetyl-CoA. Acetate is often formed unswervingly from the hydrolysis of acetyl-CoA by certain bacterial cells like *Coprococcus eutactus* and *C. comes* or through the Wood-Ljungdahl pathway from

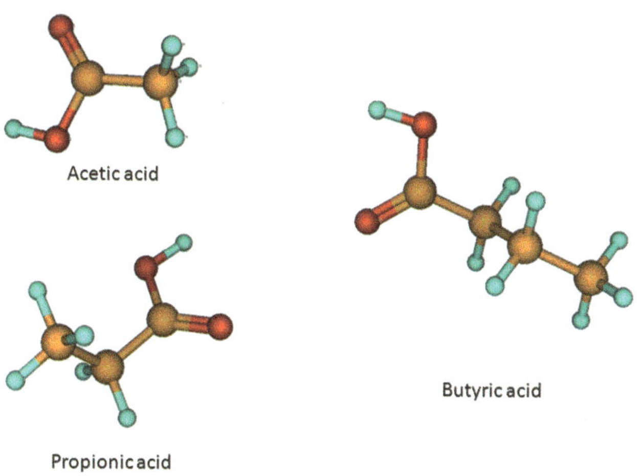

Fig. 10.1 Structure of SCFA anticancer compounds

CO2 or formate in which carbon dioxide (CO_2) is reduced to carbon monoxide (CO) and transformed into acetyl-CoA by a methyl group and by CoASH [48, 61, 62].

For the production of propionic acid (propionate, PT), colonic bacteria employ a trilogy of specific ways that includes the acrylate pathway, the succinate pathway, and the propanediol pathway [63]. The succinate route uses succinate as a PT forming substratum by utilizing a basic anaerobic electron transfer chain (ETC) for the decarboxylation of methylmalonyl-CoA into propionyl-CoA. The succinate is directly being modified through bacteria like *Phascolarctobacterium succinatutens* into succinyl-CoA and then propionyl-CoA [84]. Flint and co-workers suggested that some gut microflora species like *Eubacterium hallii, Anaerostipes* spp., and *Veillonella* spp. yields PT by pyruvate reduction to form lactate, while others like *Coprococcus catus* and *Megasphaera elsdenii* reduce lactate to PT through the 2-propenoate process, also called acrylate pathway [20]. Furthermore, some microflora avail a propanediol pathway to manufacture dihydroxyacetone phosphate (DHAP) + l-glyceraldehyde derived from rhamnose and propionate from fucose [48, 63].

BT arises out of dietary carbohydrates by dint of glycolysis via ligation of two acetyl-CoA molecules resulting in acetoacetyl-CoA and subsequent piecemeal depletion into butyryl-CoA. Two diverse metabolic pathways are identified for the concluding stage of BT production from butyryl-CoA which make headway either employing butyryl-CoA: acetate CoA-transferase or through butyrate kinase and phosphotransbutyrylase with the simultaneous generation of ATP [47]. Lately microbes, viz. *Roseburia* spp., *E. hallii, Eubacterium rectale, C. catus, Faecalibacterium prausnitzii*, and *Anaerostipes* spp., are revealed to yield BT in the butyryl-CoA: acetate CoA-transferase pathway through consumption of exogenously derived acetate [84]. Chemical characteristics of SCFAs and their microbial origins are given in Table 10.1.

In order to better understand the natal effects of SCFA on human beings, it is necessary to recognize the SCFA development site and biological gradient over the different downwind tissue. The discoveries from animal experiments that often use oral SCFA augmentation or high fibre top-up to induce SCFA development shifts are interpreted in particular. SCFAs produced in the caecum are found in hepatic, portal, and peripheral blood [15] and have a robust biological gradient from gut lumen to the periphery, leading to different exposures to the SCFA cells and tissues [53]. SCFAs affect the metabolism of lipids, glucose, and cholesterol in numerous tissues. Some research specifies that these FAs are delivered into the host's blood compartment from the intestinal lumen and absorbed by organs serving as substrates or signal molecules [15]. The interchange between usage and credibility of epithelium, splanchnic use, and peripheral accessibility involves depiction to decide whether enhanced SCFA output or limited increases in SCFA in different tissues are perceived to be responsible for any metabolic effects [53].

Table 10.1 Chemical nature and microbial origin of SCFAs

S. No.	SCFA metabolite	Chemical formula	Chemical group	Molecular weight	pKa	Microbial origin	Reference
1.	Acetic acid (acetate: AT)	$C_2H_4O_2$ (CH_3COOH)	Organic monocarboxylic acid	60.05 g/Mol	4.76 at 25 °C	*Acinetobacter*, *Bacteroides*, *Bifidobacterium*, *Enterobacter*, *Prevotella*, *Ruminococcus*, *Streptococcus*, *Staphylococcus*, *Pseudomonas*, *Proteus*, *Klebsiella*, *Escherichia*, *Enterococcus*, *Citrobacter*, *Akkermansia*	(PubChemCID-176; [79])
2.	Butyric acid (butyrate: BT)	$C_4H_8O_2$ ($CH_3CH_2CH_2COOH$)	Lipid (fatty acyl)	88.11 g/Mol	4.82 at 25 °C	*Anaerostipes*, *Eubacterium*, *Roseburia*, *Faecalibacterium*, *Coprococcus*	(PubChemCID-264; [79])
3.	Propionic acid (propionate: PT)	$C_3H_6O_2$ (CH_3CH_2COOH)	Organic carboxylic acid	74.08 g/Mol	4.88	*Propionibacterium* strains, *Phascolarctobacterium*, *Eubacterium*, *Veillonella* spp.	(PubChemCID-1032; [84])
4.	Lactic acid (lactate: LT)	$C_3H_6O_3$ ($CH_3CHOHCOOH$)	Organic acid (organic hydroxy acid)	90.08 g/Mol	3.86 at 20 °C	*Acinetobacter*, *Enterobacter*, *Corynebacterium*, *Bacillus*, *Streptococcus*, *Staphylococcus*, *Pseudomonas*, *Proteus*, *Klebsiella*, *Escherichia*, *Enterococcus*, *Citrobacter*	(PubChemCID-612; [79])

10.4 A Frenemy Alliance of Gut Integrity and CRC

In the initial chapter of life, the regular composition of the intestinal microbiota and gut microenvironment shifts swiftly. It is imperative to retain the homeostasis in the intestine/gut as metabolic and mechanical roles of the commensal microbiota prevent pathogens' intestinal colonization. A large array of maladies such as inflammatory bowel disease (IBD), colon cancer, etc. have been linked with dysbiosis disorder in the role or composition of the gut microbiota [35]. CRC is ranked third in incidence (with over 1.8 million new cases) worldwide and second for casualties (over 860,000 deaths) in 2018 among all cancers [7]. Investigations on oncogenic processes of some contagious agents also explored the aggregated microbial population of the tumour ecosystem, leading to the emergence of the gut microbiota as a critical factor for some cancers. Any alterations in the relative abundance of these tiny living forms may result in the equipoise shift and variation in GI physiology, contributing to intestinal and parietal illness like colorectal carcinogenesis [94].

Recently, Yachida and colleagues conducted a metabolomics and metagenomics investigation validating apparent swing in microbiota functional and taxonomical features in intramucosal carcinoma (IMC) and multiple colorectal adenomas (MCA) from the faecal samples of partakers through colonoscopy. Precise stage inspection showed discrete dualistic arrays of microbiome elevations. Initially, a liberal rise in density was demonstrated for some of the bacterial taxa (*F. nucleatum* and *Solobacterium moorei*) across successive stages of carcinogenesis, while in patients with MCA and IMC, *Actinomyces odontolyticus* and *Atopobium parvulum* abundance were raised at an early stage of carcinogenesis [96]. Additionally, in a report instigating people microbiome with colorectal adenomatous polyp of various stages and sizes, an increase in abundance of some fungal phyla (*Basidiomycota*) was evidenced [49].

Colorectal tumorigenesis is a dynamic and complex phenomenon with various etiological pathways affected by genetic and environmental factors. A lot of these courses such as regulation of the inflammation, immune system, dietary metabolism, and production of genotoxin are closely associated with intestinal microbiota. A significant and an essential crossing point between the host immune system and the intestinal microbiota is offered by the GI tract. Out of which, the signature and proven risk factor for CRC is persistent inflammation as patients with IBD are ominously more prone to develop cancer [94]. These facts were validated by investigation on CRC patient and healthy person faecal sample gavaged germ-free mice and normal mice with a carcinogen, azoxymethane. RT-PCR and q-PCR assay displayed an enhancement in adenomatous polyp number (histological inflammation), intestinal dysplasia levels, and inflammatory gene marker expression as a result of gut microbiota-stimulated chemotactic factors: CXCL9/10 (for type 1TH cells and CTLs) and CCL17/20 (for IL-17-producing TH cells) inducing recruitment of T cells into the site of tumour-promoting oncogenesis [12, 93].

A meta-analysis of 11 discerned human studies elucidates the link between *Helicobacter pylori* septicity and CRC risk and conveyed a 1.4 time amplified threat of CRC in patients [101], while another meta-analysis by Guo and Li, on East Asian population, suggests an oncogenic role of *H. pylori* during the earliest phase of tumorigenic transformation [27]. *E. faecalis* and *E. coli* have been recurrently found in CRC patients. Numerous inspections have proved a robust connotation among mucosa-adherent *E. coli* and CRC. Most of the isolated *E. coli* elicit genetic instability in the CRC patients by harbouring in the polyketide synthase (PKS) genomic island and encoding for colibactin, a polyketide-peptide genotoxin, which causes cell cycle interference and DNA damage mutation [35].

10.5 SCFAs: A Weak Electrolyte Test Drive

The function of SCFAs in epithelial physiologies has been re-evaluated by rumen physiologists and tissue culture scientists, establishing SCFA's swift absorption in the host epithelium. This suggests the SCFAs as an effective transformer or regulator of an eclectic range of cancer cell lines. In the existing time, the SCFAs are closely being explored for their several possible implications, counting questions on the movement of SCFAs through the epithelial system; the scope of SCFA effects as a biological response modifier; the nutritional position in SCFA; and the modification in the action of SCFA in other ways, including the intracellular pH (pHi) and the cell volume [68]. The colonocytes have been the model cell system for the major investigations on the transport mechanism of SCFA. Colonocytes were subjected to the peak concentrations of SCFA as they are crossway transported via apical and basolateral colonocyte membranes and constitute the colonic and caecal lining of the epithelium [15]. Each transporter is controlled in precise by means of its substrates themselves; in this process, SCFA as signalling molecules are involved with cell surface receptors [70, 72].

Since short-chain fatty acids are low electrolytes and majorly exist in the anionic form (A-), a balance between the charged forms, HA (protonated cation form), and A- (deprotonated anion form) in the gut epithelium intracellular, basolateral, and luminal compartments exists. Deprotonated form entails other transport proteins to move across the cellular boundary, the cell membrane, compared to lipid-soluble HA, which quickly diffuses through the cell membranes. Equipoises must be formed among the compartment sections. Therefore, the transport of any of the metabolite including SCFA will affect the concentration of the other biomolecule as fine variations in one section will mirror the shift in other [68]. Active transmission (facilitated by multiple transporting carriers of dissociated fatty acid (FA) anions) and passive diffusion (of non-dissociated SCFAs) are two different means of transporting molecules in compartments. Among these, active transport plays a significant part in the movement of SCFAs. Owing to luminal pH 5.5–6.5 (pH around 6.0) and a pKa of ~4.8 for SCFAs, these biomolecules are available in a dissociated form; hence, active transportation of these anion moieties across the apical epithelium membrane covers major proportion [15, 84].

The active transportation of dissociated anions across the apical epithelium gut lining is aided by transporters with the principal mechanism encompassing a range of anion exchangers. SCFAs cellular uptake is driven by numerous electroneutral and electrogenic transport systems. SLC16A1 (monocarboxylate transporter 1, MCT1) and SLC16A3 (MCT4) are H^+- coupled transporters, whereas SLC5A8 (sodium-coupled MCT1:SMCT1) and SLC5A12 (SMCT2) are Na^+-coupled transport system. The first one is the electroneutral transport process, which involves the exchange of imported dissociated anions with $HCO3^-$ ions by carbonic anhydrase reaction, issuing a luminal source of $HCO3^-$ anions to neutralize H^+ [1]. Numerous investigators have supplied irrefutable proof, stating short-chain fatty acids' bicarbonate anion exchange was autonomous to Na + transport and Cl–HCO3– exchange system via vesicular studies [30, 86]. Teramae et al. performed a comparative study and concluded that SLC16A1 (MCT1) carries fatty acid moieties in proton-dependent electroneutral style and also contributes to the transportation of pyruvic acid (pyruvate) and lactic acid (lactate) [80].

SLC5A8 (SMCT1) is stoichiometrically coupled to sodium ion transport in the ratio of 1:2 and induces Cl^- and absorption of water [28]. SMCT1 active transport facilitates faster mobilization of butyrate than propionate and acetate [26]. The H^+-SCFA symport and the SCFA anion-$HCO3^-$ antiport mobilize the undigested share of SCFAs, discarded by colon cells (colonocytes), to the basolateral membrane of epithelia. The apical and basolateral antiporters differ from each other as they have distinct Km values [30, 85]. Immunoblotting and immunohistochemistry studies of human intestinal mucosa indicate the occurrence of SLC16A3 (MCT4) and SLC16A4 (MCT5) in the basolateral membrane [24].

10.6 SCFA Receptors

A definite cellular reaction stems from the communication of nutrients with the host systems through transmembrane and intracellular molecules. Sensing of nutrients is an organism's environment-sensing mechanism [59]. During gut fermentation, the intestine creates an array of nutrients, i.e. short-chain fatty acids (SCFA), that are sensed by different receptors. The nutrient-sensing G protein-coupled receptors (GPCRs/GPRs) are one nifty type of nutrient sensors and can act on a range of ligands through a widespread expression of the tissue and different signalling pathways [60]. Generally, GPRs are intricated in the modulation of glucose and lipid metabolism, and among them, GPR41 and GPR43 were recognized as short-chain fatty acid receptors. The first short-chain fatty acid receptors (SCFA-Rs) were uncovered fortuitously with their ligands. A group of four intron-less genes, GPR40, GPR41, GPR42, and GPR43, were pinpointed downstream of the 19q13.1 chromosome gene CD22 in the context of a quest of human galanin receptor subtypes [67] and were categorized as orphan GPCRs [57].

Several investigations indicated that SCFAs serve as ligands of FFA2 and FFA3 receptors as well. For ligand binding and receptor stimulation, ionic bonding between the positively charged amino acid residues and negatively charged carboxylate group SCFAs is important [75]. Both FFA2 and FFA3 are expressed in brush cells of the gastric groove, spleen, etc. [16], and their distinct features of G protein alpha (G_{α}) signalling lead to discrete terminal effects. Twin signalling via Gαq/11 and Gαi/o pathways is indicated to be feasible by FFA2 inferring both activating and inhibiting cellular response, while FFA3 signals, majorly through $G_{\alpha i/o}$, have inhibitory tone [32]. Kim et al. elucidated that FFA2 and FFA3 are critical operators of intestinal penetrability [36, 59].

In carcinomas of the intestine, expression of FFA2 is downregulated or absent; the refurbishment induces G0/G1 phase cell arrest and p21 upregulation and diminishes the levels of cyclin D3 and cyclin-dependent kinases (CDKs) 1 and 2. This may stimulate programmed cell death and hinder the proliferation of cancer cells [71, 77]. Furthermore, FFA2's anti-tumour effect is not restricted to colon adenocarcinoma; it is copiously expressed in BaF3 leukaemia and countered to activate cell proliferation [3]. In contrast to FFA2, FFA3 has yet not been shown to have a function in cancer initiation or progression due to low expression in cancer cell lines compared to FFA2 [97] or its pro-cancer in vitro effects [59]. SCFAs such as PT and BT are believed to stimulate free fatty acid receptors (FFARs) specially FFAR2 (GPR43) and FFAR3 (GPR41), therefore playing part in tumour suppression and indorsing apoptosis [38, 76, 82].

The GPR109a signalling triggered by BT was reported to play a crucial role in anti-inflammatory activity in the gut. The latest data from Borthakour et al. have suggested GPR109a as a new nutrient transmitter. Improved MCT-1 function and cell surface expression through GPR109a signalling with rapid butyrate treatment (30–120 min) were also observed [6]. The BT and niacin stimulate GPR109a, and this signal has been recorded to coordinate to the development of Treg and IL-18 and IL-10 in colon cells. The expression levels of GPR109a are observed to be downregulated in colon cancer cell line, mouse models, and human cancer tissues, and its refurbishment and stimulation by their ligand may induce apoptosis [13, 81].

Olfactory receptor 78 (Olfr78) or human OR51E2(olfactory receptor family 51 subfamily E member 2) is present in numerous tissues that are less sought as compared to other receptors. These are $G_{\alpha s}$-coupled receptors shown to be stimulated by AT and PT [58]. Nevertheless, Pandora's pledge to fight severe inflammatory disorders like IBD, colon cancer, and digestive well-being encourages the interplay of intestinal microbiota, SCFAs, and cognate receptor signals.

10.7 SCFAs: A Knight in Shining Armour

The host and the microbiome communicate on the central platform of metabolism. The microbial metagenome codes genes that can metabolize many dietary foods, including undigested carbs such as galactooligosaccharides and fructo-oligosaccharides as well as bile acid-like host compounds [94]. Dietary fibre-derived short-chain fatty acids (SCFAs) are mainly ingested through the portal vein during lipid digestion and play an assorted physiological role in the body system. SCFAs are important immune and metabolic regulators and avert the headway of diseases like colitis, metabolic disorders, etc. [76]. In the bloodstream, butyrate serves as the main energy source for colonic epithelial cells, while the liver absorbs propionate, and acetate reaches the peripheral tissues. These fatty acids (FAs) are presumed to employ their upshots either by encumbering HDACs (histone deacetylases), inducing programmed cell death (apoptosis), or through G protein-coupled receptor (GPCR) stimulation. A comprehensive account of production, metabolism, and mode of action of SCFA is depicted in Fig. 10.2.

Butyrate (BT) theatres a vital role in maintaining colonic epithelial homeostasis by regulating inflammation, oxidative balance, functioning as HDAC inhibitors (HDACi), hindering DNA damage, and prevent oncogenic activation. For the initiation of CRC, APC-β-catenin-TCF4 is an imperative signalling which can be regulated by SCFAs. They amend both differentiation and proliferation of colonocytes and regulate their transformation. Butyrate oxidation in colonocytes gets influenced by exogenous factors, hence producing assorted forms of consequences on cells with varied metabolic characteristics. Interestingly, it has been perceived that it increases the proliferation of normal colonocytes and diminishes tumorigenic colonocyte proliferation [29].

In addition to the ability of BT to constrain HDAC activity, the alteration of miRNAs in cancer cells aids in anti-tumour mechanisms of butyrate. BT regulates the expression of both tumour-suppressive miRNA and oncogenic miRNA in several forms of cancers including breast, colon, and lung cancers. Lazarova et al. observed that a modification in Wnt signalling-specific gene expression has been associated with effects of butyrate including induction of apoptosis. It also controls the expression of various cell fate-related genes, such as Fas and Wnt10B, while also arbitrating FOXO3-dependent expression of Gadd45b, Cdkn1a, and Cdkn1c, subsequently leading to diminished proliferation and apoptosis in CRC [40, 95].

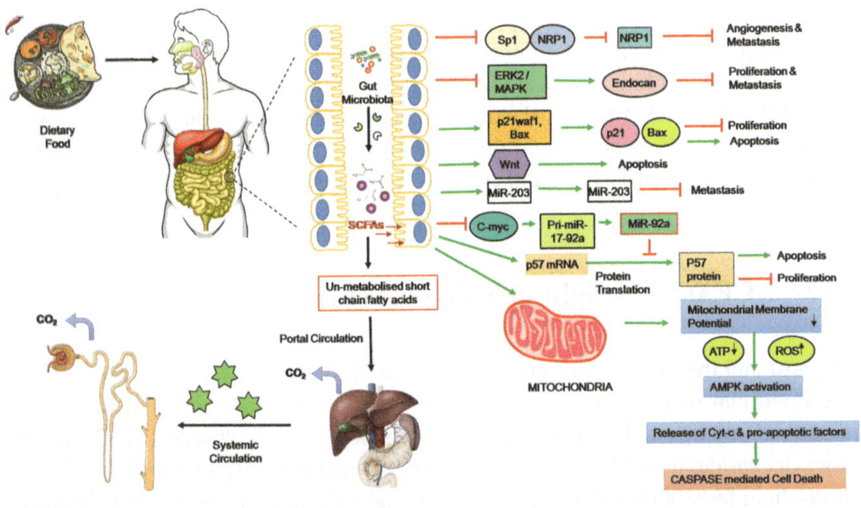

Fig. 10.2 Schematic diagram of SCFAs production, metabolism, and mode of action

To simplify the integration and assimilation of nutrients, it has been well conceded that to fulfil its energy requirements, cancer cells might shift to glycolysis. Additionally, cancer cells produce lactate through the fermentation of glucose (glycolysis-driven), refashioning the acidosis and proposing an ancestral benefit for tumour cells to upsurge their hostile phenotype. Consequently, extreme glucose ingestion in cancerous tissues leads to the reduction in expelled glucose, an escalation in the lactic acid level. This metabolic shift conquers with the rise in energy metabolism instigated by the initiation of the tumorigenic transformation of the cells. However, unlike normal colonocytes, CRC cells exhibit augmented sensitivity to SCFAs as they alone or in combination significantly heighten the consumption of glucose thru an elevation in the pentose oxidation pathway [91]. SCFAs reduce the apoptosis of non-transformed 'normal' epithelial cells through p21 activity while triggering the induction of apoptotic cell death in malignant cells. This constitutes an important defensive capability provided by SCFAs to prevent the incidence of CRC. Of late, a DARTS-based proteomics investigation by Li et al. confirmed direct binding of butyrate with PKM2 (M2 isoform of pyruvate kinase) overexpressed in neoplastic cells [42].

Other than, CRC, butyrate also shows potent anti-neoplastic activity against cervical and prostate cancer [14] and elevates the level of CDK inhibitors (CKIs) $p21^{WAF1/CIP1}$ and $p27^{KIP1}$ with a simultaneous loss of CDK2 activity, thus leading to cell cycle G1 phase growth arrest, in spite of continuing transcription of HPV [14]. Recently, investigations verified the whole transcriptome profile of CRC cells, treated with sodium butyrate via RNA sequencing, and proved participation of sodium butyrate to elicit dysregulated gene expression and cell apoptosis. qRT-PCR and sequence analysis suggest differential gene expression in treated CRC cells, i.e. out of 7192 genes, 1472 were downregulated and the rest were upregulated. Moreover, the pathway studies deduced that these genes were rich in mismatch repair, cell cycle and DNA replication, pyrimidine metabolism, etc., and among the identified factors contributing NaBT-stimulated cell death, MCM 2-7 complex may be a covert target of NaB [100].

Zhang et al. projected that sodium butyrate uplifts endoplasmic reticulum (ER) stress by tempering intracellular calcium levels, consequently, triggering autophagy. The accretion of auto-lysosomes, acidic vesicular organelles, and the expression of autophagy associated proteins, including microtubule-associated protein II light chain 3 (LC3-II), beclin-1, and Atg3 favor the autophagy. Since butyrate has a validated role in the growth inhibition and induction of cell death, it is expected to show an impact on cellular metabolic pathways and modulation in cellular metabolism [98]. Investigators recommended that though the malignant cells utilize and oxidize both butyrate and glucose into CO2, CRC cells show a higher oxidation rate for BT. Moreover, pre-treating cancer cells with BT elevates cellular capacity to oxidize butyrate and reduces glucose oxidation capacity, signifying that highly glycolytic colon cancer cells can switch to a butyrate-consuming phenotype to meet energy requirement and acetyl-CoA production. BT also orchestrate the control of the genes expression involved in glucose utilization leading to the inactivation of pyruvate dehydrogenase complex (PDC) [4]. PT-stimulated mitochondrial

Table 10.2 SCFAs and mechanism of action against colon cancer

S. No.	SCFA	Cell line/model	Signalling pathway and effects	Reference
1	Butyric acid	HCT116, HT29, Caco-2	*NRP-1/VEGF signalling*: Downturn expression of NRP-1 by impeding the transactivation of Sp1 to subdue the angiogenesis, metastasis, and survival of CRC cells	[95]
		RKO	*ERK2/MAPK signalling*: Obstruct CRC cell proliferation, clone formation, and relocation by encouraging expression of endocan	
		Dld-1, hct116	*Wnt signalling*: Endorse the apoptosis via hyper activating signalling	
		HT-29, SW48, SW1116	*p53 signalling*: Boost the P21waf1 and bax expression to prevent the proliferation and persuade apoptosis and arrest the cell cycle in G1 phase	
		SW837, HT-29, Caco-2, HCT116	*microRNA signalling*: Upstream expression of miR-203 and drop miR-92a expression to confine cellular proliferation, colony formation, cell invasion, and induce cell apoptosis	
		HCT-116 and HT-29	PERK-eIF2α *signalling pathway: acidic organelles accumulate; expression of LC3II, Atg, beclin-1, augment ER stress-associated protein expression levels (BIP, PDI,* etc.*)*	[98]
		HCT116, HT29, LOVO, and HCT8 cells	*Akt/ERK signalling*: HDAC3 silencing, deactivation of ERK1/2 and Akt1	[43]
2	Propionic acid	HCT116 cell line	*mTOR/Akt signalling*: Autophagic proteolysis and mitochondrial dysfunction-elevation in conversion of LC3-1 to LC3II, decline in expression of p62/SQSTM1 and overproduction of ROS	[77, 78]

dysfunction and autophagic proteolysis were observed in HCT116 cell line. Exposure of CRC cells to PT resulted in reduced expression of p62/SQSTM1 and overproduction of ROS leading to activation of caspases [77, 78]. Signalling pathways and subsequent effects of SCFA-derived modulations in colon cancer cells are summarized in Table 10.2.

10.8 SCFAs as Metabolic Modulators

The cancer cells exhibit an exclusive state of metabolic modification as compared to normal 'non-transformed' cells to withstand the demand for fast-dividing cells in addition to prevent immunosurveillance. Small molecules affecting cancer metabolism have been shown a promise in cancer therapy [88–90]. Butyrate was reported to modulate β-oxidation in cells of colon cancer. BT also alters glucose consumption and affects glutamine addiction in the tumour cells and, therefore, modulates lipid oxidation status in transformed cells. These metabolic alterations are critical for the survival and division of cancer cells. Several reports indicate the inactivation of PDC and modulation of PKM2. Effect of SCFAs on the metabolic state of cancer cells, especially on glycolytic metabolism and its regulation, remains largely unelucidated. Additionally, SCFAs' anti-cancer activity against a variety of cancer cells is not known along with its potential for reversal of chemoresistance [23].

Dysbiosis of metabolism in cancer cells essentially requires a unique repertoire of molecules which also bring suppression of antitumor response and skewing of immune cell activation inflator of tumour promotion. Modulation of such nexus by SCFAs is well hypothesized but remains unclear. SCFA controls the equilibrium of fatty acid production, oxidation of fatty acids, and body lipolysis magnitude. Oxidation of fatty acids can be triggered by SCFAs, whereas de novo production and lipolysis are prevented. The AMPK expression in the liver and muscular tissues has been shown to improve with the SCFAs either directly by raising AMP/ATP ratio or indirectly through the FFAR2-leptin signalling pathway [23]. Initiation of AMPK stimulates expression of PGC (peroxisome proliferator-activated receptor-gamma coactivator)-1α, known to regulate the transcriptional activity of multiple transcription factors, like (PPAR)α, PPARγ, PPARδ, liver X receptor (LXR), and farnesoid X receptor (FXR), all essential in glucose, cholesterol, and lipid metabolism regulation [34, 46]. Lately, Kimura and team disclosed that FFAR2 plays a key part in storing fats in adipose tissue [37].

Although data on the effect of SCFAs on glucose metabolism are limited, they corollary suggest its potential in the reduction of plasma glucose levels through several mechanisms. The amount of plasma glucose depends on diet intake and degree of gluconeogenesis, etc. Along with the FFARs and AMPK, the PYY (gut hormone peptide) and GLP-1 (glucagon-like peptide-1) act in tissue cross-talk. In an experiment with diabetic hyperglycaemic KK-A(y) and Sprague Dawley rats, an indirect reduction in gluconeogenesis is witnessed when AT and PT are administered orally [5, 66]. Similarly, hepatic AMPK initiation lowers the genomic expression of gluconeogenic enzymes G6Pase and PEPCK [15]. Plasma glucose rates may also be influenced by SCFAs by the induction of Ffar2 and Ffar3 receptors resulting in release of gut hormone PYY and GLP-1. PYY also enhances the insulin activity of muscle and adipose tissue on the release of glucose [15].

Cholesterol is formulated from its source, acetyl-CoA, utilizing a dynamic metabolic route in which the rate-limiting enzyme is 3-hydroxy-3-methyl-glutaryl-CoA reductase (HMGCR) [65]. The enzyme function of the 3-hydroxy-3-methylglutaryl-CoA (HMGCS) and HMGCR decreased the rate of cholesterol production in in vitro tests. A decline in the overall amount of cholesterol production by dietary PT was observed in the in vivo rat model through tritiated water (^3H_2O) as a tracer [9, 65]. Although AT role in maintaining homeostasis of cholesterol has been underrated, researchers demonstrated that AT contrived blood cholesterol level and reduces body fat mass. CYP7A1 assists in the cholesterol transformation to bile acid, as well as functions as cholesterol drain [21, 39]. In toto, short-chain fatty acids affect biochemical metabolism (glucose, lipid, and cholesterol) in a distinct way.

10.9 SCFA as an Epigenetic Modulator

Epigenetic alterations affect various cellular functions by controlling the expression of genes, especially without altering the DNA sequence of the genome directly. These dysregulated epigenomic modifications also contribute to tumour oncogenesis and enable the normal cell's transcriptome profile to vary. During an array of research, numerous types of epigenomic modifications have been recognized such as chromatin modelling, DNA methylation, histone modifications (methylation and acetylation), etc. [92]. Recent trends in scientific research highlighted epigenetics as the upcoming area of exploration due to its potent connotation with gene expression patterns [79]. Incongruous introduction or removal of acetyl/methyl groups on specific residues is commonly included in the epigenomic study. During the events of carcinogenesis, these 'epimutations' occur in proto-oncogenes and tumour suppressor genes (TSGs) at promoter or enhancer sites [8]. Gut microbiota and its metabolites stimulate epigenetic alterations and have a significant impact on the transcriptomic profile of host cells as they are critical messengers of the interplay between microbiota and host cells [33]. In CRC, many genes like LKB1, GATA4, APC, p16INK4a, MLH1, etc. and pathways are the documented targets of aberrant epigenetic mutations *[10]*. SCFAs, the chief metabolites of gut microflora, are reviewed to stimulate epigenomic modifications in histone acting as HDAC inhibitors, especially BT and AT. Because of greater bioavailability and poor accumulation in colon cells, PT shows low HDAC inhibition activity [79]. Some experimental pieces of evidence suggest, but not always, that acetate does not impede HDAC behaviour. In addition to the boosted acetylation of pro-inflammatory gene histones, for example, acetate improves LPS-6, IL-8, or TNFα development in LPS-exposed macrophages [41].

Through histone immunoblotting and flow cytometric analysis, Hinnebusch and co-workers validated that SCFA BT significantly triggered programmed cell death by downregulating CB1 (cyclin B1) and escalating the p21 (cell cycle inhibitor) expression [31]. BT regulates the expression of numerous migration-related rudiments such as TIMP-1 and TIMP-2 and quells the metastasis of CRC via deactivation of Akt/ERK signalling in HDAC3-dependent manner [43]. STAT3 activation in JAK2/STAT signalling pathway leads to an upsurge in the subsequent signalling activities of IL-8, c-myc, bcl-2, bcl-xl, VEGF, HIF, and cyclin D1, thus inferring a rise in cell proliferation, initiation of angiogenesis, and an escape from induction of apoptotic death [52].

Sodium butyrate (SB) upregulates SOCS1 and SOCS3 expression via HDAC8 inhibition and repressed JAK2/STAT signalling cascade [22]. BT-instigated HDAC inhibition also corresponds with the E2F-1 transcription factor release by a time-dependent degradation of pRb, p107, and p130. Following the preliminary G1 arrest and concomitant CKIs' upregulation in the presence of free E2F results in a 'conflicting growth situation'. This molecular cascade finally leads the cells to undergo E2F-responsive p73 pro-apoptotic isoform-induced programmed cell death interim via the mitochondrial pathway. The PI3K-Akt pathway blocked by BT via inactivation of HDAC3 resulted in a revert of tumour cell metastasis [43]. Moreover, some investigations authenticated the augmentation of PTEN by BT, which stimulated cell differentiation in gastric cells by encouraging expression of MUC2 [2]. Additionally, BT dwindled inflammation through Akt deactivation and its downflow NF-kβ signalling pathways in a colitis mouse model triggered through 2,4,6-trinitrobenzenesulfonic acid (TNBS) [11].

10.10 SCFAs in Chemoresistance and Immune Modulation

Some of the cornerstones in the treatment of certain solid tumours, including CRC, appear to be chemotherapy. The CRC-specific chemical therapeutic schemes are provided to patients with stage III or IV diseases in the context of adjuvant treatments, through the solo use or in conjunction with an individual conventional cytotoxic agent. Regardless of the amount and method of drugs or their formulations, both chemotherapy's fundamental and primary goal is easy, i.e. to prevent the deviant development and proliferation of malignant cells in the body [73]. The emergence of chemical tolerance not only raises the dosages for cancer medications but also contributes to certain adverse effects [74].

Overcoming latent aversion to treatment gained by cancer cells is a big problem as chemo(drug)-resistance induces recurrence, disease spread, and death. The chemical tolerance of malignant cells is widely agnized as a noteworthy cause of chemotherapy failures and the subsequent development of ailments accompanied by the untimely and premature death of a patient [99]. The same puddle of intestinal stem cells, for the regeneration of the intestinal epithelia, is also present in the microenvironment or tumour niche that provides development and proliferation of cancer stem cells. These cancer stem cells resist therapy and promote cancer recurrence, although they account for less than 2.5% of the tumour mass [51].

Glei et al. demonstrated the chemo-protective activity of HT29 cells from H_2O_2-triggered DNA damage by arabinoxylans via single-cell microgel electrophoresis assay [25]. Combinatorial synergistic cytotoxic activity of NaB (sodium butyrate) and artemisinin was recorded in human cancer cells [69]. Similarly, studies have validated butyrate-arbitrated procurement of chemoprotection of colon carcinoma cells in combination with irinotecan by modulating P-glycoprotein activity and bax/bcl-2 ratio to stimulate programmed cell death [17]. Another study highlighted the reverse role of BT to develop resistance to chemotherapeutics. The research involved establishing BT-resistant HCT116 colon cancer cells by treating cells to gradually increasing concentrations of BT and relating sensitivity against numerous chemotherapeutics and protein expression by immunoblotting analysis [45].

A metabolic regulator, DCA (dichloroacetate), improved the colorectal cancer cell's sensitivity to 5-FU (fluorouracil) and lowered the colony formation along with an elevated apoptosis rate. It was observed by the micro-array data that miR-149-3p was associated with the CRC chemo-resistance. The same was altered by the p53 wild form after DCA therapy which established PDK2 as a primary target for miR-149-3p. This also determine the p53/miR-149-3p/PDK2 signaling pathway as potential target for DCA [44]. The abovementioned acts suggested that there are multidimensional pathways and mechanisms operating to impart chemoprotection and chemosensitization in colorectal cancer (CRC) cells.

The latest work has shown a promising area that SCFA plays on the centre stage to control the immune and inflammatory responses. Around the turn of this century, initial research revealed the possible role of BT in immune control as butyrate was found to obstruct the macrophage activation through nuclear factor-kappa β (NF-kβ), as well as hinder histone deacetylation in acute myeloid leukaemia (AML). Inhibition of histone deacetylation theatres a crucial part in inflammatory pathways and epigenetic signalling [53]. Incidence distribution research demonstrated that the improved intake of dietary fibres mends cardiovascular efficiency and atherosclerosis risk and decreases the amount of systemic inflammation immune disorders [41, 53]. Short-chain fatty acids alter inflammation by controlling cytokine release from the immune cells. Butyrate and propionate, for instance, reduce the expression of nitric oxide synthase (NOS) and LPS-induced TNFα production in monocytes [87].

During airway inflammation, SCFAs trigger FFA2R and FFA3R on macrophages and neutrophils by plummeting the production of IL-8. LPS-stimulated TNFα secretion, activated by FFAR in mice and human mononuclear cells, is inhibited by AT inflammatory mediators, like interleukins (IL-4, IL-5, and IL-17A), which are declined significantly in the lungs in a receptor-dependent fashion when PT was administered into the allergic mouse [83]. While uncovering the underlying trigger switch of chronic inflammation, Ohira et al. supposed that the paracrine interaction in obese visceral fat tissues between adipocytes and macrophages may be the stimulating factor. Using co-culture methods with distinguished 3 T3-L1 adipocytes and RAW264.7 macrophages, they investigated the effect of BT on TNFα, MCP-1, free fatty acids, etc. and found that MAPK phosphorylation, lipase activity, and NF-kβ activation in macrophage in co-culture were inhibited by BT and hence suppressed the inflammatory responses [54].

10.11 Conclusion

SCFAs are diverse moieties of microbial origin inhabitant of the human gut. They have shown appreciable success in preclinical settings for the treatment of CRC and other malignancies. The range for their mechanistic targets and modulator patterns makes them one of the hopeful candidates for deployment against malignant disorders. SCFA, mainly BT and PT, has demonstrated key success in inhibiting cell survival, inducing programmed cell death, and preventing the spread of colon malignancies in vitro and in animal models of this deadly disease. Molecular alterations in the set of regulators of cell survival and apoptosis advocate its capabilities. Role of SCFA as metabolites also triggers cascades of enzyme-catalysed reaction, skewing metabolic output and affecting existing tempo of tumour catabolic and anabolic balance. Moreover, the ligand nature of SCFA to stimulate a repertoire of receptors also prompts the modulation of tumour cell physiology. Intracellular existence of SCFA and its act is not limited to the role of metabolite; these also play epigenetic modulators affecting on/off switch of (proto-)oncogenes and TSG. Modulation of HDAC and HAT activities is established, and many other epigenetic effects are suggested. Surprisingly, a group of molecules have many dimensions in cancer biology; these also influence the anti-tumour immune responses. Augmenting anti-tumour activation as well maturation will also contribute to its clinical applications. Strikingly, SCFA has distinct effects on non-transformed 'normal' colonocytes, where they protect them from metabolic injury and promote their regeneration and maintenance. This makes SCFAs as promising candidates for clinical utilization; however, further investigation is required.

References

1. Aschenbach JR, Bilk S, Tadesse G, Stumpff F, Gäbel G. Bicarbonate-dependent and bicarbonate-independent mechanisms contribute to nondiffusive uptake of acetate in the ruminal epithelium of sheep. Am J Physiol Gastrointest Liver Physiol. 2009;296:G1098–G107.
2. Bai Z, Zhang Z, Ye Y, Wang S. Sodium butyrate induces differentiation of gastric cancer cells to intestinal cells via the PTEN/phosphoinositide 3-kinase pathway. Cell Biol Int. 2010;34:1141–5.
3. Bindels LB, Porporato P, Dewulf EM, Verrax J, Neyrinck AM, Martin JC, Scott KP, Calderon PB, Feron O, Muccioli GG, Sonveaux P, Cani PD, Delzenne NM. Gut microbiota-derived propionate reduces cancer cell proliferation in the liver. Br J Cancer. 2012;107:1337–44.
4. Blouin J-M, Penot G, Collinet M, Nacfer M, Forest C, Laurent-Puig P, Coumoul X, Barouki R, Benelli C, Bortoli S. Butyrate elicits a metabolic switch in human colon cancer cells by targeting the pyruvate dehydrogenase complex. Int J Cancer. 2011;128:2591–601.
5. Boillot J, Alamowitch C, Berger A, Luo J, Bruzzo F, Bornet F, Slama G. Effects of dietary propionate on hepatic glucose production, whole-body glucose utilization, carbohydrate and lipid metabolism in normal rats. Br J Nutr. 1995;73:241–51.
6. Borthakur A, Priyamvada S, Kumar A, Natarajan AA, Gill RK, Alrefai WA, Dudeja PK. A novel nutrient sensing mechanism underlies substrate-induced regulation of monocarboxylate transporter-1. Am J Physiol Gastrointest Liver Physiol. 2012;303:G1126–33.
7. Bray F, Ferlay J, Soerjomataram I, Siegel RL, Torre LA, Jemal A. Global cancer statistics 2018: GLOBOCAN estimates of incidence and mortality worldwide for 36 cancers in 185 countries. CA Cancer J Clin. 2018;68:394–424.
8. Bultman SJ. Interplay between diet, gut microbiota, epigenetic events, and colorectal cancer. Mol Nutr Food Res. 2017;61(1):10.1002/mnfr.201500902.
9. Bush RS, Milligan LP. Study of the mechanism of inhibition of Ketogenesis by propionate in bovine liver. Can J Anim Sci. 1971;51:121–7.
10. Carmona FJ, Esteller M. Epigenomics of human colon cancer. Mutat Res. 2010;693:53–60.
11. Chen G, Ran X, Li B, Li Y, He D, Huang B, Fu S, Liu J, Wang W. Sodium butyrate inhibits inflammation and maintains epithelium barrier integrity in a TNBS-induced inflammatory bowel disease mice model. EBioMedicine. 2018;30:317–25.
12. Cremonesi E, Governa V, Garzon JFG, Mele V, Amicarella F, Muraro MG, Trella E, Galati-Fournier V, Oertli D, Däster SR, Droeser RA, Weixler B, Bolli M, Rosso R, Nitsche U, Khanna N, Egli A, Keck S, Slotta-Huspenina J, Terracciano LM, Zajac P, Spagnoli GC, Eppenberger-Castori S, Janssen K-P, Borsig L, Iezzi G. Gut microbiota modulate T cell trafficking into human colorectal cancer. Gut. 2018;67:1984–94.

13. Cresci GA, Thangaraju M, Mellinger JD, Liu K, Ganapathy V. Colonic gene expression in conventional and germ-free mice with a focus on the butyrate receptor GPR109A and the butyrate transporter SLC5A8. J Gastrointest Surg. 2010;14:449–61.
14. Decrion-Barthod A-Z, Bosset M, Plissonnier M-L, Marchini A, Nicolier M, Launay S, Prétet J-L, Rommelaere J, Mougin C. Sodium butyrate with UCN-01 has marked antitumour activity against cervical cancer cells. Anticancer Res. 2010;30:4049–61.
15. den Besten G, van Eunen K, Groen AK, Venema K, Reijngoud D-J, Bakker BM. The role of short-chain fatty acids in the interplay between diet, gut microbiota, and host energy metabolism. J Lipid Res. 2013;54:2325–40.
16. Eberle JA, Widmayer P, Breer H. Receptors for short-chain fatty acids in brush cells at the "gastric groove". Front Physiol. 2014;5
17. Encarnação JC, Pires AS, Amaral RA, Gonçalves TJ, Laranjo M, Casalta-Lopes JE, Gonçalves AC, Sarmento-Ribeiro AB, Abrantes AM, Botelho MF. Butyrate, a dietary fiber derivative that improves irinotecan effect in colon cancer cells. J Nutr Biochem. 2018;56:183–92.
18. Etxeberria U, Fernández-Quintela A, Milagro FI, Aguirre L, Martínez JA, Portillo MP. Impact of polyphenols and polyphenol-rich dietary sources on gut microbiota composition. J Agric Food Chem. 2013;61:9517–33.
19. Feng W, Ao H, Peng C. Gut microbiota, short-chain fatty acids, and herbal medicines. Front Pharmacol. 2018;9:1354.
20. Flint HJ, Duncan SH, Scott KP, Louis P. Links between diet, gut microbiota composition and gut metabolism. Proc Nutr Soc. 2015;74(1):13–22.
21. Fushimi T, Suruga K, Oshima Y, Fukiharu M, Tsukamoto Y, Goda T. Dietary acetic acid reduces serum cholesterol and triacylglycerols in rats fed a cholesterol-rich diet. Br J Nutr. 2006;95:916–24.
22. Gao S-m, Chen C-q, Wang L-y, Hong L-l, Wu J-b, Dong P-h, Yu F-j. Histone deacetylases inhibitor sodium butyrate inhibits JAK2/STAT signaling through upregulation of SOCS1 and SOCS3 mediated by HDAC8 inhibition in myeloproliferative neoplasms. Exp Hematol. 2012;41:261–70.
23. Gao Z, Yin J, Zhang J, Ward RE, Martin RJ, Lefevre M, Cefalu WT, Ye J. Butyrate improves insulin sensitivity and increases energy expenditure in mice. Diabetes. 2009;58:1509–17.
24. Gill RK, Saksena S, Alrefai WA, Sarwar Z, Goldstein JL, Carroll RE, Ramaswamy K, Dudeja PK. Expression and membrane localization of MCT isoforms along the length of the human intestine. Am J Physiol Gastrointest Liver Physiol. 2005;289:C846–52.
25. Glei M, Hofmann T, Küster K, Hollmann J, Lindhauer MG, Pool-Zobel BL. Both wheat (Triticum aestivum) bran Arabinoxylans and gut Flora-mediated fermentation products protect human Colon cells from genotoxic activities of 4-Hydroxynonenal and hydrogen peroxide. J Agric Food Chem. 2006;54:2088–95.
26. Gonçalves P, Araújo JR, Martel F. Characterization of butyrate uptake by nontransformed intestinal epithelial cell lines. J Membr Biol. 2011;240:35–46.
27. Guo Y, Li HY. Association between helicobacter pylori infection and colorectal neoplasm risk: a meta-analysis based on east Asian population. J Cancer Res Ther. 2014:263–6.
28. Gupta N, Martin PM, Prasad PD, Ganapathy V. SLC5A8 (SMCT1)-mediated transport of butyrate forms the basis for the tumor suppressive function of the transporter. Life Sci. 2006;78:2419–25.
29. Han A, Bennett N, Ahmed B, Whelan J, Donohoe DR. Butyrate decreases its own oxidation in colorectal cancer cells through inhibition of histone deacetylases. Oncotarget. 2018; 9(43):27280–292.
30. Harig JM, Ng Ek Fau - Dudeja PK, Dudeja Pk Fau - Brasitus TA, Brasitus Ta Fau - Ramaswamy K, Ramaswamy K. Transport of n-butyrate into human colonic luminal membrane vesicles. Am J Physiol Gastrointest Liver Physiol. 1996;271:G415–22.
31. Hinnebusch BF, Meng S, Wu JT, Archer SY, Hodin RA. The effects of short-chain fatty acids on human colon cancer cell phenotype are associated with histone Hyperacetylation. J Nutr. 2002;132:1012–7.

32. Hudson BD, Pandey SKTIF, Ulven TPSF, Milligan GUTF, Milligan G. Extracellular ionic locks determine variation in constitutive activity and ligand potency between species orthologs of the free fatty acid receptors FFA2 and FFA3. J Biol Chem. 2012;287:41195–209.
33. Hullar MA, Fu BC. Diet, the gut microbiome, and epigenetics. Cancer J. 2014;20:170–5.
34. Jäger S, Handschin C, St-pierre J, Spiegelman B. AMP-activated protein kinase (AMPK) action in skeletal muscle via direct phosphorylation of PGC-1alpha. Proc Natl Acad Sci. 2007;104(29):12017–22.
35. Jahani-Sherafat S, Alebouyeh M, Moghim S, Amoli HA, Ghasemian-Safaei H. Role of gut microbiota in the pathogenesis of colorectal cancer; a review article. Gastroenterol Hepatol Bed Bench. 2018;11:101–9.
36. Kim MH, Kang SG, Park JH, Yanagisawa M, Kim CH. Short-chain fatty acids activate GPR41 and GPR43 on intestinal epithelial cells to promote inflammatory responses in mice. Gastroenterology. 2013;145:396–406.e1-10.
37. Kimura I, Ozawa K, Inoue D, Imamura T, Kimura K, Maeda T, Terasawa K, Kashihara D, Hirano K, Tani T, Takahashi T, Miyauchi S, Shioi G, Inoue H, Tsujimoto G. The gut microbiota suppresses insulin-mediated fat accumulation via the short-chain fatty acid receptor GPR43. Nat Commun. 2013;4:1829.
38. Kobayashi M, Mikami D, Uwada J, Yazawa T, Kamiyama K, Kimura H, Taniguchi T, Iwano M. A short-chain fatty acid, propionate, enhances the cytotoxic effect of cisplatin by modulating GPR41 signaling pathways in HepG2 cells. Oncotarget. 2018;9(59):31342–354.
39. Kondo T, Kishi M, Fushimi T, Ugajin S, Kaga T. Vinegar intake reduces body weight, body fat mass, and serum triglyceride levels in obese Japanese subjects. Biosci Biotechnol Biochem. 2009;73:1837–43.
40. Lazarova DL, Chiaro C, Bordonaro M. Butyrate induced changes in Wnt-signaling specific gene expression in colorectal cancer cells. BMC Res Notes. 2014;7:226.
41. Li M, van Esch BCAM, Wagenaar GTM, Garssen J, Folkerts G, Henricks PAJ. Pro- and anti-inflammatory effects of short chain fatty acids on immune and endothelial cells. Eur J Pharmacol. 2018a;831:52–9.
42. Li Q, Cao L, Tian Y, Zhang P, Ding C, Lu W, Jia C, Shao C, Liu W, Wang D, Ye H, Hao H. Butyrate suppresses the proliferation of colorectal cancer cells via targeting pyruvate kinase M2 and metabolic reprogramming. Mol Cell Proteomics. 2018b;17:1531–45.
43. Li Q, Ding C, Meng T, Lu W, Liu W, Hao H, Cao L. Butyrate suppresses motility of colorectal cancer cells via deactivating Akt/ERK signaling in histone deacetylase dependent manner. J Pharmacol Sci. 2017;135:148–55.
44. Liang Y, Hou L, Li L, Li L, Zhu L, Wang Y, Huang X, Hou Y, Zhu D, Zou H, Gu Y, Weng X, Wang Y, Li Y, Wu T, Yao M, Gross I, Gaiddon C, Luo M, Wang J, Meng X. Dichloroacetate restores colorectal cancer chemosensitivity through the p53/miR-149-3p/PDK2-mediated glucose metabolic pathway. Oncogene. 2020;39:469–85.
45. Lim S-j, Choi HG, Jeon CK, Kim SH. Abstract 900: chemoresistance is induced by butyrate in colon cancer cells. Cancer Res. 2013;73:900.
46. Lin J, Handschin C, Spiegelman BM. Metabolic control through the PGC-1 family of transcription coactivators. Cell Metab. 2005;1:361–70.
47. Louis P, Flint HJ. Diversity, metabolism and microbial ecology of butyrate-producing bacteria from the human large intestine. FEMS Microbiol Lett. 2009;294:1–8.
48. Louis P, Hold GL, Flint HJ. The gut microbiota, bacterial metabolites and colorectal cancer. Nat Rev Microbiol. 2014;12:661–72.
49. Luan C, Xie L, Yang X, Miao H, Lv N, Zhang R, Xiao X, Hu Y, Liu Y, Wu N, Zhu Y, Zhu B. Dysbiosis of fungal microbiota in the intestinal mucosa of patients with colorectal adenomas. Sci Rep. 2015;5:7980.
50. Martin AM, Sun EW, Rogers GB, Keating DJ. The influence of the gut microbiome on host metabolism through the regulation of gut hormone release. Front Physiol. 2019;10:428.

51. Mathonnet M, Perraud A, Christou N, Akil H, Melin C, Battu S, Jauberteau M-O, Denizot Y. Hallmarks in colorectal cancer: angiogenesis and cancer stem-like cells. World J Gastroenterol. 2014;20:4189–96.
52. Mehta A, Soni VK, Shukla D, Vishvakarma NK. Chapter 24 – cyanobacteria: a potential source of anticancer drugs. In: Singh PK, Kumar A, Singh VK, Shrivastava AK, editors. Advances in cyanobacterial biology: Academic Press (United States). 2020;369–384.
53. Morrison DJ, Preston T. Formation of short chain fatty acids by the gut microbiota and their impact on human metabolism. Gut Microbes. 2016;7(3):189–200.
54. Ohira H, Fujioka Y, Katagiri C, Mamoto R, Aoyama-Ishikawa M, Amako K, Izumi Y, Nishiumi S, Yoshida M, Usami M, Ikeda M. Butyrate attenuates inflammation and lipolysis generated by the interaction of adipocytes and macrophages. J Atheroscler Thromb. 2013;20:425–42.
55. Oliphant K, Allen-Vercoe E. Macronutrient metabolism by the human gut microbiome: major fermentation by-products and their impact on host health. Microbiome. 2019;7(1):91.
56. Parada Venegas D, De la Fuente MK, Landskron G, González MJ, Quera R, Dijkstra G, Harmsen HJM, Faber KN, Hermoso MA. Short chain fatty acids (SCFAs)-mediated gut epithelial and immune regulation and its relevance for inflammatory bowel diseases. Front Immunol. 2019;10:277.
57. Pierce KL, Premont RT, Lefkowitz RJ. Seven-transmembrane receptors. Nat Rev Mol Cell Biol. 2002;3:639–350.
58. Pluznick JL, Protzko RJ, Gevorgyan H, Peterlin Z, Sipos A, Han J, Brunet I, Wan L-X, Rey F, Wang T, Firestein SJ, Yanagisawa M, Gordon JI, Eichmann A, Peti-Peterdi J, Caplan MJ. Olfactory receptor responding to gut microbiota-derived signals plays a role in renin secretion and blood pressure regulation. Proc Natl Acad Sci. 2013;110:4410–5.
59. Priyadarshini M, Kotlo KU, Dudeja PK, Layden BT. Role of short chain fatty acid receptors in intestinal physiology and pathophysiology. Compr Physiol. 2019;8(3):1091–115.
60. Priyadarshini M, Wicksteed B, Schiltz GE, Gilchrist A, Layden BT. SCFA receptors in pancreatic β cells: novel diabetes targets? Trends Endocrinol Metab. 2016;27:653–64.
61. Pryde SE, Duncan SH, Hold GL, Stewart CS, Flint HJ. The microbiology of butyrate formation in the human colon. FEMS Microbiol Lett. 2002;217:133–9.
62. Ragsdale SW, Pierce E. Acetogenesis and the Wood–Ljungdahl pathway of CO2 fixation. Biochim Biophys Acta. 2008;1784:1873–98.
63. Reichardt N, Duncan SH, Young P, Belenguer A, Leitch CMW, Scott KP, Flint HJ, Louis P. Phylogenetic distribution of three pathways for propionate production within the human gut microbiota. ISME J. 2014;8:1323–35.
64. Rinninella E, Raoul P, Cintoni M, Franceschi F, Miggiano GAD, Gasbarrini A, Mele MC. What is the healthy gut microbiota composition? A changing ecosystem across age, environment, diet, and diseases. Microorganisms. 2019;7:14.
65. Rodwell VW, Nordstrom JL, Mitschelen JJ. Regulation of HMG-CoA reductase. Adv Lipid Res. 1976;14:1–74.
66. Sakakibara S, Yamauchi T, Oshima Y, Tsukamoto Y, Kadowaki T. Acetic acid activates hepatic AMPK and reduces hyperglycemia in diabetic KK-A(y) mice. Biochem Biophys Res Commun. 2006;344:597–604.
67. Sawzdargo M, George SR, Nguyen T, Xu S, Kolakowski LF, O'Dowd BF. A cluster of four novel human G protein-coupled receptor genes occurring in close proximity to CD22 gene on chromosome 19q13.1. Biochem Biophys Res Commun. 1997;239:543–7.
68. Sellin JH. SCFAs: the enigma of weak electrolyte transport in the colon. Physiology. 1999;14:58–64.
69. Singh NP, Lai HC. Synergistic cytotoxicity of artemisinin and sodium butyrate on human cancer cells. Anticancer Res. 2005;25(6B):4325–31.
70. Sivaprakasam S, Bhutia YD, Yang S, Ganapathy V. Short-chain fatty acid transporters: role in colonic homeostasis. Compr Physiol. 2011;8:299–314.

71. Sivaprakasam S, Gurav A, Paschall AV, Coe GL, Chaudhary K, Cai Y, Kolhe R, Martin P, Browning D, Huang L, Shi H, Sifuentes H, Vijay-Kumar M, Thompson SA, Munn DH, Mellor A, McGaha TL, Shiao P, Cutler CW, Liu K, Ganapathy V, Li H, Singh N. An essential role of Ffar2 (Gpr43) in dietary fibre-mediated promotion of healthy composition of gut microbiota and suppression of intestinal carcinogenesis. Oncogenesis. 2016a;5:e238.
72. Sivaprakasam S, Prasad PD, Singh N. Benefits of short-chain fatty acids and their receptors in inflammation and carcinogenesis. Pharmacol Ther. 2016b;164:144–51.
73. Skarkova V, Kralova V, Vitovcova B, Rudolf E. Selected aspects of Chemoresistance mechanisms in colorectal carcinoma-a focus on epithelial-to-mesenchymal transition, autophagy, and apoptosis. Cell. 2019;8:234.
74. Soni VK, Shukla D, Kumar A, Vishvakarma NK. Curcumin circumvent lactate-induced Chemoresistance in hepatic cancer cells through modulation of Hydroxycarboxylic acid receptor-1. Int J Biochem Cell Biol. 2020;123:105752.
75. Stoddart LA, Smith NJ, Jenkins L, Brown AJ, Milligan G. Conserved polar residues in transmembrane domains V, VI, and VII of free fatty acid receptor 2 and free fatty acid receptor 3 are required for the binding and function of short chain fatty acids. J Biol Chem. 2008;283:32913–24.
76. Sun M, Wu W, Liu Z, Cong Y. Microbiota metabolite short chain fatty acids, GPCR, and inflammatory bowel diseases. J Gastroenterol. 2017;52:1–8.
77. Tang Y, Chen Y, Jiang H, Robbins GT, Nie D. G-protein-coupled receptor for short-chain fatty acids suppresses colon cancer. Int J Cancer. 2011b;128:847–56.
78. Tang Y, Chen Y, Jiang H, Nie D. Short-chain fatty acids induced autophagy serves as an adaptive strategy for retarding mitochondria-mediated apoptotic cell death. Cell Death Differ. 2011a;18:602–18.
79. Tarashi S, Siadat SD, Badi SA, Zali M, Biassoni R, Ponzoni M, Moshiri A. Gut Bacteria and their metabolites: which one is the defendant for colorectal cancer? Microorganisms. 2019;7:561.
80. Teramae H, Yoshikawa T, Inoue R, Ushida K, Takebe K, Nio-Kobayashi J, Iwanaga T. The cellular expression of SMCT2 and its comparison with other transporters for monocarboxylates in the mouse digestive tract. Biomed Res (Tokyo, Japan). 2010;31:239–49.
81. Thangaraju M, Cresci GA, Liu K, Ananth S, Gnanaprakasam JP, Browning DD, Mellinger JD, Smith SB, Digby GJ, Lambert NA, Prasad PD, Ganapathy V. GPR109A is a G-protein-coupled receptor for the bacterial fermentation product butyrate and functions as a tumor suppressor in colon. Cancer Res. 2009;69:2826–32.
82. Thirunavukkarasan M, Wang C, Rao A, Hind T, Teo YR, Siddiquee AA-M, Goghari MAI, Kumar AP, Herr DR. Short-chain fatty acid receptors inhibit invasive phenotypes in breast cancer cells. PLoS One. 2017;12:e0186334.
83. Trompette A, Gollwitzer ES, Yadava K, Sichelstiel AK, Sprenger N, Ngom-Bru C, Blanchard C, Junt T, Nicod LP, Harris NL, Marsland BJ. Gut microbiota metabolism of dietary fiber influences allergic airway disease and hematopoiesis. Nat Med. 2014;20:159–66.
84. Tungland B. Chapter 2 – short-chain fatty acid production and functional aspects on host metabolism. In: Tungland B, editor. Human microbiota in health and disease: Academic Press (United States). 2018;37–106.
85. Tyagi S, Venugopalakrishnan J, Ramaswamy K, Dudeja PK. Mechanism of n-butyrate uptake in the human proximal colonic basolateral membranes. Am J Physiol Gastrointest Liver Physiol. 2002;282:G676–82.
86. Vidyasagar S, Barmeyer C, Geibel J, Binder HJ, Rajendran VM. Role of short-chain fatty acids in colonic HCO(3) secretion. Am J Physiol Gastrointest Liver Physiol. 2005;288:G1217–26.
87. Vinolo MAR, Rodrigues HG, Hatanaka E, Sato FT, Sampaio SC, Curi R. Suppressive effect of short-chain fatty acids on production of proinflammatory mediators by neutrophils. J Nutr Biochem. 2011;22:849–55.

88. Vishvakarma NK, Singh SM. Immunopotentiating effect of proton pump inhibitor pantoprazole in a lymphoma-bearing murine host: implication in antitumor activation of tumor-associated macrophages. Immunol Lett. 2010;134:83–92.
89. Vishvakarma NK, Singh SM. Augmentation of myelopoiesis in a murine host bearing a T cell lymphoma following in vivo administration of proton pump inhibitor pantoprazole. Biochimie. 2011a;93:1786–96.
90. Vishvakarma NK, Singh SM. Mechanisms of tumor growth retardation by modulation of pH regulation in the tumor-microenvironment of a murine T cell lymphoma. Biomed Pharmacother. 2011b;65:27–39.
91. Wang GA-O, Yu Y, Wang YZ, Wang JJ, Guan R, Sun Y, Shi F, Gao J, Fu XL. Role of SCFAs in gut microbiome and glycolysis for colorectal cancer therapy. J Cell Physiol. 2019;234:17023–49.
92. Wang X, Wang J, Rao B, Deng L. Gut flora profiling and fecal metabolite composition of colorectal cancer patients and healthy individuals. Exp Ther Med. 2017;13:2848–54.
93. Wong SH, Zhao L, Zhang X, Nakatsu G, Han J, Xu W, Xiao X, Kwong TNY, Tsoi H, Wu WKK, Zeng B, Chan FKL, Sung JJY, Wei H, Yu J. Gavage of fecal samples from patients with colorectal cancer promotes intestinal carcinogenesis in germ-free and conventional mice. Gastroenterology. 2017;153:1621–33.
94. Wong SH, Yu J. Gut microbiota in colorectal cancer: mechanisms of action and clinical applications. Nat Rev Gastroenterol Hepatol. 2019;16:690–704.
95. Wu X, Wu Y, He L, Wu L, Wang X, Liu Z. Effects of the intestinal microbial metabolite butyrate on the development of colorectal cancer. J Cancer. 2018;9:2510–7.
96. Yachida S, Mizutani S, Shiroma H, Shiba S, Nakajima T, Sakamoto T, Watanabe H, Masuda K, Nishimoto Y, Kubo M, Hosoda F, Rokutan H, Matsumoto M, Takamaru H, Yamada M, Matsuda T, Iwasaki M, Yamaji T, Yachida T, Soga T, Kurokawa K, Toyoda A, Ogura Y, Hayashi T, Hatakeyama M, Nakagama H, Saito Y, Fukuda S, Shibata T, Yamada T. Metagenomic and metabolomic analyses reveal distinct stage-specific phenotypes of the gut microbiota in colorectal cancer. Nat Med. 2019;25:968–76.
97. Yonezawa T, Kobayashi Y, Obara Y. Short-chain fatty acids induce acute phosphorylation of the p38 mitogen-activated protein kinase/heat shock protein 27 pathway via GPR43 in the MCF-7 human breast cancer cell line. Cell Signal. 2007;19:185–93.
98. Zhang J, Yi M, Zha L, Chen S, Li Z, Li C, Gong M, Deng H, Chu X, Chen J, Zhang Z, Mao L, Sun S. Sodium butyrate induces endoplasmic reticulum stress and autophagy in colorectal cells: implications for apoptosis. PLoS One. 2016;11:e0147218.
99. Zheng HC. The molecular mechanisms of chemoresistance in cancers. Oncotarget. 2017;8:59950–64.
100. Zhou Q, Li G, Zuo S, Zhu W, Yuan X. RNA sequencing analysis of molecular basis of sodium butyrate-induced growth inhibition on colorectal cancer cell lines. Biomed Res Int. 2019
101. Zumkeller N, Brenner H, Zwahlen M, Rothenbacher D. Helicobacter pylori infection and colorectal cancer risk: a meta-analysis. J Cancer Res Therap. 2016;12(Supplement):15–18.

Chapter 11
Targeting Angiogenesis for Colorectal Cancer Therapy

Vaishali Gupta, Taha Bharmal, Vineeta Dixit, Naveen Kumar Vishvakarma, Atul Kumar Tiwari, Dhananjay Shukla, and Shirish Shukla

Abstract Recent years have witnessed the development of a large number of agents that have proven to manage colorectal cancer (CRC) effectively. Angiogenic growth factors such as VEGF and EGFR play an eminent role in the regulation of tumor angiogenesis and are predominantly overexpressed in patients with colorectal cancer. The growing understanding of the role of angiogenic signalling pathways in the development of cancer has led to its exploitation to restrict tumor progression. Targeting angiogenesis has emerged as an important therapeutic approach for the treatment of cancer. A large number of targeted therapies consisting of monoclonal antibodies and tyrosine kinase inhibitors have been developed to specifically inhibit the molecular pathways mediating tumor cell growth and proliferation. Clinical trials have confirmed the efficiency of targeted anti-angiogenic therapies for the treatment of patients with metastatic CRC. Currently, a large number of anti-angiogenic drugs in combination with chemotherapy have been approved for the treatment of CRC. However, the current anti-angiogenic drugs are far from obtaining the desired results. The arising subsidiary limitations and drug administration-related toxicities cannot be ignored. Researches are being conducted to develop new antiangiogenic agents in order to overcome various pre-existing limitations of anti-angiogenic therapy. Better strategies are needed to evaluate the therapeutic response in CRC to ensure maximum clinical advantage. In the present chapter, we aim to explore the role of tumor angiogenesis in the progression of CRC and its therapeutic intervention. It highlights the role of the VEGF and EGFR signalling pathways in CRC biology and discusses the current anti-angiogenic treatment modalities for

V. Gupta · T. Bharmal · N. K. Vishvakarma · D. Shukla (✉)
Department of Biotechnology, Guru Ghasidas Vishwavidyalaya, Bilaspur, CG, India

V. Dixit
Department of Botany, Guru Ghasidas Vishwavidyalaya, Bilaspur, CG, India

A. K. Tiwari
Department of Zoology, Dr. Bhanvar Singh Porte Govt. College, Pendra, CG, India

S. Shukla (✉)
Discovery Oncology, The Janssen Pharmaceuticals, Spring House, PA, USA
e-mail: sshukla11@its.jnj.com

G. P. Nagaraju et al. (eds.), *Colon Cancer Diagnosis and Therapy*,
https://doi.org/10.1007/978-3-030-63369-1_11

CRC. Further, it outlines the toxicities and limitations of the available anti-angiogenic drugs.

Keywords Anti-angiogenesis · Metastatic colorectal cancer · Vascular endothelial growth factor · Epidermal growth factor receptor · Monoclonal antibodies · Tyrosine kinase inhibitors

11.1 Introduction

Angiogenesis is a physiological process of the formation of the new blood vessels from pre-existing vasculature [1–4]. It is a well-regulated process that occurs in both healthy and the diseased state and requires an adequate balance between endogenous stimulators and inhibitors [2, 5]. A number of dynamic factors such as low oxygen levels, low pH, inflammatory stimuli affects angiogenic equalibrium and a slight imbalance leads to the development of various pathological conditions like cancer [2, 6]. Judah Folkman, an American scientist, laid the foundation of the modern history of angiogenesis by hypothesizing that tumor growth depends on angiogenesis. Folkman proposed the term "anti-angiogenesis" and hypothesized that the inhibition of angiogenesis in tumor cells can be used to restrict tumor growth. Various studies have revealed the significant role of angiogenesis in colorectal cancer (CRC) progression and considered it as one of the best-studied angiogenesis-dependent solid tumors [7–10]. Tumor growth and metastasis in CRC are influenced by multiple signalling pathways however vascular endothelial growth factor (VEGF) and epidermal growth factor receptor (EGFR) signalling pathways are mainly involved in regulating the angiogenic process [11, 12]. VEGF is a key regulator in angiogenesis and plays a central role in the regulation of CRC biology [7]. Various researchers have focused on the development of targeted therapeutic agents by using anti-angiogenic molecules for the treatment of cancer. It has been reported that the successful inhibition of VEGF suppresses cell proliferation and inhibits tumor angiogenesis [13]. In 2004, the Food and Drug Administration approved the usage of bevacizumab (anti-VEGF monoclonal antibody) for the first- and second-line treatment of metastatic CRC in combination with chemotherapy. Since then, numerous anti-angiogenic agents have been identified and approved by various agencies for the treatment of different solid tumors. These targeted therapies consist of monoclonal antibodies against receptors, growth factors, and tyrosine kinase inhibitors. Some of the monoclonal antibodies against VEGF include ramucirumab, regorafenib, bevacizumab, and fusion protein aflibercept, whereas VEGFR tyrosine kinase inhibitors include vatalanib and sunitinib. Likewise, many EGFR targeting therapies have been recommended for the treatment of mCRC. Some of the monoclonal antibodies targeting EGFR include cetuximab and panitumumab, whereas the EGFR-targeted tyrosine kinase inhibitors include gefitinib and erlotinib. The monotherapy has shown positive outcomes. However, despite the positive results, studies have pointed out that not all patients respond to the anti-EGFR treatment. Further, presence of genetic mutations and alterations contributes to the development of primary and adaptive resistance in patients leading to reduced efficiency and enhanced toxicity as the major limitations of the current angiogenic inhibitors. To overcome this limitation, combination of standard chemotherapy with the targeted agents becomes the treatment of choice and has conferred survival advantage to patients with mCRC. The present chapter summarizes the current research on anti-angiogenic targeted therapies for the treatment of CRC. Development of anti-angiogenic molecules to overcome the pre-existing limitations of angiogenic inhibitors is also reviewed.

11.2 Tumor Angiogenesis

Tumor cells possess the ability to penetrate the vascular system and surrounding tissues through which they spread to different sites resulting in metastasis. Like any other cell, tumor cells also require access to oxygen, nutrients, and growth factors for its unhindered growth and metastatic spread which is fulfilled by tumor angiogenesis. The process of cancer cell invasion initiates when a motile metastatic cell infiltrates the extracellular matrix (ECM) and basement membrane (BM) reaching the vascular system. The metastatic cells also invade neighboring tissues by the process of extravasation and proliferate in a different site leading to the formation of secondary tumors [14, 15]. A large number of angiogenic growth factors stimulate the process of blood vessel formation by activating the underlying signalling pathways affecting angiogenesis [16]. The imbalance between the angiogenic stimulators and inhibitors under certain conditions causes a drastic increase in endothelial cell proliferation that leads to the activation of the angiogenic switch. The signalling occurs between the endothelial cells and extracellular matrix components and is influenced by many other angiogenic factors [1]. The genetic mutation in the tumor cells is an important factor that is known to set off the angiogenic switch which triggers transcriptional responses resulting in the elevated synthesis of stimulators and leads to increased cell proliferation or responding to tumor-associated inflammation and immune cell recruitment [17]. The other factor that regulates angiogenic switches is the tumor microenvironment. The proliferating tumor often outgrows the capacity of host vasculature leading to a reduced supply of nutrients and oxygen [18]. The oxygen-deprived cells trigger a transcriptional response resulting in the development of the hypoxic conditions. Under hypoxic conditions, the stabilized hypoxia-inducible factor 1 (HIF-1) heterodimer binds to the hypoxia response element (HRE) and increases the expression of genes required for hypoxic adaptation. The hypoxic microenvironment induced angiogenic and metastatic signals to allow the prolonged survival of the cells by adapting to a reduced supply of oxygen and nutrients. Endothelial cell (EC) receptors bind to the angiogenic factors produced by the tumor cells and initiate angiogenesis. These substances also stimulate neighboring cells to further produce and secrete angiogenic signalling molecules [18].

The stimulated ECs produce proteases and various other digestive enzymes to digest the basement membrane surrounding the blood vessel. The matrix metalloproteinases (MMPs) secreted by the tumor cells initiate degradation of the basement membrane and ECM surrounding the pre-existing blood vessels. This permits the release of pro-angiogenic substances from the matrix and alteration of endothelial cell junctions leading to the sprouting of blood vessels towards the stimulus. The newly formed ECs are organized into hollow tubes, and blood starts flowing through the newly formed blood vessels [18]. Hypoxia induces a potent response in the poorly perfused tissue until the pressure of the oxygen is normalized by the flow of blood, which brings the oxygen, required nutrients, and growth factors via newly formed blood vessels [16, 19]. The newly formed blood vessel penetrates the tumor and serves the function of "feeding" tumor cells. This allows the tumor to proliferate and invade nearby tissues. The resulting tumor vessels are thin-walled and highly unorganized. They are hyperpermeable and are often described as "leaky" due to the loss of adherence between endothelial junctions and discontinuous basement membrane. The discontinuous basement membrane varies in thickness [18, 20]. These blood vessels are involved in the diffusion exchange of metabolites, nutrients, oxygen, growth factors, and removal of waste products [14, 20]. Thus, tumor growth is angiogenesis dependent, and an underlying mechanism can be used to identify the anti-angiogenic molecules for therapeutic purposes [21].

11.3 Angiogenesis and CRC

Neovascularization is essential for the growth of solid tumors. In CRC, the angiogenic switch occurs early in the neoplastic tumor progression [22, 23]. The oxygen and nutrient-deprived tumor trigger a transcriptional response to initiate the adaptation to adverse conditions. Hypoxia-inducible factor 1 (HIF-1) – a heterodimer – is considered as the main transcriptional factor responsible for sensing oxygen and driving angiogenesis. HIF-1 comprises two DNA-binding proteins, namely, HIF-1 α that senses oxygen and HIF-1 β that activates transcription. Together they function as a global regulator of oxygen homeostasis. Under hypoxic conditions, HIF-1 α is stabilized, and it forms a heterodimer with HIF-1 β. The formed HIF-1 heterodimer binds to the hypoxia response elements (HRE) leading to an upregulation of expression of various hypoxia-induced genes. An extensive body of literature shows that HIF-1 governs the adaptive phenotype in cancer cells. The overexpression of the HIF-1α subunit is observed in CRC. Further, it was recognized that the increased expression of HIF-1α is an independent prognostic marker of CRC and its increased expression correlates with the transcription of genes including VEGF-A. It was established that the stabilized HIF-1α induces the mRNA expression of cyclooxygenase-2 (COX-2), which enhances the levels of prostaglandin E2 linked with the increased vessel formation in CRC. Thus, prostaglandin E2 was proposed as the prognostic marker in CRC [22, 24].

Tumor angiogenesis begins with the release of pro-angiogenic growth factors stimulating endothelial cell proliferation, migration, and formation of new capillaries leading to tumor perfusion, growth, and metastases [23]. A large number of angiogenic stimulators are secreted in response to the development of hypoxic conditions. These stimulators like vascular endothelial growth factor (VEGF), platelet-derived growth factor (PDGF), fibroblast growth factor (FGF), epidermal growth factor (EGF), transforming growth factor (TGF), matrix metalloproteinases (MMPs), angiopoietins (Ang), COX-2, tumor necrosis factor (TNF), and ephrin are expressed concomitantly, resulting in elevated angiogenesis [16, 17, 24–28]. Their expression corresponds to the advancement in the tumor stages and a significant decrease in patient survival rate. Among these, VEGF is predominantly the prime growth factor regulating angiogenesis [4, 29]. Various ongoing studies aim to establish a prominent relationship between COX-2 expression and colon cancer and its role in tumor progression [30]. The level of expression of angiogenic factors in the tissue directly correlates to the tumor aggressiveness depicting the speed with which it spreads [14]. Some of the common molecular markers involved in angiogenesis on mCRC include VEGF, cell adhesion molecules (CAMs), and platelet-derived endothelial cell growth factor (PD-ECGF) [30]. The CRC patients with high expression of PD-ECGF were found with increased mortality rate. However, the role of PD-ECGF remains unclear till date. The tumor growth and metastasis in CRC are influenced by multiple cellular pathways; however, a large number of preclinical and clinical studies identify VEGF and EGFR signalling pathways for the growth and proliferation of mCRC [11, 12].

11.3.1 VEGF Pathway

VEGF is considered as the main inducer that stimulates endothelial cell proliferation, sprouting, migration, and tube formation. VEGF inhibits the apoptosis of endothelial cells, activates enzymes involved in the degradation of ECM, and is actively involved in the regulation of vascular leakage and permeability [16, 31]. Various studies have identified the central role of VEGF in the regulation of colorectal cancer (CRC) biology [7]. It enhances cell proliferation by activating the members of MAP kinase (MAPK) and protein kinase C (PKC) pathway, thereby augmenting the expression of the EGFR signalling pathway [23].

VEGF's family comprises of VEGF-A, VEGF-B, VEGF-C, VEGF-D, VEGF-E, and placental growth factor (PlGF-1 and PlGF-2) with VEGF-A being the predominant isoform [4, 5, 26, 29, 32]. These isoforms mediate their angiogenic effect by binding to specific surface cell receptors, i.e., tyrosine kinase (TK) receptors (VEGF 1/2) [4, 33]. Vascular endothelial growth factor receptors (VEGFR-1 and VEGFR-2) are expressed on the surface of the endothelial cell, whereas VEGFR-3 is expressed on the lymphatic vessel [34]. VEGFR-1 binds to VEGF-A, VEGF-B, and PlGF, whereas VEGFR-2 binds to VEGF-A, VEGF-C, and VEGF-D [26]. The receptor

VEGFR-3 binds to VEGF-C and VEGF-D and is involved in controlling the growth and maintenance of the lymphatic vessel [34]. The VEGF-D is involved in the tumor metastasization of the lymph nodes [31]. Neuropilin-1 (NP-1) is a non-kinase receptor present on the endothelial cell surface which enhances the binding efficiency of VEGF-A to VEGFR-2 and facilitates the proliferative effects of VEGF-A [4, 8]. VEGF signalling along with other signalling pathways like angiopoietin/tie, integrin, and Notch is involved in triggering the angiogenic growth of blood vessels. The overexpression of VEGF is observed in colorectal cancer [1]. Several studies have revealed the prominent role of VEGF in the growth and proliferation of cells in colon cancer. Reports indicate a surge in the expression of VEGF mRNA in CRC with an upregulated expression of VEGFR [31]. This overexpression of VEGF, its receptor VEGFR, and PlGF in tumors correspond to its poor prognosis and metastasis [31]. The occurrence of angiogenesis in CRC makes it a potential therapeutic target for the treatment of cancer [7]. Since VEGF stands at the center of the angiogenic pathway, targeting the VEGF signalling pathway has become a key target for the novel therapeutic agents treating cancer. The results from the preclinical and clinical trials have shown that the successful inhibition of VEGF suppresses cell proliferation and tumor angiogenesis. As a result, the improved prognosis is observed for patients with non-resectable CRC [13]. Various drugs have been developed to inhibit VEGF signalling pathway to prevent tumor angiogenesis. A large number of antibodies neutralizing VEGF by blocking VEGFR and tyrosine kinase inhibitors have been identified to obstruct the VEGF signalling pathway [7]. Numerous antiangiogenic agents have been approved, and many are still undergoing clinical trials for the treatment of patients with mCRC. Bevacizumab (a monoclonal antibody inhibiting VEGF) accounts as the first anti-angiogenic drug approved for the treatment of mCRC. It is currently being used in the first-line treatment of patients with mCRC [35]. Some other approved drugs for the treatment of mCRC include aflibercept, ramucirumab, and regorafenib [11, 36].

11.3.2 EGFR Pathway

Epidermal growth factor is a pro-angiogenic growth factor that induces cell proliferation, thereby aiding to angiogenesis [3, 16]. The EGF family encompasses 11 members and 4 epidermal growth factor receptors (EGFR) [3]. The EGF molecule binds to the tyrosine kinase receptor EGFR [37]. The transmembrane receptor family comprises ErbB1, ErbB2, ErbB3, and ErbB4 [12]. EGFR popularly known as HER (human EGF receptor) comprises an extracellular cysteine-rich domain that consists of a ligand-binding region, a membrane-spanning region, and a cytoplasmic domain [38, 39]. The alpha-helix transmembrane domain of the receptor attaches the ligand-binding region to the intracellular receptor that comprises three domains. Domain 1 assists in serving as the site for providing feedback attenuation by MAPK and PI3K-PTEN-Akt pathway; Domain 2 corresponds to tyrosine kinase activity, whereas Domain 3 acts as a carboxy-terminal tail [39]. These receptors are expressed on epithelial, stromal, glial, and smooth muscle cells. They play a pivotal role in inducing cell proliferation, migration, and metastasis. It is also involved in the inhibition of apoptosis and stimulation of tumor cell survival [39]. The ligands of EGFR are inclusive of transforming growth factor alpha (TGF-α), EGF, heparin-binding EGF-like growth factor (HB-EGF), betacellulin (BTC), epigen, amphiregulin (AR), and epiregulin (EPR) [12, 37]. The EGFR signalling cascade begins with its ligand activation that occurs as a consequence of the binding of ligand and EGFR, which activates the tyrosine kinase [38]. Once the ligand binds to the EGFR, it undergoes dimerization and continues to elevate its intracellular tyrosine kinase activity [37]. The activated EGFR in turn activates various other underlying signalling pathways like the MAPK pathway and PI3K-AKT pathway that stimulate tumor angiogenesis and cell survival [12, 38].

In the mitogen-activated protein kinase (MAPK) pathway, a number of proteins like Src homology 2 (SH2) proteins are recruited to activate EGFR. The adaptor molecule Grb2 (growth factor receptor-bound protein 2) recruits SOS (son of sevenless) to the membrane which then activates Ras which is actively involved in the recruitment and activation of B-Raf that triggers activation of MEK1 and MEK2. The subsequent phosphorylation of MEKs triggers the extracellular signal-regulated kinase (ERK 1/2). The phosphorylated ERK translocate to the nucleus and initialize the activation of various transcription factors in the nucleus that affects cell growth, proliferation, and migration [38, 40]. In the PI3K-PTEN-Akt pathway, activated PI3K is involved in the conversion of PIP2 (phosphatidylinositol 4, 5 bisphosphate) to PIP3 (phosphatidylinositol 3, 4, 5 triphosphate). PIP3 binds to AKT and activates it [38, 40]. The tumor suppressor phosphatase and tensin homologue gene (PTEN) acts on PIP3 and negatively regulates it [12]. RAS homolog enriched in the brain (RHEB) enables the activation of mTOR that plays an eminent role in the regulation of cellular function and angiogenesis [38, 40]. The study demonstrates that the PI3K-AKT pathway is involved in inhibiting cell apoptosis [12, 38, 40]. The pathway inactivates pro-apoptotic protein BAD (BCL2-associated agonist of cell death) that causes the inhibition of apoptosis [39]. Data from numerous experimental studies indicate overexpression of EGFR in around 60–80% of tumors [39]. In addition, studies demonstrate the eminent role of EGFR in tumorigenesis, especially in CRC [13]. Its overexpression is related to poor prognosis of the tumor [39]. EGFR ligands also promote the expression of VEGF [39]. EGFR contributes to both prognosis and carcinogenesis of CRC [38]. This makes EGFR a potential target for cancer treatment [39]. The recent years have witnessed the development of new anti-cancer drugs targeting angiogenic signalling pathways for treating mCRC. The EGFR is being targeted with small molecule inhibitors or monoclonal antibodies [39]. The therapeutic EGFR targeting monoclonal antibodies either targets EGFR or its ligand by binding to the receptor or the molecule and inhibiting the EGFR signalling pathway [41]. These anti-cancer drugs have demonstrated promising results with increased efficiency in treating cancers. Some of the most commonly used FDA-approved anti-EGFR monoclonal antibodies include cetuximab and panitumumab. They have proven their effectiveness in treating patients with wild-type RAS in mCRC [42].

11.4 Targeted Therapies

The treatment strategy for solid tumors depends on their stage of diagnosis. Surgery is the preferred choice for the tumor localized to their site of origin, which is used along with chemotherapy and radiotherapy to limit the chances of reoccurrence. Currently, chemotherapy is the most widely used for the first- and second-line treatments for solid tumors. There are several limitations of chemotherapy as most chemotherapeutic drugs affect normal cells along with the cancer cells. The limitations and serious toxicities of chemotherapy prompted the search for better alternative therapeutic strategies. This led to the development of targeted therapies aiming to specifically target the subpopulation of cells that directly influence the disease progression, i.e., cancer cells without hampering the growth of normal cells thereby causing minimal side effects. The molecules used in targeted therapy have the ability to specifically inhibit the target. These targeted therapies interfere with the growth, division, repair, and communication of cancer cells [43]. With a better understanding of the mechanism of blood vessel formation and its role in the progression of cancer cells, the search for anti-angiogenesis molecules is increased. Several monoclonal antibodies and tyrosine kinase inhibitors have been developed to target VEGF, VEGFR, EGFR, and EGFR ligands for the treatment of mCRC [12]. Angiogenic inhibitors are chemicals that block the growth of the blood vessels by interfering at various steps of vasculature formation [44], for example, monoclonal antibodies targeting angiogenic factors like VEGF by bevacizumab and VEGFR-2 receptor by ramucirumab. Human recombinant fusion protein aflibercept binds both VEGF-A and VEGF-B functions as decoy receptors and has anti-angiogenic effects. Sunitinib and sorafenib are other multi-targeted tyrosine kinase inhibitors that inhibit angiogenesis and are used in the treatment of solid tumors [45]. Angiogenic inhibitors can be used as a monotherapy or in combination with other therapies to inhibit angiogenesis and tumor progression. Several preclinical and clinical studies of combination therapies have shown promising results with an increase in therapeutic effect [46]. The combination of chemotherapy with anti-angiogenic drugs has yielded better outcomes conferring survival advantage to the patients, and therefore, anti-angiogenic agents are being used to prevent or retard the fast progression of solid tumors. The following are the different anti-angiogenic molecules currently used for the treatment of solid tumors.

11.4.1 Monoclonal Antibodies

Monoclonal antibodies specifically bind to the specific domains of the receptors expressed on surface tumor cells [43]. Monoclonal antibodies are designed to inhibit the interaction between the ligand and receptor, thereby preventing the downstream of the signalling cascade. Studies have identified a varied mechanism of action by which binding of monoclonal antibodies induces cytotoxicity in tumors. The most common mechanism is antibody-dependent cell-mediated cytotoxicity and complement-mediated cytotoxicity [47]. In the present chapter, we have disused inhibition of VEGF and EGFR angiogenic signalling pathway by monoclonal antibodies.

11.4.1.1 Monoclonal Antibodies Against VEGF

Bevacizumab

Bevacizumab (Avastin) is the first recombinant humanized anti-VEGF monoclonal immunoglobulin G1 (IgG_1) having an anti-angiogenic effect and is successfully used for the treatment of mCRC [7, 48]. It specifically binds to the VEGF-A molecule and prevents its interaction with the VEGF receptor. Studies have demonstrated an enhanced response of bevacizumab in combination with other chemotherapeutic drugs benefiting patient with an increased overall survival and progression-free survival [49]. An important randomized placebo-controlled trial investigating the bevacizumab plus oxaliplatin as first-line treatment for CRC showed an improved PFS. However, no significant changes were observed in response rates and OS. Another study showed the effect of bevacizumab along with fluorouracil (FU), and leucovorin in a placebo-controlled trial for first-line treatment demonstrated an improved PFS compared to the administration of irinotecan alone. The successful outcomes from these studies established bevacizumab as a standard first-line treatment for mCRC in combination with the other chemotherapeutics [50]. A set of contrasting results was also observed from studies using the combination of bevacizumab with mFOLFOX6, which does not show improvement in survival rate. However, the delayed progression of disease was observed, although the cytostatic effect diminished as the dosage of bevacizumab was discontinued [49]. Based on evident advantages of bevacizumab in combination with chemotherapeutics, the FDA and European Medicines Agency approved its usage in patients with mCRC [12].

Ramucirumab

Ramucirumab (Cyramza) is a fully human IgG1 monoclonal antibody that has been tested for the treatment of metastatic cancer. So far, it has been trailed for lung cancer, gastric cancer, and colorectal cancer. It is designed to block the binding of VEGF ligands with the VEGFR-2 receptor [7, 49]. In phase I clinical trials, patients with advanced solid tumors on receiving a dosage of 16 mg/kg body weight experienced dosage toxicity with effects such as hypertension, abdominal pain, anorexia, headache, vomiting, and deep venous thrombosis. In April 2015, FDA approved ramucirumab in second-line treatment of mCRC in combination with FOLFIRI along with first-line treatment with FOLFOX and either bevacizumab or oxaliplatin [7, 49, 51].

Regorafenib

Regorafenib (Stivarga) is the first oral multikinase inhibitor against VEGFR-2, VEGFR-3, TIE-2, FGFR, PDGFR, RAF, and RET. It is the only approved medication to be given to patients after failure of standard anti-angiogenic therapies in advanced mCRC stage [49, 51]. In phase I trial, a study on patients with advanced tumors receiving a dose between 10 and 200 mg experienced a grade 3 or 4 toxicity effects showing hand-foot skin reaction, fatigue, diarrhea, hypertension, rash, or desquamation. A study has shown better response in disease control with 160 mg dosage in 28 days schedule [51]. Along with controversies of adverse effects of regorafenib, it continued to phase III trials. A large, international, multicenter, randomized, double-blind, placebo-controlled trial (CORRECT trial) was performed with a recommended dose of 160 mg. The primary endpoint was OS with 6.4 months and 5 months for regorafenib and placebo, respectively. However, adverse effects continued as of in phase I trials, adding some others such as oral mucositis, anorexia, voice change, and liver dysfunction. In September 2012, the US FDA approved the use of regorafenib in the treatment of mCRC in patients, previous treated with anti-angiogenic therapies. In year 2016 regorafenib lost its approval in Germany due to various adverse effect after treatment [7, 31, 49, 51].

11.4.1.2 Monoclonal Antibodies Against EGFR

Cetuximab

Cetuximab (Erbitux) is a recombinant monoclonal IgG1 antibody that acts as an EGFR inhibitor. This chimeric human-mouse antibody binds with a higher affinity to the extracellular domain of EGFR expressed on cells and competitively inhibits the binding of ligands to EGFR. The inactive EGFR exists as a monomer until it undergoes ligand activation. Cetuximab further aids in the internalization of the receptor followed by degradation without receptor phosphorylation and activation. Binding of cetuximab with EGFR blocks the ligand-induced phosphorylation of EGFR [12]. Multiple studies have concluded that cetuximab is capable of causing a significant level of reduction in VEGF, bFGF, and interleukin-8 [52]. The phase II trials of cetuximab monotherapy in first-line treatment were capable of inducing significant anti-tumor activity in the patients suffering from mCRC and not responding to chemotherapeutic drugs like oxaliplatin, irinotecan, and fluoropyrimidine [12]. However, the combinatorial strategies of cetuximab with other chemotherapeutic regimens have shown more promising results [47]. Many patients do not respond to anti-EGFR-related drugs such as cetuximab mainly due to the mutation in the KRAS gene which makes mCRC resistant to respond to the therapy, which is also associated with poor prognosis of the disease [12, 53]. Hence, the mutation in KRAS is used as a biomarker for predicting the response in patients [47]. Mutation in B-Raf does not show any resistance related to therapy in the CRYSTAL study [12]. Cetuximab is well tolerated in patients with mCRC at all the stages in different line settings, and its the administration is associated with an improvement in overall survival [54]. Experimental studies indicate that cetuximab is capable of augmenting the effect of radiotherapy and chemotherapeutic drugs like irinotecan, thereby producing better results [53].

Panitumumab

Panitumumab (Vectibix) is a recombinant IgG2 mAb known to specifically bind to the extracellular domain of EGFR with high affinity. It competitively inhibits the binding of EGFR ligand to its receptors, thereby preventing the activation of EGFR. It was observed that panitumumab enhanced the progression-free survival in patients who showed resistance to the prior best supportive care and paved its path to approval for the treatment of mCRC in Europe and the USA in 2006. A phase II study revealed the influence of panitumumab along with irinotecan-containing regimens as first-line therapy in patients with mCRC. Panitumumab and FOLFIRI were efficiently tolerated with 10.9 months as a median-free progression time and a survival time of 22.5 months. The phase III trial, comparative study – PRIME, estimated the first-line treatment therapy of panitumumab with FOLFOX-4 against that of FOLFOX-4 alone in patients with mCRC wherein the combination therapy indicated a notable improvement in the progression-free survival time. However, the second-line treatment of panitumumab with FOLFIRI is still under investigation. The successful and beneficial outcomes of panitumumab in patients with mCRC with wild-type KRAS led to its approval for usage by the European Medicines Agency [12].

11.4.2 Tyrosine Kinase Inhibitors

Tyrosine kinase inhibitors (TKIs) are drugs with a low molecular weight that specifically function to inhibit the kinase activity of receptors. They competitively inhibit the ATP-binding site of the tyrosine kinase receptor, thereby preventing the phosphorylation of tyrosine residue. As a result, the downstream signalling pathway is hindered [55, 56]. Thus, tyrosine kinase inhibitors are capable of regulating blood vessel growth. TKIs are effective in the targeted treatment of various cancers. Imatinib was the first TKI to be approved for the treatment of cancer. Since then, various TKIs have been approved for the same as sunitinib, erlotinib, gefitinib, dasatinib, sorafenib, etc. At present, 28 kinase inhibitors have been approved by the FDA [55, 57]. These TKIs vary greatly in the pharmacokinetics and substance-specific effects [56]. TKIs also exhibit minimal side effects and are well tolerated in patients.

11.4.2.1 Tyrosine Kinase Inhibitor Against VEGF

Sunitinib

Sunitinib (Sutent) is an orally administered multi-targeted tyrosine kinase inhibitor that specifically targets vascular endothelial growth factor receptor (VEGFR) and several other growth factor receptors like platelet-derived growth factor receptor (PDGFR), c-Kit, RET, and flt3 [12]. Sunitinib exhibits both anti-VEGF and antitumor effects [58]. Various studies have revealed the efficiency of sunitinib alone to manage mCRC causing amplification of flt3 in patients [58, 59]. The phase I trial aimed to determine the dosage, pharmacokinetic profiles of sunitinib along with mFOLFOX-6 in patients with mCRC. The primary results of the combination were quite promising and well tolerated in patients [12]. The administration of sunitinib is also associated with adverse side effects like fatigue, diarrhea, nausea, internal bleeding, etc. Thus, detailed studies are needed to analyze the toxicity profiles. Results from ongoing researches evaluating the efficiency of chemotherapeutic combinatorial drugs like fluorouracil, leucovorin, oxaliplatin, and irinotecan regimens for patients with mCRC are still awaited [58].

Vatalanib

Vatalanib is a small molecule TKI that blocks the VEGFR-1, VEGFR-2, and VEGFR-3. A phase I trial was conducted to evaluate the efficiency and safety of vatalanib in combination with FOLFOX-4, where the drug was well tolerated in the first-line treatment for patients with mCRC showing an ORR of 48.6% and a median PFS of 11.4 months. This was followed by a phase III clinical trial that aimed to comparatively analyze the vatalanib plus FOLFOX4 against FOLFOX4 plus placebo wherein an improved PFS and OS of (7.7 months; 21.4 months) and (7.6 months; 20.5) were observed, respectively. The latter results from the study showed that patients with advanced CRC were benefited from the combination of FOLFOX4 and vatalanib [12, 60]. Table 11.1 summarizes the current anti-angiogenic drug and their targets along with drug administration-related toxicities.

11.4.2.2 Tyrosine Kinase Inhibitor Against EGFR

Gefitinib

It is an anilinoquinazoline derived orally administered TKI that inhibits the autophosphorylation of EGFR and further prevents the downstream signalling [12]. Gefitinib (Iressa) possesses a greater affinity towards the EGFR and is a noncompetitive inhibitor with EGFR-specific ligand. Studies have revealed that this inhibition of EGFR resulted in a 70% increase in the patient's response [47]. The preliminary results from phase I and II trial showed little activity; however, the pre-

Table 11.1 Angiogenic inhibitors, their targets, and associated side effects

Angiogenesis inhibitors	Inhibitory target	Associated toxicity	Ref.
Bevacizumab (Avastin)	VEGF-targeted mAb	Diarrhea, epistaxis, hemoptysis, hemorrhages, thrombosis, poor wound healing, GI perforation, irregular bleeding, constipation	[7, 12, 65, 68, 73–77]
Aflibercept (Zaltrap)	Fusion protein against VEGF ligands (VEGF-A, VEGF-B, and PIGF)	Diarrhea, hypertension, proteinuria, hemorrhages, delayed wound healing, neutropenia, infections, abdominal pain	[7, 12, 26, 32, 65, 74, 75, 78, 79]
Ramucirumab (Cyramza)	Anti-VEGFR-2 mAb	Excessive bleeding, gastrointestinal perforations, impaired wound healing	[7, 12, 32, 74, 80]
Regorafenib (Stivarga)	Multi-target TKI (VEGF, TIE2 VEGFR-2)	Hand-foot syndrome, hemorrhages, proteinuria, GI perforations, thromboembolic events, diarrhea, wound healing complications, skin rash, and liver problems like hepatotoxicities	[7, 12, 26, 32, 75, 76, 81, 82]
Vatalanib	TKI (VEGFR, PDGF-β, and c-kit)	Hypertension, proteinuria, abdominal pain, hypercalcemia, pain	[12, 19, 26, 83]
Sunitinib (Sutent)	Multi-target TKI (VEGFR, PDGFR, c-kit, RET, and flt3)	Anemia, fever, hand-foot syndrome, bleeding, constipation, abdominal pain, blood clots, neutropenia	[12, 19, 26, 32, 84, 85]
Cetuximab (Erbitux)	EGFR-targeted mAbs	Diarrhea, fever, abdominal pain, skin rash, electrolyte disturbance, stomatitis, fatigue, infusion reactions	[12, 53, 74, 86, 87]
Panitumumab (Vectibix)	EGFR-targeted mAbs	Diarrhea, hypomagnesemia, dermatological toxicities, vomiting, infusion reaction, electrolyte imbalance, acneiform rash	[12, 74, 86, 88]
Gefitinib (Iressa)	EGFR-TKI	Diarrhea, anorexia, mouth ulcers, rash, pruritus, interstitial disease	[1, 12]
Erlotinib (Tarceva)	EGFR-targeted TKI	Skin rashes, diarrhea, poor appetite, fatigue, vomiting, abdominal pain	[1, 12, 89]

clinical trials suggested a supra-additive inhibitory effect on the tumor angiogenesis when combined with other chemotherapeutic drugs [61]. The results from preclinical trials reveal the synergistic activity of gefitinib in combination with oxaliplatin in patients with mCRC [62]. The encouraging preliminary results from randomized phase II trials have established the eminent ability of gefitinib to cause therapeutic relief for mCRC [47, 62]. It was also observed that gefitinib is capable of inhibiting other tyrosine kinase receptors [47]. The detailed analysis of in vitro cell lines reveals the EGFR-targeted TKI like gefitinib and erlotinib possessed the capacity to inhibit the tumor growth in cetuximab-resistant cell lines further adding to the advantages of TKIs possess over mAb [61]. Despite promising results, patients often experience diarrhea, nausea, fatigue, and neutropenia, and therefore further studies are needed in this regard [12, 62].

Erlotinib

Erlotinib (Tarceva) consists of a small quinazolinamine molecule that acts as a reversible tyrosine kinase inhibitor. This orally administered drug serves as an ATP analog that competes with the ATP molecule for the intracellular tyrosine kinase domain ATP-binding pockets in the EGFRs. Thus, erlotinib selectively inhibits the EGFR autophosphorylation and prevents its downstream signalling [12, 47, 61]. Erlotinib possesses anti-proliferative effects and is capable of arresting cell cycle at the G1 phase [47]. Studies have revealed that the monotherapy of erlotinib is capable of effectively managing CRC. However, the combination of erlotinib along with other therapeutic regimes like oxaliplatin and fluoropyrimidine has shown quite promising results with a RR of 25% [12, 61].

11.4.3 Fusion Protein

11.4.3.1 Aflibercept

Aflibercept (Zaltrap) is a recombinant fusion protein decoy receptor designed to block VEGF-A and VEGF-B. This decoy fusion protein consists of an extracellular domain – second Ig domain of VEGFR-1 and third Ig domain of VEGFR-2 fused with the Fc domain of IgG1 [12, 49]. It selectively traps the VEGF-A and binds to it with higher affinity. This inhibits the binding of VEGF-A to their respective tyrosine kinase cell surface receptors, thereby preventing the stimulation of angiogenesis [7, 12, 50, 63]. The preclinical trials of aflibercept have shown promising results [12]. A phase I trial evaluating the aflibercept along with irinotecan, 5-fluorouracil, and leucovorin for patients with mCRC showed partial response. Exposure to several anti-angiogenic inhibitors tends to elevate the level of PlGF, whereas aflibercept was hypothesized to overcome this resistance compared to other therapeutic drugs [49]. Studies have indicated that unlike other VEGF and VEGFR inhibitors, aflibercept induces limited hypoxia and thus does not stimulate an angiogenic escape program. This results in reduced incidences of drug resistance [31]. In the year 2012, FDA approved aflibercept in combination with FOLFIRI regimen for the treatment of mCRC in patients that were previously treated with oxaliplatin-containing regimen [63]. However, studies have reported grade 3 and 4 levels of toxicities associated with the administration of aflibercept [49].

11.5 Conclusion

The classical anti-angiogenic therapy specifically aims to reduce neovascularization by inhibiting endothelial cell proliferation. The last decades witnessed a remarkable increase in the number of researches focusing on the development of anti-angiogenic drugs and molecules to specifically target the signalling pathway in order to inhibit tumor progression and metastasis. The result from various studies demonstrates overexpression of EGFR in around 60–80% of tumors. As of now, targeting EGFR and its ligand has become a prime focus for the treatment of mCRC. However, data from the preclinical and clinical trials reveal that 80% of mCRCs have not been benefited from anti-EGFR therapy. The clinical trials revealed that only a small portion of patients with mCRC responded to the anti-EGFR therapy and those who responded were likely to develop resistance to it. The reports indicate the development of primary resistance in most of the CRCs depicting the limitation of the therapy [42]. Only 20–23% of patients with wild-type RAS respond to the anti-EGFR monotherapy treatment. Around 65–70% of patients with wild-type RAS depicted the response to the combination of anti-EGFR and chemotherapy [64]. These mutations are known to activate the EGFR downstream signalling pathway irrespective of the EGFR blockade [42]. Thus, only a fraction of patients with the wild-type RAS responds to anti-EGFR therapy [64]. Due to the frequent occurrence of these mutations, sequencing has become mandatory before the drug administration. The phenomenon of development of resistance to the angiogenic inhibitors has become a major concern in the long-term experimental studies and clinical trials. It was further established that the epigenetic alterations in the genes contribute to the development of such resistance [64]. Thus, it has become necessary to overcome these challenges in order to increase the efficiency of the drug. The combination of anti-angiogenic drugs targeting specific multiple molecules and signalling pathways along with chemotherapy has shown promising results [42]. Several combinatorial chemotherapeutic drugs with anti-angiogenic drugs are currently under preclinical and clinical trials [30]. As the studies continue to explore and exploit molecular angiogenic pathways against cancer, a wide range of new unexpected toxicities have surfaced [65]. Several researchers have pointed out the drawbacks and limitations of anti-angiogenic therapies [46]. Some mild side effects include fatigue, low blood count, bleeding, proteinuria, poor wound healing, thromboembolic events, diarrhea, nausea, vomiting, constipation, skin rashes, hypertension, dizziness, dry skin, loss of appetite, weight loss, fatigue, weakness, headaches, depression, hypertension, etc. Some rare and serious side effects include high blood pressure, heart attacks, gastrointestinal perforations, severe bleeding, heart failure, blood clot, intestinal bleeding, electrolyte imbalance, and bowel perforations [55, 66–68]. The use of chemotherapy for the treatment of cancers sometimes results in serious toxicities including hypersensitivity reactions, nausea, vomiting, fatigue, constipation, diarrhea, myelosuppression, neuropathy, and hand-foot syndrome [68]. As investigations continue to explore the combination therapies utilizing anti-angiogenic agents and chemotherapeutic drugs, it is expected that patients experience toxicities related to both the treatment strategies [46]. Experimental studies conducted on mouse models using VEGF inhibitors on tumors demonstrate how these inhibitors promote invasiveness in the primary tumor cells and induce metastasis [69]. The employment of anti-angiogenic drugs can also exacerbate tumor aggressiveness [70]. Some studies claim that the combination of chemotherapy with the anti-VEGF drug like bevacizumab increases the risk of serious side effects and may even lead to death. Furthermore, administration of anti-angiogenic drugs, especially anti-VEGF and anti-EGFR therapy, affects the vasculature of various organs [55]. The development of resistance against the targeted therapies remains a major concern for the application of anti-angiogenic drugs [69]. The tumor cell growth is not entirely based on single angiogenic growth factors. Therefore, obstructing a single angiogenic factor will result in little or almost no effect on tumor growth. However, other studies contradict this by demonstrating that inhibiting pro-angiogenic factor VEGF alone can suppress angiogenesis and tumor growth [71]. Therefore anti-angiogenic drug administration-related toxicities require urgent attention [72].

References

1. Yoo SY, Kwon SM. Angiogenesis and its therapeutic opportunities. Mediat Inflamm. 2013;2013 https://doi.org/10.1155/2013/127170.
2. Rajabi M, Mousa SA. The role of angiogenesis in cancer treatment. Biomedicine. 2017;5 https://doi.org/10.3390/biomedicines5020034.
3. Yadav L, Puri N, Rastogi V, et al. Tumour angiogenesis and angiogenic inhibitors: a review. J Clin Diagn Res. 2015;9:XE01–5. https://doi.org/10.7860/JCDR/2015/12016.6135.
4. Folkman J. Angiogenesis. 2006; 57: 1-18.
5. Ucuzian AA, Gassman AA, East AT, Greisler HP. Molecular mediators of angiogenesis. J Burn Care Res. 2010;31:158–75. https://doi.org/10.1097/BCR.0b013e3181c7ed82.
6. Deveza L, Choi J, Yang F. Therapeutic angiogenesis for treating cardiovascular diseases. Theranostics. 2012;2:801–14. https://doi.org/10.7150/thno.4419.
7. Seeber A, Gunsilius E, Gastl G, Pircher A. Anti-angiogenics: their value in colorectal cancer therapy. Oncol Res Treat. 2018;41:188–93. https://doi.org/10.1159/000488301.
8. Adair T, Montani J. Overview of angiogenesis. Angiogenesis. 2010:1–10.
9. S.M. Sagar, D. Yance, MH and R.K. Wong. Natural health products that inhibit angiogenesis: a potential source for investigational new agents to treat cancer—Part 1. Curr Oncol. 2006 Feb; 13(1): 14–26.
10. Cohen MM. Judah Folkman, MD, 1933–2008: father of angiogenesis. J Craniofac Surg. 2009;20:590–1. https://doi.org/10.1097/SCS.0b013e3181927e8a.
11. Mousa L, Salem ME, Mikhail S. Biomarkers of angiogenesis in colorectal Cancer. Biomarkers Cancer. 2015;7s1:BIC.S25250. https://doi.org/10.4137/bic.s25250.
12. Winder T, Lenz HJ. Vascular endothelial growth factor and epidermal growth factor signaling pathways as therapeutic targets for colorectal cancer. Gastroenterology. 2010;138:2163–76. https://doi.org/10.1053/j.gastro.2010.02.005.
13. Ding C, Li L, Yang T, et al. Combined application of anti-VEGF and anti-EGFR attenuates the growth and angiogenesis of colorectal cancer mainly through suppressing AKT and ERK signaling in mice model. BMC Cancer. 2016;16:1–13. https://doi.org/10.1186/s12885-016-2834-8.
14. Nishida N, Yano H, Nishida T, et al. Angiogenesis in cancer. Vasc Health Risk Manag. 2006;2:213–9. https://doi.org/10.2147/vhrm.2006.2.3.213.
15. Martin T, Ye L, Sanders A, et al. Cancer invasion and metastasis: molecular and cellular perspective. 2014.
16. Loizzi V, del Vecchio V, Gargano G, et al. Biological pathways involved in tumor angiogenesis and bevacizumab based anti-angiogenic therapy with special references to ovarian cancer. Int J Mol Sci. 2017;18:1–11. https://doi.org/10.3390/ijms18091967.

17. Lugano R, Ramachandran M, Dimberg A. Tumor angiogenesis: causes, consequences, challenges and opportunities. Cell Mol Life Sci. 2020;77:1745–70. https://doi.org/10.1007/s00018-019-03351-7.
18. Tonini T, Rossi F, Claudio PP. Molecular basis of angiogenesis and cancer. Oncogene. 2003;22:6549–56. https://doi.org/10.1038/sj.onc.1206816.
19. Makarevich PI, Parfyonova YV. Therapeutic angiogenesis: foundations and practical application. Physiologic and pathologic angiogenesis – signaling mechanisms and targeted therapy. 2017. p. 343–64.
20. Angiogenesis inhibitors. https://www.cancer.gov/about-cancer/treatment/types/immunotherapy/angiogenesis-inhibitors-fact-sheet.
21. Ribatti D. History of research on angiogenesis. Chem Immunol Allergy. 2014;99:1–14. https://doi.org/10.1159/000353311.
22. Angelucci A, Delle Monache S, Cortellini A, et al. "Vessels in the storm": searching for prognostic and predictive angiogenic factors in colorectal cancer. Int J Mol Sci. 2018;19 https://doi.org/10.3390/ijms19010299.
23. Konda B. Anti-angiogenic agents in metastatic colorectal cancer. World J Gastrointest Oncol. 2015;7:71. https://doi.org/10.4251/wjgo.v7.i7.71.
24. Pang RWC, Poon RTP. Clinical implications of angiogenesis in cancers. Vasc Health Risk Manag. 2006;2:97–108. https://doi.org/10.2147/vhrm.2006.2.2.97.
25. Ribatti D. The discovery of angiogenic growth factors: the contribution of Italian scientists. Vascular Cell. 2014;6:1–6. https://doi.org/10.1186/2045-824X-6-8.
26. Crivellato E. The role of angiogenic growth factors in organogenesis. Int J Dev Biol. 2011;55:365–75. https://doi.org/10.1387/ijdb.103214ec.
27. Bisht M, Dhasmana DC, Bist SS. Angiogenesis: future of pharmacological modulation. Indian J Pharmacol. 2010;42:2–8. https://doi.org/10.4103/0253-7613.62395.
28. Cook KM, Figg WD. Angiogenesis inhibitors: current strategies and future prospects. CA Cancer J Clin. 2010;60:222–43. https://doi.org/10.3322/caac.20075.
29. Huang Z, Bao SD. Roles of main pro- and anti-angiogenic factors in tumor angiogenesis. World J Gastroenterol. 2004;10:463–70. https://doi.org/10.3748/wjg.v10.i4.463.
30. Mihalache A, Rogoveanu I. Angiogenesis factors involved in the pathogenesis of colorectal cancer. Curr Health Sci J. 2014;40:5–11. https://doi.org/10.12865/CHSJ.40.01.01.
31. Giordano G, Febbraro A, Venditti M, et al. Targeting angiogenesis and tumor microenvironment in metastatic colorectal cancer: role of Aflibercept. Gastroenterol Res Pract. 2014;2014 https://doi.org/10.1155/2014/526178.
32. Inampudi C, Akintoye E, Ando T, Briasoulis A. Angiogenesis in peripheral arterial disease. Curr Opin Pharmacol. 2018;39:60–7. https://doi.org/10.1016/j.coph.2018.02.011.
33. Marech I, Leporini C, Ammendola M, et al. Classical and non-classical proangiogenic factors as a target of antiangiogenic therapy in tumor microenvironment. Cancer Lett. 2016;380:216–26. https://doi.org/10.1016/j.canlet.2015.07.028.
34. Gupta K, Zhang J. Angiogenesis: a curse or cure? Postgrad Med J. 2005;81:236–42. https://doi.org/10.1136/pgmj.2004.023309.
35. Zouhairi M El, Charabaty A, Pishvaian MJ (2011) Molecularly targeted therapy for metastatic colon cancer: proven treatments and promising new agents. Gastrointest Cancer Res 4:15–21.
36. Kanat O, Ertas H. Existing anti-angiogenic therapeutic strategies for patients with metastatic colorectal cancer progressing following first-line bevacizumab-based therapy. World J Clin Oncol. 2019;10:52–61. https://doi.org/10.5306/wjco.v10.i2.52.
37. Pache JC. Epidermal growth factors. Encyclopedia of Respiratory Medicine, Four-Volume Set 2. 2006:129–133. https://doi.org/10.1016/B0-12-370879-6/00138-1.
38. Krasinskas AM. EGFR signaling in colorectal carcinoma. Pathol Res Int. 2011;2011:1–6. https://doi.org/10.4061/2011/932932.
39. Pabla B, Bissonnette M, Konda VJ. Colon cancer and the epidermal growth factor receptor: current treatment paradigms, the importance of diet, and the role of chemoprevention. World J Clin Oncol. 2015;6:133–41. https://doi.org/10.5306/wjco.v6.i5.133.

40. Koveitypour Z, Panahi F, Vakilian M, et al. Signaling pathways involved in colorectal cancer progression. Cell Biosci. 2019;9:1–14. https://doi.org/10.1186/s13578-019-0361-4.
41. Zhang W, Gordon M, Lenz HJ. Novel approaches to treatment of advanced colorectal cancer with anti-EGFR monoclonal antibodies. Ann Med. 2006;38:545–51. https://doi.org/10.1080/09546630601070812.
42. Zhao B, Wang L, Qiu H, et al. Mechanisms of resistance to anti-EGFR therapy in colorectal cancer. Oncotarget. 2017;8:3980–4000. https://doi.org/10.18632/oncotarget.14012
43. Cetuximab. In: Chemocare. 2020. http://chemocare.com/chemotherapy/drug-info/cetuximab.aspx.
44. Cohen AB, Lessell S. Angiogenesis and pituitary tumors. Semin Ophthalmol. 2009;24:185–9. https://doi.org/10.1080/08820530902805651.
45. Katayama Y, Uchino J, Chihara Y, et al. Tumor neovascularization and developments in therapeutics. Cancers. 2019;11 https://doi.org/10.3390/cancers11030316.
46. El-Kenawi AE, El-Remessy AB. Angiogenesis inhibitors in cancer therapy: mechanistic perspective on classification and treatment rationales. Br J Pharmacol. 2013;170:712–29. https://doi.org/10.1111/bph.12344.
47. Seshacharyulu P, Ponnusamy MP, Haridas D, et al. Targeting the EGFR signaling pathway in cancer therapy. Expert Opin Ther Targets. 2012;16:15–31. https://doi.org/10.1517/14728222.2012.680957.
48. Kazazi-Hyseni F, Beijnen JH, Schellens JHM. Bevacizumab. Oncologist. 2012;15:819–25. https://doi.org/10.1634/theoncologist.2011-0227.
49. Ciombor KK, Goldberg RM. Update on anti-angiogenesis therapy in colorectal cancer. Curr Colorect Cancer Rep. 2015;11:378–87. https://doi.org/10.1007/s11888-015-0292-3.
50. Rosen LS, Jacobs IA, Burkes RL. Bevacizumab in colorectal cancer: current role in treatment and the potential of Biosimilars. Target Oncol. 2017;12:599–610. https://doi.org/10.1007/s11523-017-0518-1.
51. Battaglin F, Puccini A, Intini R, et al. The role of tumor angiogenesis as a therapeutic target in colorectal cancer. Expert Rev Anticancer Ther. 2018;18:251–66. https://doi.org/10.1080/14737140.2018.1428092.
52. Maiello E, Giuliani F, Gebbia V, et al. Cetuximab: clinical results in colorectal cancer. Annals of oncology. 2007;18:vi8–vi10. https://doi.org/10.1093/annonc/mdm216.
53. Chidharla A, Parsi M, Kasi A. Cetuximab. In: StatPearls [Internet]. StatPearls Publishing. 2020.
54. Yazdi MH, Faramarzi MA, Nikfar S, Abdollahi M. A comprehensive review of clinical trials on EGFR inhibitors such as cetuximab and panitumumab as monotherapy and in combination for treatment of metastatic colorectal cancer. Avicenna J Med Biotechnol. 2015;7:134–44.
55. Maj E, Papiernik D, Wietrzyk J. Antiangiogenic cancer treatment: the great discovery and greater complexity (review). Int J Oncol. 2016;49:1773–84. https://doi.org/10.3892/ijo.2016.3709.
56. Hartmann J, Haap M, Kopp H-G, Lipp H-P. Tyrosine kinase inhibitors – a review on pharmacology, metabolism and side effects. Curr Drug Metab. 2009;10:470–81. https://doi.org/10.2174/138920009788897975.
57. Wu P, Nielsen TE, Clausen MH. FDA-approved small-molecule kinase inhibitors. Trends Pharmacol Sci. 2015;36:422–39. https://doi.org/10.1016/j.tips.2015.04.005.
58. Saltz LB, Rosen LS, Marshall JL, et al. Phase II trial of sunitinib in patients with metastatic colorectal cancer after failure of standard therapy. J Clin Oncol. 2007;25:4793–9. https://doi.org/10.1200/JCO.2007.12.8637.
59. Alvarez RH, Garrett-Mayer E, Halabi S, et al. Sunitinib in patients with metastatic colorectal cancer with FLT-3 alterations: results from the Targeted Agent and Profiling Utilization Registry (TAPUR) Study. https://doi.org/10.1158/1538-7445.sabcs18-ct146.
60. Grothey A, Allegra C. Antiangiogenesis therapy in the treatment of metastatic colorectal cancer. Therap Adv Med Oncol. 2012;4:301–19. https://doi.org/10.1177/1758834012454464.

61. Ponz-Sarvisé M, Rodríguez J, Viudez A, et al. Epidermal growth factor receptor inhibitors in colorectal cancer treatment: what's new? World J Gastroenterol. 2007;13:5877–87. https://doi.org/10.3748/wjg.v13.i44.5877.
62. Zampino MG, Lorizzo K, Massacesi C, Rizzi A, Crispino S, Boselli S, Pelosi G, Zorzino L, Fazio N, de Braud F. First-line gefitinib combined with simplified FOLFOX-6 in patients with epidermal growth factor receptor- positive advanced colorectal cancer. J Clin Oncol. 2005;23 https://doi.org/10.1200/jco.2005.23.16_suppl.3659.
63. Perkins SL, Cole SW. Ziv-aflibercept (Zaltrap) for the treatment of metastatic colorectal Cancer. Ann Pharmacother. 2014;48:93–8. https://doi.org/10.1177/1060028013506562.
64. Lièvre A, Ouine B, Canet J, et al. Protein biomarkers predictive for response to anti-EGFR treatment in RAS wild-type metastatic colorectal carcinoma. Br J Cancer. 2017;117:1819–27. https://doi.org/10.1038/bjc.2017.353.
65. Elice F, Rodeghiero F. Side effects of anti-angiogenic drugs. Thromb Res. 2012;129:S50–3. https://doi.org/10.1016/S0049-3848(12)70016-6.
66. Angiogenesis and Angiogenesis Inhibitors to Treat Cancer. https://www.cancer.net/navigating-cancer-care/how-cancer-treated/personalized-and-targeted-therapies/angiogenesis-and-angiogenesis-inhibitors-treat-cancer.
67. Ribatti D. The discovery of antiangiogenic molecules: a historical review. Curr Pharm Des. 2009;15:345–52. https://doi.org/10.2174/138161209787315855.
68. Grenon NN. Managing toxicities associated with antiangiogenic biologic agents in combination with chemotherapy for metastatic colorectal cancer. Clin J Oncol Nurs. 2013;17:425–33. https://doi.org/10.1188/13.CJON.425-433.
69. Abdalla AME, Xiao L, Ullah MW, et al. Current challenges of cancer anti-angiogenic therapy and the promise of nanotherapeutics. Theranostics. 2018;8:533–49. https://doi.org/10.7150/thno.21674.
70. Moserle L, Jiménez-Valerio G, Casanovas O. Antiangiogenic therapies: going beyond their limits. Cancer Discov. 2014;4:31–41. https://doi.org/10.1158/2159-8290.cd-13-0199.
71. Ribatti D. The history of angiogenesis inhibitors. Leukemia. 2007;21:1606–9. https://doi.org/10.1038/sj.leu.2404756.
72. Zirlik K, Duyster J. Anti-angiogenics: current situation and future perspectives. Oncol Res Treat. 2018;41:166–71. https://doi.org/10.1159/000488087.
73. Avastin. In: Chemocare. 2020. http://chemocare.com/chemotherapy/drug-info/avastin.aspx.
74. Pinto MP, Sotomayor P, Carrasco-Avino G, et al. Escaping antiangiogenic therapy: strategies employed by cancer cells. Int J Mol Sci. 2016;17:1–20. https://doi.org/10.3390/ijms17091489.
75. Al-Abd AM, Alamoudi AJ, Abdel-Naim AB, et al. Anti-angiogenic agents for the treatment of solid tumors: potential pathways, therapy and current strategies – a review. J Adv Res. 2017;8:591–605. https://doi.org/10.1016/j.jare.2017.06.006.
76. Jitawatanarat P, Ma WW. Update on antiangiogenic therapy in colorectal cancer: Aflibercept and regorafenib. J Gastrointest Oncol. 2013;4:231–8. https://doi.org/10.3978/j.issn.2078-6891.2013.008.
77. Taugourdeau-Raymond S, Rouby F, Default A, Jean-Pastor MJ. Bevacizumab-induced serious side-effects: a review of the French pharmacovigilance database. Eur J Clin Pharmacol. 2012;68:1103–7. https://doi.org/10.1007/s00228-012-1232-7.
78. Tang PA, Moore MJ. Aflibercept in the treatment of patients with metastatic colorectal cancer: latest findings and interpretations. Ther Adv Gastroenterol. 2013;6:459–73. https://doi.org/10.1177/1756283X13502637.
79. Saif MW, Relias V, Syrigos K, Gunturu KS. Incidence and management of ZIv-aflibercept related toxicities in colorectal cancer. World J Clin Oncol. 2014;5:1028–35. https://doi.org/10.5306/wjco.v5.i5.1028.
80. Ramucirumab. In: Chemocare. https://chemocare.com/chemotherapy/drug-info/ramucirumab.aspx.
81. Regorafenib. In: Chemocare. 2020. http://chemocare.com/chemotherapy/drug-info/regorafenib.aspx.

82. Krishnamoorthy SK, Relias V, Sebastian S, et al. Management of regorafenib-related toxicities: a review. Ther Adv Gastroenterol. 2015;8:285–97. https://doi.org/10.1177/1756283X15580743.
83. Joensuu H, De Braud F, Grignagni G, et al. Vatalanib for metastatic gastrointestinal stromal tumour (GIST) resistant to imatinib: final results of a phase II study. Br J Cancer. 2011;104:1686–90. https://doi.org/10.1038/bjc.2011.151.
84. Sunitinib. In: Chemocare. http://chemocare.com/chemotherapy/drug-info/Sunitinib.aspx.
85. Schwandt A, Wood LS, Rini B, Dreicer R. Management of side effects associated with sunitinib therapy for patients with renal cell carcinoma. Onco Targets Ther. 2009;2:51–61. https://doi.org/10.2147/ott.s4052.
86. Ciftci R, Tural D. Anti-epidermal growth factor receptor (EGFR) treatment in patients with metastatic colorectal cancer. Colorectal Cancer - From Pathogenesis to Treatment. 2016. https://doi.org/10.5772/62304.
87. Cetuximab. In: Chemocare. http://chemocare.com/chemotherapy/drug-info/cetuximab.aspx.
88. Panitumumab. In: Chemocare. http://chemocare.com/chemotherapy/drug-info/Panitumumab.aspx.
89. Erlotinib. In: Chemocare. http://chemocare.com/chemotherapy/drug-info/erlotinib.aspx.

Chapter 12
Anti-Inflammatory Molecular Mechanism and Contribution of Drug Transport Molecules in Colorectal Cancer Cells

Dowluru S. V. G. K. Kaladhar and Srinivasan Tantravahi

Abstract Colorectal cancer (CRC) is a third most common malignant neoplasm arising from the lining of colon and rectum of the large intestine. The molecular mechanisms provide some fundamental effects and activities of molecules as chemopreventive, anti-inflammatory, and antioxidative agents in CRC. The expressions and regulation of COX-2, HER-2, Oct4, Sox2, p53, MDR1/P-glycoprotein, CXCR4, VEGF-C, etc. are important to understand the anti-inflammatory molecular mechanisms and inhibitory effect on cell growth and in induction of apoptosis in colorectal cancer. Nonsteroidal anti-inflammatory drugs (NSAIDs) and several drug inhibitors can act against colorectal tumorigenesis. The present literature and experimentation provide the precise information on anti-inflammatory molecular mechanisms that regulate apoptosis in colorectal cancer cells and on proliferation and on induction of apoptosis by nonsteroidal anti-inflammatory inhibitors as transport molecules in colorectal cancer cells. The gene superfamilies that are involved in the transport of drugs are the solute carrier (SLC) family and the ATP-binding cassette (ABC) family. The effects of selective COX-2 inhibitors (COXIBs) and nonsteroidal anti-inflammatory drugs (NSAIDs) may be the most promising chemopreventive agents for CRC prevention and treatment.

Keywords Colorectal cancer · Anti-inflammatory molecular mechanisms · Molecular inhibitors · Transport molecules

D. S. V. G. K. Kaladhar
Microbiology and Bioinformatics, UTD, Atal Bihari Vajpayee University, Bilaspur, CG, India

S. Tantravahi (✉)
Botany, Indira Gandhi National Tribal University, Amarkantak, MP, India

G. P. Nagaraju et al. (eds.), *Colon Cancer Diagnosis and Therapy*,
https://doi.org/10.1007/978-3-030-63369-1_12

12.1 Introduction

Colorectal cancer (CRC), also known as colon cancer or bowel cancer or rectal cancer, is a type of cancer from the parts of the large intestine like colon or rectum. Colorectal cancer (CRC) is a heterogeneous disease that results from the stepwise accumulation of multiple genetic and epigenetic alterations that promote the transformation of normal colonic mucosa into cancer. Colorectal cancer will often begin as small growth or as polyp inside the colon or rectum of the digestive system. It is the third most frequent and the fourth leading cause of cancer-related deaths worldwide; it is primarily due to the failure of (a) approved targeted therapies and (b) development of resistance to the approved drugs. Besides, poor understanding of therapeutic targets and the drug resistance mechanisms is also contributing to the failure of therapies and increasing incidence and mortality rates. The environmental and genetic factors influence the development of CRC; broadly age, diet, lifestyle, and metabolic disorders play a significant role. Over 70% of CRC cases are sporadic and the remaining cases influenced by genetic predisposition with or without the part of environmental factors. The risk of developing CRC increases with age, and over 90% of sporadic CRCs occur in individuals over the age of 50 [1, 2].

Cancer is a single or group of diseases in living organisms that are involving in abnormal cell growth at one or more locations with the potential to invade or spread to various parts of the systems and cause abnormal function (Fig. 12.1). CRC is reported as the second most common cause of death in the Western countries next to heart disease [3, 4]. CRC occurs from the colorectal epithelium and causes genetic alterations in several oncogenes and tumor suppressor genes (TSG). Mechanisms of genomic instability by K-ras and inactivation of TSG like p53, DCC/Smad4, and APC [5], DNA mismatch repair genes like MLH1 and/or MSH2 hypermethylation of promoter, mutation of genes with coding microsatellites like transforming growth factor receptor II (TGF-RII) and BAX, and mutation in the tumor suppressor gene like APC on chromosome 5q in FAP and mutated DNA mismatch repair genes in the HNPCC have been identified majorly in sporadic CRC progression [6].

Hereditary, sporadic, and colitis-associated CRC are the three major forms of colorectal cancer. The risk of CRC may be due to genetic mutations, chronic inflammation, epigenetic changes, diet, and lifestyle [7]. The effects of selective COX-2 inhibitors (COXIBs) and nonsteroidal anti-inflammatory drugs (NSAIDs) may be the most promising chemopreventive agents for CRC prevention and treatment.

The genetic and epigenetic alterations developed in the colon or rectum dysregulate conserved signalling pathways of cellular metabolism, proliferation, differentiation, survival, apoptosis, etc. leading to initiation of CRC. In general, three diverse pathways are responsible for these effects. These are the chromosomal instability (CIN) pathway, the microsatellite instability (MSI) pathway, and the CpG island methylator phenotype (CIMP) pathway. The alterations induced by the first two pathways change the DNA sequence of the gene or region, whereas the latter pathway does not change the DNA sequence but leads to suppression in the gene expression [8, 9].

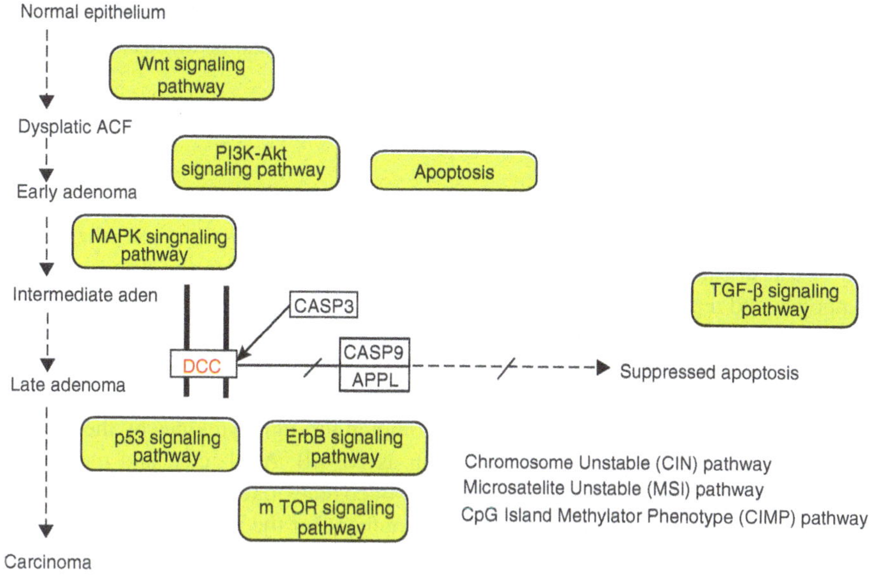

Fig. 12.1 Cellular processes for formation of carcinoma

The hereditary CRC is caused by germline mutations, whereas sporadic CRC is caused by progressive accumulation of genetic and epigenetic aberrations. In this regard, the role of external or environmental factors is more dominant than that of the genetic factors where specifically environmental and food-borne mutagens and intestinal commensals and pathogens along with chronic intestinal inflammation play a substantial role [10–12]. The inflammation and cancer are inseparable, and inflammation is triggered by infections, mutagens, carcinogens, obesity, etc. It is reported that the incidence of CRC is 60% more in patients with inflammatory bowel disease (IBD) over the normal population. Inflammation is said to be involved in sporadic as well as heritable CRC [2].

Inflammation plays a key role in the induction, promotion, and invasion of cancer. In IBD patients, chronic inflammation initiates colitis-associated cancer, a subtype of CRC. Similarly, chronic inflammation also generates free radicals like reactive oxygen species (ROS) and reactive nitrogen intermediates (RNI) that can induce DNA damage. The alterations in the DNA may mutate tumor suppressor genes, protooncogenes, etc. that can also cause initiation and further development of tumors. The accumulation of additional mutations and epigenetic changes will promote the uncontrolled growth of cancer cells. Thus, the inflammation influences many vital stages of metastasis, starting from enhancing mobility to the invasion of tissues [11, 13].

Inflammation plays a significant role in every facet of tumor development, and hence, anti-inflammatory drugs can reduce the risk of CRC. In this chapter, we will describe different anti-inflammatory drugs and molecular mechanisms of their control in the mitigation of colorectal cancer. Further, the effect of transport molecules on the efficacy and efficiency of the drug will also be discussed.

12.2 Inflammation

Inflammation is the sum of host defense responses against infections and other stimuli to translocate immune cells to the location, thus leading to the destruction of pathogen and repair of the tissue. Inflammation is initially known for its role in host defense against pathogens, but it is equally important in tissue repair and regeneration and maintenance of homeostasis [14]. It turns out to be chronic in conditions where its regulatory mechanism fails or the inflammatory stimulus persists. Under these conditions, the cell proliferation is promoted through cytokines by the activation of various downstream effectors, such as NF-κB, AP-1, etc., and mutations induced in tumor suppressor genes and protooncogenes like p53, KRASF, BRCA, BCL2, etc., often creating a conducive environment for the induction and development of cancer.

An increased risk of developing colorectal cancer in patients is observed with long-standing of human disease like inflammatory bowel disease (IBD) [15]. Cyclooxygenase-2 (COX-2) and nuclear factor kappaB (NF-κB) ate the two key genes involved in the inflammatory process that provide a process link between inflammation and cancer. The factors such as IL-6- and TNF-α-induced signalling were recently identified that promote tumor growth in colitis-associated cancer. The microbiota, chemicals in the ingested food, etc. can cause inflammation in the GI tract, and injury is a common phenomenon in all these stress conditions. The inflammation is primarily caused by damaged cells and various immune cells that are present in the area of damage. The wound or injury in the tissue initiates coagulation, platelet activation, and aggregation along with the release of various proteins like cell growth factors (platelet-derived growth factor (PDGF), platelet-derived angiogenesis factor, transforming growth factor-α (TGF-α), TGF-β, etc.). The release of TGF-β1, PDGF, platelet-activating factor, etc. facilitates chemotaxis of neutrophils, monocytes, fibroblasts, and myofibroblasts along with tissue repair mechanisms [13]. The neutrophils further recruit and activate other effector cells and also participate in wound healing by the release of pro-inflammatory cytokines like TNF-α, interleukin (IL)-1α, and IL-1β [16, 17]. These cytokines further influence the expression of matrix metalloproteinases (MMPs) and keratinocyte growth factor (KGF/FGF-7) that initiate the repair of damaged tissue and are also involved in angiogenesis and metastasis.

The monocytes migrate to the injured area and are transformed into macrophages due to the effect of TGF-β, PDGF, IL-1β, TNF-α, MCP-1/CCL2, MCP-2/CCL8, etc. The mature and activated macrophages secrete TGF-α, TGF-β1, PDGF, bFGF, insulin-like growth factor (IGF)-I and IGF-II, TNF-α, and IL-1 that promote tissue repair through the initiation of cell proliferation and angiogenesis [18]. Mast cells upon activation also release various growth factors, and all these responses lead to the early phase of inflammation. The profile of cytokines present dictates the influence of the inflammation and, thus, the fate of the cell. If the pro-inflammatory cytokines persist for a longer period of time, it can lead to the conversion of a normal cell into adenoma. For example, TNF plays important roles in cell survival, proliferation, differentiation, and death through activating distinct signalling pathways such as nuclear factor-κB (NF-κB) and c-Jun N-terminal kinase (JNK) [19]. TGF-α and TGF-β1, in specific, regulate many aspects of inflammation and repair, helping the affected tissue to defend and recover, but, if these self-limiting steps are dysregulated, it leads to abnormalities and thus the pathogenesis.

In case if the infestation of microorganisms does not develop the injury, inflammation is established by a different series of events. The pathogen like *H. pylori* would be identified by sensors like Toll-like receptor 2 (TLR2) and TLR4, stimulator of interferon genes (STING), which initiates downstream signalling and activates the nuclear transcriptional factor-kappa B (NF-κB) signalling pathway [20]. Further, induction of pro-inflammatory gene expression occurs leading to the inflammation. Moreover, variations in intestinal microbiota composition can disturb the homeostasis as the new microorganisms and their products can induce inflammation. These conditions, if persist for a longer period of time, will play a significant role in tumor induction as well as its progression [12].

In the scenario of chronic inflammation, the other factor that can trigger tumor formation is free radicals. Macrophages and neutrophils serve as a source of free radicals especially reactive oxygen species (ROS) and reactive nitrogen intermediates (RNI). Parallelly, the cytokines also influence the release of free radicals from the neighboring epithelial cells [21]. The free radicals can induce DNA damage and affect the response mechanism also. The DNA damage includes base modification, rearrangement of DNA sequence, DNA miscoding lesions, gene amplification, activation of oncogenes, and suppression of tumor suppressor genes, whose consequence is genomic instability. The mutation of a single gene does not form cancer, especially CRC, as it requires mutation of multiple genes to initiate and progress. Thus, the disease stands as a progressive disease and develops through a series of events that lead to the transformation of normal mucosa to adenoma and then to carcinoma. Three distinct pathways are recognized that leads to genomic instability. They are the chromosomal instability (CIN) pathway, the microsatellite instability (MSI) pathway, and the CpG island methylator phenotype (CIMP) pathway [8, 9].

The CIN is characterized by gain or loss of chromosome(s) or its regions leading to aneuploidy, telomere dysfunction, or defects in the DNA damage response mechanisms. This is the major cause of genomic instability and accounts for 65–70% of sporadic CRC [22]. The cancer was reported when the large amplifications in chromosomes 7, 8q, 13q, 20, and X and deletions on chromosomes 1, 4, 5, 8p, 14q, 15q, 17p, 18, 20p, and 22q occurred. Moreover, the gain or loss in regions containing important cancer genes, e.g., VEGF, MYC, MET, LYN, PTEN, and others, have also contributed to the cause [23]. Further, the accumulation of mutations specifically in oncogenes and tumor suppressor genes has also induced CRC mostly commonly in APC, p53, and K-ras genes [8].

The MSI comes into play when the enzymes in the DNA mismatch repair (MMR) system are mutated. The repetitive nature of the microsatellites makes them prone to errors during the replication process, and the MMR system is supposed to rectify the alterations. Microsatellites are dispersed throughout the genome including vital genes involved in cell cycle and regulation like K-ras, p53, BRAF, TGFbRII, etc. In case of chronic inflammation, the MMR genes MSH2, MLH1, MSH6, PMS2, MLH3, MSH3, etc. are mutated or silenced [24]. Hence the errors in the microsatellites are left unattended leading to frameshift mutations and loss of function.

CIMP is an epigenetic way of gene silencing. The free radicals activate DNA modification enzymes that can lead to methylation, histone modifications, etc. [25]. The methylation of DNA commonly occurs at the 5′-CG-3′ (CpG) dinucleotide, and if the promoter region is methylated, it leads to gene silencing. The genes like APC, MCC, MLH1, MGMT, etc. are identified to be hypermethylated in cases of CRC [8, 26].

The environmental factors and microorganisms can induce inflammation, where chronic inflammation can produce chemokines persistently that can influence the normal cell to convert to a cancerous cell. Further, free radicals like ROS and RNI are generated during chronic inflammation, and they can cause genomic instability or epigenetic changes which affect the functioning of oncogenes and tumor suppressor genes leading to malignancy.

12.3 Signalling Pathways of Cancer

In colorectal cancer, the genetic predisposition or environmental factors either individually or cumulatively will mutate or silence certain tumor suppressor genes and/or oncogenes. Depending on the genes mutated or silenced, the cell initiates different molecular mechanisms and overcomes the cell cycle regulation and progresses into cancer. These signalling pathways might overlap, and tumors exhibit features of one or more pathways. The possible signalling pathways and their aberrations are discussed in this section.

Multiple genes like *p53*, *EGFR*, *RAS*, *RAF*, *Notch-1*, *APC*, *Jagged-1*, *PIK3CA*, *PTEN*, etc. belonging to various pathways are said to be frequently dysregulated leading to enhanced cell proliferation, invasion, progression, or inhibition of apoptosis. Therefore, the epidermal growth factor receptor (EGFR), PI3K/AKT, Notch, transforming growth factor-β (TGF-β), and Wnt signalling pathways are considered.

12.3.1 Notch Signalling Pathway

The Notch signalling pathway is highly conserved and helps in the maintenance of intestinal development and homeostasis. It is involved in the normal cell development, differentiation, proliferation, and apoptosis [27, 28]. The pathway comprises four receptors, namely, *Notch*-1, *Notch*-2, *Notch*-3, and *Notch*-4, and at least five ligands, namely, *Jagged-1*, *Jagged-2*, Delta-*like-1* (*Dll-1*), *Delta-like-3* (*Dll-3*), and *Delta-Like-4* (*Dll-4*). These are transmembrane single pass heterooligomer proteins where the ligands belong to the DSL family of proteins containing EGF-like repeats. The signalling pathway gets activated as the ligand binds to the respective receptors on the target cell through the activation of a γ-secretase protein complex. The complex induces cleavage and release of the intracellular domain of the receptor; thus, the active form is known as Notch intracellular domain (NICD) [29]. The NICD translocates into the nucleus and activates CSL (CBF-1/suppressor of the hairless/LAG1) transcription factor by releasing the co-repressors and forming a complex. The co-activators like histone acetyltransferase (HAT), p300, and mastermind-like proteins (MAML) will be bound to CSL. The downstream target genes of the Notch signalling pathway including *p21*, *Hes-1*, and *Deltex* have activated the CSL complex. If this pathway is dysregulated, it leads to the transformation of a normal cell to adenoma and then to carcinoma through the regulation of p21 and PUMA genes, prominently [30]. The Notch ligands, Notch receptors, and some downstream targets of the pathway are overexpressed in colorectal cancer cells, where the expression is relatively higher in the primary stage than the later stages.

12.3.2 PI3K-Akt Signalling Pathway

This is an intracellular signalling pathway that promotes metabolism, survival, and growth of the cell in response to extracellular signals through PI3K (phosphatidylinositol 3-kinase) and Akt (protein kinase B) [31]. The pathway can be activated by the extracellular factors through receptor tyrosine kinases (RTK) or RAS protein. This is also activated by EGFR signalling. PI3K is a heteromeric protein consisting of two domains, namely, a catalytic domain (p110) and a regulatory domain (p85). In the process of activation by RTK or RAS, the p85 domain gets dissociated, and PI3K gets activated. Upon activation, the PI3K phosphorylates phosphatidylinositol 4,5-biphosphate (PIP2) to phosphatidylinositol 3,4,5-triphosphate (PIP3). PIP3 activates Akt, a serine/threonine protein which translocates to the nucleus and mediates the activities of cell survival and growth [32]. Akt has many substrates and regulates them by phosphorylation. Akt inhibits TSC2 and activates mTOR complex 1 (mTORC1) that aids in metabolism and growth. Further, it negatively regulates the function or expression of BH3, Bcl-2, Bax, and Bim proteins and can induce the degradation of p53 leading to the inhibition of apoptosis and thus the survival of the cell. The pathway is regulated by phosphatase and tensin homologue protein (PTEN) through dephosphorylating of PIP3 apart from its feedback mechanism mediated by NF-κB [33]. The dysregulation of this pathway leads to carcinoma.

12.3.3 Wnt Signalling Pathway

Wnt signalling is also a conserved pathway that serves important roles in tissue maintenance and regeneration by regulating cell proliferation, migration, and asymmetric cell division [34, 35]. The pathway is subclassified into the canonical β-catenin-dependent and the non-canonical β-catenin-independent pathways where the former plays a significant role in the physiology and pathology of the cell. Therefore, the mutation in the canonical β-catenin-dependent pathway is crucial in the development of CRC. There are 19 secretory cysteine-rich glycoproteins that are Wnt ligands which can activate the Wnt pathway by binding to the Frizzled receptors. Further, co-receptor like the low-density-lipoprotein-related protein5/6 (LRP5/6) is required to mediate the canonical Wnt signal, activating the phosphoprotein Dishevelled (Dsh). The activated Dsh inhibits the activity of glycogen synthase kinase 3 (GSK3), a key component of β-catenin destruction complex (APC/Axin/GSK3 complex), thus dissociating β-catenin from the complex. The β-catenin accumulates in the cytoplasm and translocates to the nucleus, where it binds with T-cell transcription factor (TCF) or the lymphoid enhancer factor (LEF) and acts as transcriptional co-activator [36–38]. The complex activates many genes involved in proliferation and transmission, such as *CCND1* (the gene encoding *cyclin D1*), *c-MYC*, *c-Jun*, *CD133*, *EGFR*, *CD44*, and leucine-rich repeat-containing receptor 5 (*LGR5*). The abnormal activation of Wnt can lead to CRCs [35, 39] (Figs. 12.2 and 12.3).

12.3.4 TGF-β Signalling Pathway

TGF-β signalling pathway plays a critical role in the regulation of cell growth, differentiation, and development apart from the other biological processes. In specific, it curtails the proliferation of colon epithelial cells and promotes apoptosis.

The receptors involved in the pathway are type I TGF-β receptors (TGFBR1) and type II TGF-β receptors (TGFBR2). TGFBR2 is a serine/threonine receptor kinase that phosphorylates TGFBR1 where each class of ligand binds to a specific TGFBR2 [40]. The ligands are TGFβs, anti-Müllerian hormone (AMH), Nodal, activin, etc.

The signalling is initiated by the binding of TGF-β ligands to TGFBR2 dimer; thereby, TGFBR2 recruits and phosphorylates the TGFBR1. The activated TGFBR1 phosphorylates the downstream transcription factors known as receptor-associated SMAD proteins (R-SMAD proteins), and this process is mediated by SMAD anchor for receptor activation (SARA). The activated R-SMAD (SMAD2 and SMAD3) dissociates and forms a complex with coSMAD (SMAD4). This complex translocates to the nucleus and regulates the transcription of the target genes [41, 42]. The cell cycle checkpoint genes like p21, p27, and p15 are some of the downstream targets which upon activation cause growth arrest [43]. Therefore, TGF-β acts as a tumor suppressor gene even in the normal intestinal epithelium. The CRCs mostly loose TGF-β in the initiation step itself and at times in the later stages [42] (Fig. 12.4).

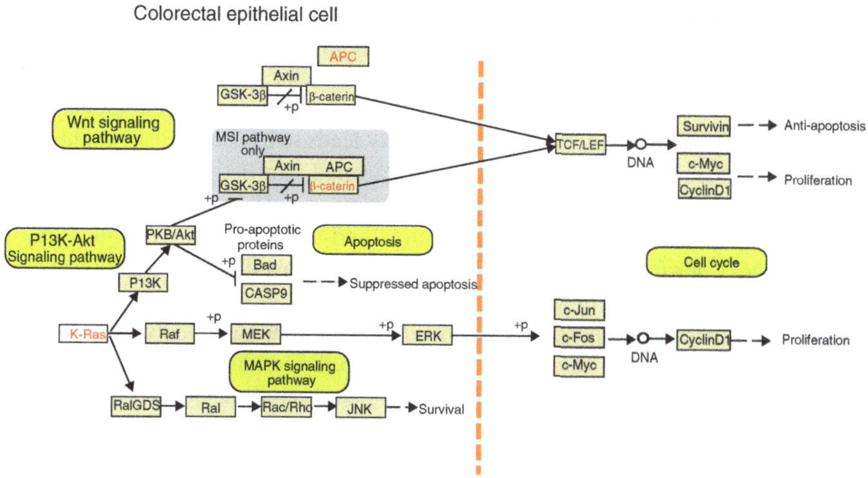

Fig. 12.2 PI3K-Akt signalling and Wnt signalling pathways

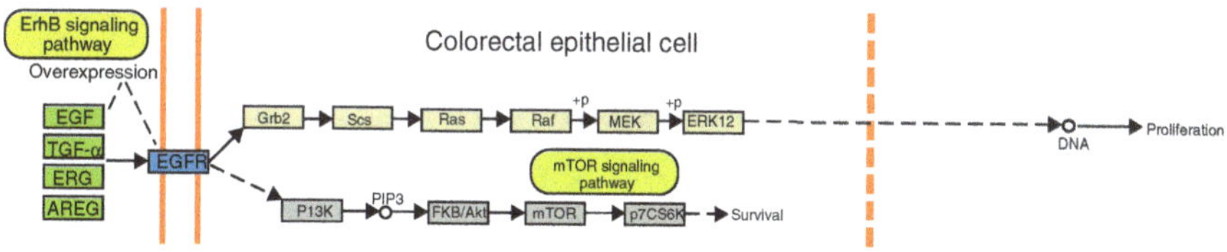

Fig. 12.3 ErhB and mTOR signalling pathway

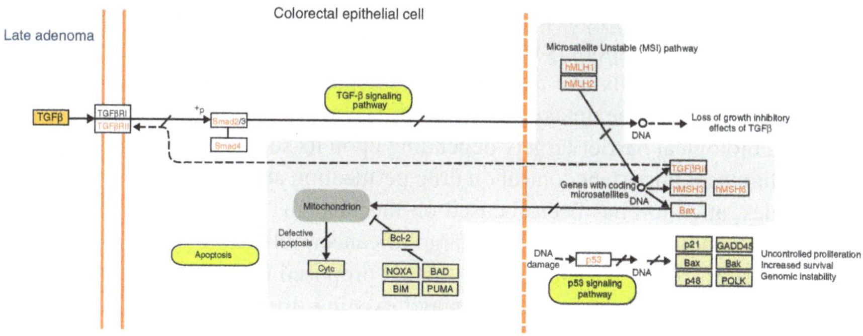

Fig. 12.4 TGF-β signalling pathway

12.3.5 EGFR/MAPK Signalling Pathway

The EGFR signalling pathway is involved in the growth, proliferation, and survival of normal cells. The EGFR is a transmembrane protein which functions as a receptor tyrosine kinase (RTK). A MAPK is a downstream effector of EGFR and acts as an extracellular signal-regulated kinase. The signalling is initiated by the binding of ligands to EGFR receptor which gets dimerized and autophosphorylates selected tyrosine residues on it. It further recruits a growth factor receptor-bound protein 2 (Grb2) and the son of seven-less (SOS) which is an adaptor protein complex [44]. This complex activates Ras-GTP that eventually leads to a cascade of phosphorylation events where RAF, MEK, and ERK are activated. The activated ERK mediates the expression of target genes, namely, *myc*, *cyclins*, *c-FOS*, *c-JUN*, etc., that play a significant role in cell growth, differentiation, and survival. The dysregulation of this pathway leads to enhanced cell proliferation, prolonged survival, angiogenesis, anti-apoptosis, etc. that will lead to malignancy [33].

The mutations in oncogenes and tumor suppressor genes lead to dysregulation in the abovementioned pathways which also overlap in the tumor initiation and progression. There are multiple cross-talks reported between Wnt and Notch signalling which leads to CRC [45]. Notch also stimulates EGFR and PI3/AKT pathway in CRC and suppresses TGF-β pathway [46]. Equally, TGF-β can activate several CRC oncogenic pathways like PI3K/AKT, MAPK/ERK, Wnt, and Notch [47, 48]. The dysregulations in the signalling pathways lead to unchecked cell cycle progression leading to cancer.

12.4 Molecular Transport System

Drugs that are ingested into the living systems are generally transported through the *cellular* membranes' surface. Transporter proteins are present in living systems that are expressed throughout in different vital organs and play an important role as therapeutic molecules. Drugs generally undergo four stages within the living system: absorption, distribution, metabolism, and excretion [49]. Drugs need the carrier proteins called transporters for their transmembrane transport plays an important role in cellular functions like absorption and hepatobiliary and urinary excretion. Drug transporters are the uptake and efflux transporters that are carrying molecules through a biological barrier largely depending upon its solubility [50]. Solubility of drugs exhibits an important control on drug permeation and absorption. In the present decades, attention has been focused on mechanisms and drug transport molecules that promote resistance by discharge of cancer cells from the mechanism of apoptosis. Most of the pharmaceutical sectors proposed that advances in drug discovery from the novel drug candidates and existing drug molecules may provide major solubility problems. Protein-based drug transporters are generally present in most of the tissues including the liver, intestine, kidney, and brain. The gene superfamilies that are involved in the transport of drugs are the solute carrier (SLC) family and the ATP-binding cassette (ABC) family [51]. The overexpression of ATP-binding cassette (ABC) transporters and shirking of apoptosis provide therapeutic strategies for cancer.

Transporter ligand identification studies for the pharmaceutically significant transporters hPepT1, BCRP, P-gp, MRP1, and DAT are a significant step in drug discovery and development. Yttrium 90 (Y90), cetuximab, aflibercept, regorafenib, bevacizumab, capecitabine, oxymetholone, vandetanib, vinorelbine, ledipasvir, erlotinib, axitinib, clofarabine, curcumin, vemurafenib, and abemaciclib are some of the inhibitors of colorectal cancers and act as antitumor agents [52, 53]. The inhibitors of BCL-2/BCL-XL with TORC1/2 inhibitors show a promising targeted therapy strategy in the treatment of colorectal cancers [54].

Methotrexate (MTX) in combination with nonsteroidal anti-inflammatory drugs (NSAIDs) effects on MTX transport in membrane vesicles transported by overexpressing human multidrug resistance protein 2 (MRP 2/ABCC2) and multidrug resistance protein 4 (MRP4/ABCC4) by one-site competition model [55]. Zinc (Zn) homeostasis is regulated by proteins that are belonging to the Solute Carrier Family 30 (ZnT) and Solute Carrier Family 39 (ZIP) in acute and chronic airway inflammation linking to asthma. Alteration in the expression of Zn transporter during acute inflammation increases concentrations of ZIP1 and ZIP14 proteins and decreases concentrations of ZIP4 and ZnT4 proteins [56].

Fatty acid binding proteins (FABPs) like FABP5 and FABP7 which are intracellular transporters for the endocannabinoid anandamide (AEA) that provide beneficial effects on pain, stress, and inflammation are excellent pharmacological targets. Truxillic acids and their derivatives which are active components of a Chinese herbal medicine (*Incarvillea sinensis*) show anti-inflammatory and anti-nociceptive effects in the treatment of rheumatism and pain in humans [57]. Nonsteroidal anti-inflammatory drugs (NSAIDs) like diflunisal, ketoprofen, indomethacin, flurbiprofen, ibuprofen, and naproxen inhibit membrane transport protein and human renal organic anion transporter 1 (hOAT1)-specific transport of adefovir efficiently and provide nephroprotective effects [58]. NSAIDs suppress colorectal tumorigenesis used to treat inflammatory illnesses due to expression of *MRP1* and *MRP3* as encoded membrane transporters [59].

Breast Cancer Resistance Protein (*BCRP/ABCG2*) and Xenobiotic protein transporters, Multidrug Resistance 1 (*MDR1/ABCB1*) may control intestinal absorption of assorted carcinogens, including polycyclic aromatic hydrocarbons (PAH) and heterocyclic amines (HCA). Polymorphisms in these genes due to lifestyle factors, such as meat consumption, smoking, and NSAID use, may be associated with risk of colorectal cancer (CRC). Cyclooxygenase-2 (COX-2) promotes gastrointestinal carcinogenesis, but *BCRP* and *COX-2* polymorphisms were not associated with CRC risk [60].

Butyrate (BT) which is one of the end products produced due to anaerobic bacterial fermentation is a dietary fiber in the human colon. BT which is generally transported by two specific carrier-mediated transport systems, the sodium-coupled monocarboxylate transporter 1 (SMCT1) and the monocarboxylate transporter 1 (MCT1), into colonic epithelial cells provides the ability to prevent/inhibit carcinogenesis [61]. Dietary polyphenols (quercetin, rutin, chrysin, myricetin, epicatechin, epigallocatechin-3-gallate, catechin, xanthohumol, and resveratrol) and foods containing these compounds (vegetables and fruits) interfere with colorectal cancer initiation, promotion, and progression and control CRC [62].

Patients due to a germline mutation in one of the alleles of the tumor suppressor gene known as adenomatous polyposis coli (*APC*) which produces adenomatous

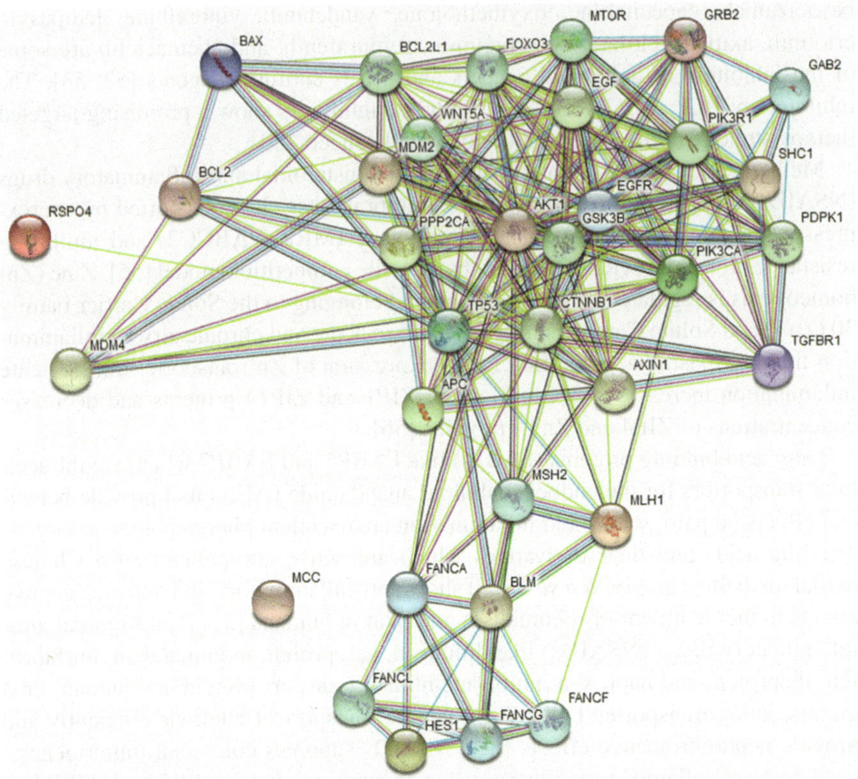

Fig. 12.5 Protein-protein interaction networks

polyposis (FAP) are having 100% risk of developing CRC. Inherited mutations like DNA mismatch repair in genes *MLH1*, *MSH2*, and *MSH6* may develop hereditary nonpolyposis colorectal cancer. Chronic inflammation and aging are also the two major risk factors that are associated with CRC development [7].

Some of the genes like PI3K, AKT, Grb2, EGFR, GSK3, Wnt, TGFBR1, TGFBR1, Bcl-2, Bax, Akt, Hes-1, Dll-4, p53, APC, MCC, and MLH1 that are involved in colorectal cancer are tested for protein-protein interaction. The genes except MCC and RSPO4 have shown multiple interactions (Fig. 12.5).

12.4.1 *Ligand Transporters*

HLA Class I and NKG2D ligands and genes encoding peptide transporters or proteasomal genes provide controlling immune recognition in colorectal cancer cells [63]. The large neutral amino acid transporter 1 (LAT1 or SLC7A5) plays an important role at the blood-brain barrier (BBB) and is believed to be an important drug

Table 12.1 Ligand/inhibitor showing activity of transporter in colorectal cancer

Inhibitor	Cancer	Ligand transporter	Reference
Regorafenib	Metastatic colorectal cancer and gastrointestinal stromal tumors	ABCB1	[64]
Apple polyphenol phloretin (Ph)	Colorectal cancer	GLUT2 and p53	[65]
Cisplatin, carboplatin, and oxaliplatin	Colorectal tumors	OCT1 and 2	[66]
5-fluorouracil (5-FU), leucovorin, and oxaliplatin	Colorectal cancer (CRC)	ABC transporters (BCRP/ABCG2, MRP2/ABCC2, or MRP3/ABCC3)	[67]
Riboflavin	Colorectal cancer	RFVT1, RFVT2, and RFVT3	[68]

target for cancer treatment. Novel chemotypes of ligands of LAT1 supply essential amino acids (e.g., leucine, phenylalanine) to cells. Some of the ligands/inhibitors that express influx or efflux activity of transporters and are used in the treatment of metastatic colorectal cancer are shown in Table 12.1.

12.4.2 Protein Transporters

ABC transporters for the efflux of drugs and drug-like molecules with gene names like MDR1/P-gp, ABCB1, BCRP, ABCG2 (ABCP/MXR/BCRP), BSEP, ABCB1, MRP, and ABCC. SLCs have more diverse functions compared to ABC that mediates cellular influx and efflux of drugs like SLCO, SLC15, SLC22, and SLC47. These proteins protect living cells and tissues and play a crucial role in the intestine, placenta, liver, and blood-brain barrier. The drug transporters are applicable as selectable markers in stem cell-based gene therapy [69].

12.5 Conclusion

Colorectal cancer (CRC) is the most common malignancy and heterogeneous disease that is accumulated with genetic changes with more incidence rates that developed regionally and across countries. The present work showed recent advances in knowledge of the molecular mechanisms of colorectal cancer and drug molecular transporters.

Acknowledgments The authors like to thank administration of Atal Bihari Vajpayee University and IGNTU for providing assistance and support.

References

1. Terzić J, Grivennikov S, Karin E, Karin M. Inflammation and colon cancer. Gastroenterology. 2010;138(6):2101–2114.e5.
2. Long AG, Lundsmith ET, Hamilton KE. Inflammation and colorectal cancer. Curr Colorectal Cancer Rep. 2017;13(4):341–51.
3. Husseini A, Abu-Rmeileh NM, Mikki N, Ramahi TM, Ghosh HA, Barghuthi N, Khalili M, Bjertness E, Holmboe-Ottesen G, Jervell J. Cardiovascular diseases, diabetes mellitus, and cancer in the occupied Palestinian territory. Lancet. 2009;373(9668):1041–9.
4. Fuchs CS, Giovannucci EL, Colditz GA, Hunter DJ, Speizer FE, Willett WC. 1994. A prospective study of family history and the risk of colorectal cancer. N Engl J Med. 1994;331(25):1669–74.
5. Shu S, Cheng JQ. Mechanisms of carcinogenesis in colorectal cancer. In: Mechanisms of oncogenesis, vol. 2010. Dordrecht: Springer; 2010. p. 269–77.
6. Søreide K. Molecular testing for microsatellite instability and DNA mismatch repair defects in hereditary and sporadic colorectal cancers–ready for prime time? Tumor Biol. 2007;28(5):290–300.
7. Wang D, DuBois RN. The role of COX-2 in intestinal inflammation and colorectal cancer. Oncogene. 2010a;29(6):781–8.
8. Al-Sohaily S, Biankin A, Leong R, Kohonen-Corish M, Warusavitarne J. Molecular pathways in colorectal cancer. J Gastroenterol Hepatol. 2012;27(9):1423–31.
9. Nguyen HT, Nguyen HT. The molecular characteristics of colorectal cancer: implications for diagnosis and therapy (review). Oncol Lett. 2018;16:9–18.
10. Colussi D, Brandi G, Bazzoli F, Ricciardiello L. Molecular pathways involved in colorectal cancer: implications for disease behavior and prevention. Int J Mol Sci. 2013;14(8):16365–85.
11. Singh N, Baby D, Rajguru JP, Patil PB, Thakkannavar SS, Pujari VB. Inflammation and cancer. Ann Afr Med. 2019;18(3):121–6.
12. De Waal GM, de Villiers WJS, Forgan T, et al. Colorectal cancer is associated with increased circulating lipopolysaccharide, inflammation and hypercoagulability. Sci Rep. 2020;10:8777.
13. Coussens LM, Werb Z. Inflammation and cancer. Nature. 2002;420(6917):860–7.
14. Medzhitov R. Origin and physiological roles of inflammation. Nature. 2008;454:428–35.
15. Kraus S, Arber N. Inflammation and colorectal cancer. Curr Opin Pharmacol. 2009;9(4):405–10.
16. Feiken E, Rømer J, Eriksen J, Lund LR. Neutrophils express tumor necrosis factor-alpha during mouse skin wound healing. J Invest Dermatol. 1995;105(1):120–3.
17. Hübner G, Brauchle M, Smola H, Madlener M, Fässler R, Werner S. Differential regulation of pro-inflammatory cytokines during wound healing in normal and glucocorticoid-treated mice. Cytokine. 1996;8(7):548–56.
18. DiPietro LA. Wound healing: the role of the macrophage and other immune cells. Shock. 1995;4(4):233–40.
19. Wang X, Lin Y. Tumor necrosis factor and cancer, buddies or foes? Acta Pharmacol Sin. 2008;29(11):1275–88.
20. Woo SR, Corrales L, Gajewski TF. Innate immune recognition of cancer. Annu Rev Immunol. 2015;33:445–74.
21. Hussain SP, Hofseth LJ, Harris CC. Radical causes of cancer. Nat Rev Cancer. 2003;3(4):276–85.
22. Pino MS, Chung DC. The chromosomal instability pathway in colon cancer. Gastroenterology. 2010;138:2059–72.
23. Sheffer M, Bacolod MD, Zuk O, et al. Association of survival and disease progression with chromosomal instability: a genomic exploration of colorectal cancer. Proc Natl Acad Sci U S A. 2009;106:7131–6.
24. Boland CR, Goel A. Microsatellite instability in colorectal cancer. Gastroenterology. 2010;138:2073–87.
25. Wong JJL, Hawkins NJ, Ward RL. Colorectal cancer: a model for epigenetic tumorigenesis. Gut. 2007;56:140–8.

26. Toyota M, Ahuja N, Ohe-Toyota M, Herman JG, Baylin SB, Issa JP. CpG island methylator phenotype in colorectal cancer. Proc Natl Acad Sci U S A. 1999;96:8681–6.
27. Carulli AJ, Keeley TM, Demitrack ES, Chung J, Maillard I, Samuelson LC. Notch receptor regulation of intestinal stem cell homeostasis and crypt regeneration. Dev Biol. 2015;402(1):98–108.
28. Previs RA, Coleman RL, Harris AL, Sood AK. Molecular pathways: translational and therapeutic implications of the Notch signaling pathway in cancer. Clin Cancer Res. 2015;21(5):955–61.
29. Ziouti F, Ebert R, Rummler M, Krug M, Müller-Deubert S, Lüdemann M, Jakob F, Willie BM, Jundt F. NOTCH signaling is activated through mechanical strain in human bone marrow-derived mesenchymal stromal cells. Stem Cells Int. 2019;2019:5150634.
30. Liao W, Li G, You Y, Wan H, Wu Q, Wang C, Lv N. Antitumor activity of Notch-1 inhibition in human colorectal carcinoma cells. Oncol Rep. 2018;39(3):1063–71.
31. Świderska E, Strycharz J, Wróblewski A, Szemraj J, Drzewoski J, Śliwińska A. Role of PI3K/AKT pathway in insulin-mediated glucose uptake. In: Glucose transport. Rijeka: IntechOpen; 2018.
32. Papadatos-Pastos D, Rabbie R, Ross P, Sarker D. The role of the PI3K pathway in colorectal cancer. Crit Rev Oncol Hematol. 2015;94(1):18–30.
33. Koveitypour Z, Panahi F, Vakilian M, et al. Signaling pathways involved in colorectal cancer progression. Cell Biosci. 2019;9:97.
34. Clevers H, Nusse R. Wnt/β-catenin signaling and disease. Cell. 2012;149(6):1192–205.
35. Jeong WJ, Ro EJ, Choi KYNPJ. Interaction between Wnt/β-catenin and RAS-ERK pathways and an anti-cancer strategy via degradations of β-catenin and RAS by targeting the Wnt/β--catenin pathway. Precis Oncol. 2018;2(1):5.
36. Niehrs C. The complex world of WNT receptor signalling. Nat Rev Mol Cell Biol. 2012;13(12):767–79.
37. Polakis P. Wnt signaling in cancer. Cold Spring Harb Perspect Biol. 2012;4(5): a008052.
38. Novellasdemunt L, Antas P, Li VS. Targeting Wnt signaling in colorectal cancer. A review in the theme: cell signaling: proteins, pathways and mechanisms. Am J Physiol Cell Physiol. 2015;309(8):C511–21.
39. Jardé T, Evans RJ, McQuillan KL, Parry L, Feng GJ, Alvares B, Clarke AR, Dale TC. In vivo and in vitro models for the therapeutic targeting of Wnt signaling using a Tet-OΔN89β-catenin system. Oncogene. 2013;32(7):883–93.
40. Alberts B, Johnson A, Lewis J, Raff M, Roberts K, Walter P. Molecular biology of the cell. New York: Garland Science; 2002.
41. Bailey KL, Agarwal E, Chowdhury S, Luo J, Brattain MG, Black JD, Wang J. PLoS One. 2017;12(4):e0176096.
42. Jung B, Staudacher JJ, Beauchamp D. Transforming growth factor β superfamily signaling in development of colorectal cancer. Gastroenterology. 2017;152(1):36–52.
43. Zhao M, Mishra L, Deng CX. The role of TGF-β/SMAD4 signaling in cancer. Int J Biol Sci. 2018;14(2):111.
44. Saletti P, Molinari F, De Dosso S, Frattini M. EGFR signaling in colorectal cancer: a clinical perspective. Gastrointest Cancer. 2015;5:21–38.
45. Bertrand FE, Angus CW, Partis WJ, Sigounas G. Developmental pathways in colon cancer: crosstalk between WNT, BMP, Hedgehog and Notch. Cell Cycle. 2012;11(23):4344–51.
46. Rajendran DT, Subramaniyan B, Ganeshan M. Colorectal cancer in role of transcription factors in gastrointestinal malignancies. In: Role of Notch signaling. Singapore: Springer; 2017. p. 307–14.
47. Roy S, Majumdar APJ. Signaling in colon cancer stem cells. Mol Signal. 2012;7(1):11.
48. Staudacher JJ, Bauer J, Jana A, Tian J, Carroll T, Mancinelli G, Özden Ö, Krett N, Guzman G, Kerr D, Grippo P, Jung B. Activin signaling is an essential component of the TGF-β induced pro-metastatic phenotype in colorectal cancer. Sci Rep. 2017;7(1):5569.

49. Lin J, Sahakian DC, De Morais SM, Xu JJ, Polzer RJ, Winter SM. The role of absorption, distribution, metabolism, excretion and toxicity in drug discovery. Curr Top Med Chem. 2003;3(10):1125–54.
50. Oostendorp RL, Beijnen JH, Schellens JH. The biological and clinical role of drug transporters at the intestinal barrier. Cancer Treat Rev. 2009;35(2):137–47.
51. Matsson P, Bergström CA. Computational modeling to predict the functions and impact of drug transporters. In Silico Pharmacol. 2015;3(1):8.
52. Corcoran RB, Ebi H, Turke AB, Coffee EM, Nishino M, Cogdill AP, Brown RD, Della Pelle P, Dias-Santagata D, Hung KE, Flaherty KT. EGFR-mediated reactivation of MAPK signaling contributes to insensitivity of BRAF-mutant colorectal cancers to RAF inhibition with vemurafenib. Cancer Discov. 2012;2(3):227–35.
53. Temraz S, Mukherji D, Shamseddine A. Dual inhibition of MEK and PI3K pathway in KRAS and BRAF mutated colorectal cancers. Int J Mol Sci. 2015;16(9):22976–88.
54. Faber AC, Coffee EM, Costa C, Dastur A, Ebi H, Hata AN, Yeo AT, Edelman EJ, Song Y, Tam AT, Boisvert JL. mTOR inhibition specifically sensitizes colorectal cancers with KRAS or BRAF mutations to BCL-2/BCL-XL inhibition by suppressing MCL-1. Cancer Discov. 2014;4(1):42–52.
55. El-Sheikh AA, Van Den Heuvel JJ, Koenderink JB, Russel FG. Interaction of nonsteroidal anti-inflammatory drugs with multidrug resistance protein (MRP) 2/ABCC2-and MRP4/ABCC4-mediated methotrexate transport. J Pharmacol Exp Ther. 2007;320(1):229–35.
56. Lang C, Murgia C, Leong M, Tan LW, Perozzi G, Knight D, Ruffin R, Zalewski P. 2007. Anti-inflammatory effects of zinc and alterations in zinc transporter mRNA in mouse models of allergic inflammation. Am J Phys Lung Cell Mol Phys. 2007;292(2):L577–84.
57. Berger WT, Ralph BP, Kaczocha M, Sun J, Balius TE, Rizzo RC, Haj-Dahmane S, Ojima I, Deutsch DG. 2012. Targeting fatty acid binding protein (FABP) anandamide transporters–a novel strategy for development of anti-inflammatory and anti-nociceptive drugs. PLoS One. 2012;7(12):e50968.
58. Mulato AS, Ho ES, Cihlar T. Nonsteroidal anti-inflammatory drugs efficiently reduce the transport and cytotoxicity of adefovir mediated by the human renal organic anion transporter 1. J Pharmacol Exp Ther. 2000;295(1):10–5.
59. Tatebe S, Sinicrope FA, Kuo MT. Induction of multidrug resistance proteins MRP1 and MRP3 and γ-glutamylcysteine synthetase gene expression by nonsteroidal anti-inflammatory drugs in human colon cancer cells. Biochem Biophys Res Commun. 2002;290(5):1427–33.
60. Andersen V, Østergaard M, Christensen J, Overvad K, Tjønneland A, Vogel U. Polymorphisms in the xenobiotic transporter multidrug resistance 1 (MDR1) and interaction with meat intake in relation to risk of colorectal cancer in a Danish prospective case-cohort study. BMC Cancer. 2009;9(1):407.
61. Gonçalves P, Martel F. Butyrate and colorectal cancer: the role of butyrate transport. Curr Drug Metab. 2013;14(9):994–1008.
62. Araújo JR, Gonçalves P, Martel F. Chemopreventive effect of dietary polyphenols in colorectal cancer cell lines. Nutr Res. 2011;31(2):77–87.
63. Sers C, Kuner R, Falk CS, Lund P, Sueltmann H, Braun M, Buness A, Ruschhaupt M, Conrad J, Mang-Fatehi S, Stelniec I. Down-regulation of HLA class I and NKG2D ligands through a concerted action of MAPK and DNA methyltransferases in colorectal cancer cells. Int J Cancer. 2009;125(7):1626–39.
64. Wang YJ, Zhang YK, Zhang GN, Al Rihani SB, Wei MN, Gupta P, Zhang XY, Shukla S, Ambudkar SV, Kaddoumi A, Shi Z. Regorafenib overcomes chemotherapeutic multidrug resistance mediated by ABCB1 transporter in colorectal cancer: in vitro and in vivo study. Cancer Lett. 2017;396:145–54.
65. Lin ST, Tu SH, Yang PS, Hsu SP, Lee WH, Ho CT, Wu CH, Lai YH, Chen MY, Chen LC. Apple polyphenol phloretin inhibits colorectal cancer cell growth via inhibition of the type 2 glucose transporter and activation of p53-mediated signaling. J Agric Food Chem. 2016;64(36):6826–37.

66. Zhang S, Lovejoy KS, Shima JE, Lagpacan LL, Shu Y, Lapuk A, Chen Y, Komori T, Gray JW, Chen X, Lippard SJ. Organic cation transporters are determinants of oxaliplatin cytotoxicity. Cancer Res. 2006;66(17):8847–57.
67. Theile D, Grebhardt S, Haefeli WE, Weiss J. Involvement of drug transporters in the synergistic action of FOLFOX combination chemotherapy. Biochem Pharmacol. 2009;78(11):1366–73.
68. Tutino V, Defrancesco ML, Tolomeo M, De Nunzio V, Lorusso D, Paleni D, Caruso MG, Notarnicola M, Barile M. The expression of riboflavin transporters in human colorectal cancer. Anticancer Res. 2018;38(5):2659–67.
69. Sarkadi B, Özvegy-Laczka C, Német K, Váradi A. ABCG2–a transporter for all seasons. FEBS Lett. 2004;567(1):116–20.

[illegible]

Chapter 13
Emerging Role of Circulating Tumour DNA in Treatment Response Prognosis in Colon Cancer

Eveline M. Anto, Anaga Nair, and Jayamurthy Purushothaman

Abstract Colon cancer is the fourth most commonly diagnosed and second deadliest cancer globally (Bray et al., CA Cancer J Clin. 68:394–424, 2018). Recurrence is found to be the most common reason behind the increasing mortality rate in this disease. Customized treatment is recommended due to heterogeneity of the disease which can be attributed to its pathogenesis involving mutations, epigenetic alterations and DNA methylation. Efficacy of the treatment has to be timely monitored to avoid recurrence, and hence a lot of focus has been put into studies involving liquid biopsies wherein blood collected from the patient contain cell-free nucleic acids which can be residual tumour tissue DNA fragments (ctDNA). ctDNA is exquisitely specific for an individual's tumour at its primary site or even if it has metastasized. Many advantages like non-invasive nature, drawing of samples multiple times and guidance to therapy especially in colon cancer have attracted many clinical studies recently. Based on the evidences, this chapter involves significance of ctDNA in treatment prognosis in colon cancer.

Keywords ctDNA · Prognosis · Personalized therapy · Non-invasive · Liquid biopsy

Abbreviations

CAPP-Seq	CAncer Personalized Profiling by deep Sequencing
CC	Colon cancer
CEA	Carcinoembryonic antigen

Eveline M. Anto and Anaga Nair contributed equally with all other contributors.

E. M. Anto · A. Nair · J. Purushothaman (✉)
Agroprocessing and Technology Division, CSIR-National Institute for Interdisciplinary Science and Technology, Thiruvananthapuram, India
e-mail: pjayamurthy@niist.res.in

G. P. Nagaraju et al. (eds.), *Colon Cancer Diagnosis and Therapy*,
https://doi.org/10.1007/978-3-030-63369-1_13

CRC	Colorectal cancer
ctDNA	Circulating tumour DNA
dPCR	Digital polymerase chain reaction
FAST-SeqS	Fast Aneuploidy Screening Test-Sequencing System
NGS	Next-generation sequencing
PARE	Personalized analysis of rearranged ends
SERS	Surface-enhanced Raman spectroscopy
TAm-Seq	Tagged Amplicon deep Sequencing
WGS	Whole genome sequencing

13.1 Introduction

Colon cancer (CC) or colorectal cancer (CRC) is the fourth most (6.1%) commonly diagnosed and second most (9.2%) deadly cancer globally [1]. The 5-year survival rate is 90% when disease is diagnosed at stage I, 70% for stage II and 14% for advanced stage [2]. The increased fatality can be attributed to the heterogeneity of the disease resulting in poor prognosis, treatment resistance and ultimately recurrence. The pathogenesis of colon cancer involves epigenetic alterations such as hypermethylation of CpG islands and mutations in predominantly APC, KRAS and TP53 genes and less commonly in RAS and RAF genes. The disease progresses mainly through two main pathways, adenoma-carcinoma pathway or chromosome instability pathway which accounts for 70–90% cases and the serrated neoplasia pathway which accounts for 10–20% cases [3]. The conventional treatment strategy for colon cancer comprises surgical resection followed by adjuvant chemotherapy and post-operative monitoring to check the remission of the cancer [2].

As mentioned above, due to the heterogeneous nature of the disease, in order to prevent remission, the post-operative treatment in patients should be personalized by using effective prognostic biomarkers. Radiological imaging, solid or tissue biopsy and carcinoembryonic antigen (CEA) are the clinically used prognostics for disease monitoring in CC, but these approaches have their limitations [4]. The drawback associated with radiological imaging is the hazard posed to patients due to the frequent exposure to radiation, and also the image obtained depicts only a part of the tumour and hence is not representative of the entire tumour burden [5]. Tissue biopsy involves the removal of part of the tumour tissue by a needle. Even though it is a gold standard in oncology, it is not very suitable for post-operative surveillance in patients due to its invasive nature and repeated requirement of adequate tissue sample which may not be available every time. Also, since tissue biopsy examines a particular area, it only gives a static information about the tumour which may lead to misguided treatment strategies. CEA, a high molecular weight glycoprotein detected in serum, is a clinically used liquid biopsy method for detection of disease progression in colon cancer [6]. But it may also be elevated in response to conditions other than cancer such as smoking, inflammatory bowel disease, hepatic diseases and obstructive pulmonary disease which tend to lower its specificity [4]. It is important to know that even during treatment, a tumour is ever-evolving which may lead to resistance to treatment. So there is a need for a biomarker which can detect the mutations in the tumour in a time-effective manner for better treatment response.

Circulating tumour DNA (ctDNA) is an emerging liquid biopsy biomarker for colon cancer. ctDNAs are small DNA fragments released into the bloodstream from apoptotic or necrotic tumour cells [7]. ctDNA contains information about the mutation profile of the tumour including the epigenetic changes. Therefore, measurement of ctDNA provides a comprehensive snapshot of intra-tumour heterogeneity [8].

13.2 Circulating Tumour DNA

Nucleic acids are known to us since long, and this easy application was dawn to Leon et al. in 1977, who discovered the presence of ctDNA in the serum samples of patients diagnosed with different types of cancer [9]. His experiments led to the prediction of probable use of ctDNA as a biomarker and prognosis of treatment efficacy in cancer patients [9]. ctDNA has been considered to be a subset of genomic DNA and especially an individual's tumour DNA profile before and after treatment. Consequently, the quantity of DNA obtained from blood collected from healthy and cancer patients should differ as the latter will have most DNA released due to apoptosis. This has been correctly correlated in several studies, and some suggest this can also be considered as a very early stage diagnostic procedure, complimentary to the usual screening [10].

Colon cancer is a result of mainly genetic alterations; those involved in common disease progression pathways are described in Fig. 13.1. Surgical resection is usually the foremost step of treatment. The relapse can be monitored using blood samples and checked for the said mutations. The two major genomic changes expected are chromosomal instability pathway and microsatellite instability. Another cases being reported are due to changes in the epigenetic level, precisely in the methylation patterns at CpG islands of certain genes, for example, of MLH1. Studies tracing back to almost three decades back have proved the usefulness of ctDNA in recognizing aforementioned genetic alterations [11–13]. Wang et al. (2004) showed a serum sample analysis of levels of mutation in tumour suppressor genes of APC, p53 and K-ras which is a proto-oncogene predicting their applicability as biomarkers in colon cancer [14].

13.3 Methods for Detection of ctDNA

ctDNA levels are usually better detected in plasma than serum as the latter is contaminated by other cells such as the neutrophils [15]. The ctDNA detection involves the detection of mutations. Sanger sequencing is not a reliable technique for detection of mutations in ctDNA due to the infiltration of wild-type DNA from the

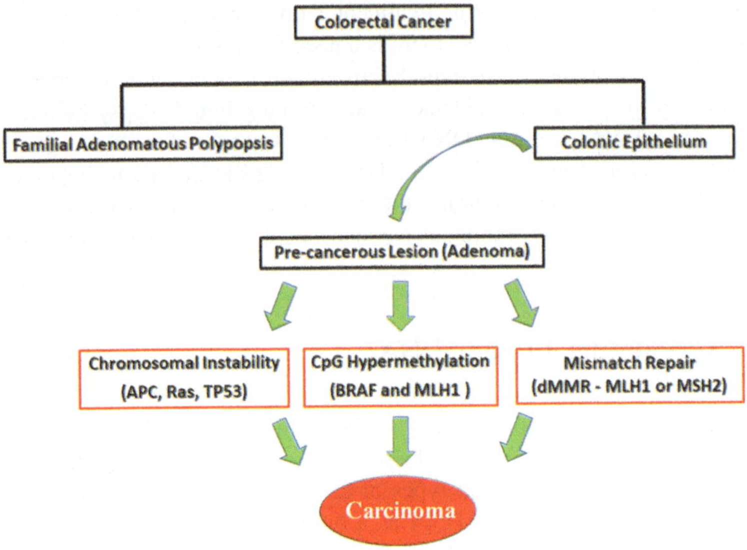

Fig. 13.1 Adenocarcinoma is the most prevalent pathway in case of colon cancer (70–90%). A normal colonic epithelium transforms into pre-cancerous lesion (adenoma) followed by progression to invasive carcinoma due to accumulation of mutation which can be either somatic or germline. Detection of these hallmark genetic mutations often found in colon cancer through ctDNA sample using various techniques based on sensitivity is the aim of the studies

leukocytes which leads to high background [16]. Detection of ctDNA requires techniques with high sensitivity and specificity; few such techniques are mentioned below.

13.3.1 Digital PCR

Digital PCR (dPCR) involves the simultaneous detection of multiple mutations from a single sample [17]. The term digital PCR came into use due to the ability of this technique to detect rare mutants containing the single nucleotide polymorphisms which are otherwise undetectable by the qPCR because of the predominance of wild-type sequences [18]. In this method, DNA sample is partitioned into different compartments; standard PCR reaction is run in each compartment separately followed by detection of amplified targets by fluorescence and quantification by Poisson statistics [19]. There are several dPCR subtypes based on the partitioning method.

13.3.1.1 Droplet Digital PCR

In this method, the DNA sample is partitioned into approximately 20,000 droplets made of water in oil emulsion [20]. Each droplet acts as a micro-reactor where PCR reaction takes place. It has advantage over other dPCR techniques due to its smaller sample requirement which also reduces the cost [21]. Taly et al. used droplet digital PCR technique to detect seven mutations in KRAS oncogene from plasma samples of patients with metastatic colon cancer, thereby confirming its clinical utility [17].

13.3.1.2 BEAMing

BEAMing (beads, emulsion, amplification and magnetic) is a highly sensitive (0.02%) dPCR technique developed by Bert Vogelstein and team. In this method, primer-bound magnetic beads and template DNA are distributed into microemulsions; following amplification by PCR reaction, the magnetic beads containing thousands of copies are released. The variant DNA are then stained with fluorescent probes followed by quantification using flow cytometry [22]. The only drawback is the relatively high cost and complex mechanism which limits its clinical utility.

13.3.2 Amplification Refractory Mutation System PCR

Amplification refractory mutation system PCR (ARMS PCR) or allele-specific PCR is a method for detection of known single nucleotide polymorphism (SNP) or point mutations by using sequence-specific PCR primers which specifically amplify DNA segments containing the target allele [23]. This technique was pioneered by Newton et al. (1989) [24]. In this technique, two sets of specific primers are designed for both normal and mutant alleles with a mismatch at the 3′ end of one of the primers. The mismatch increases the specificity of this technique by altering the annealing temperature and thereby degree of amplification. An internal PCR control is also included in ARMS PCR which acts as a quality control mechanism [25]. Splindler et al. (2014) have reportedly applied this method for the detection of KRAS and BRAF mutations in plasma ctDNA of patients with metastatic colorectal cancer [26]. An upgraded version of ARMS PCR is tetra-primer ARMS PCR (T-ARMS PCR) which is a combination of tetra-primer PCR and ARMS PCR [27]. T-ARMS PCR involves introducing additional mismatches at position-2 from 3′ end of inner primers which improves allele specificity [28]. T-ARMS PCR, although a gold standard for SNP genotyping, is limited by its complex and lengthy optimization step [29].

13.3.3 Mass Spectrometry-Based PCR

The mass spectrometry-based PCR method is known for its enhanced multiplexing ability which enables the detection of several ctDNA mutations from a single sample. The two mass spectrometry-based PCR methods developed are surface-enhanced Raman spectroscopy (*SERS*) and *UltraSEEK* [30].

In PCR/SERS technology, nanotags such as gold nanoparticles coated with Raman reporters and DNA probes on the surface are utilized [31]. SERS has better sensitivity (3 orders of magnitude) than fluorescence-based methods for detection of labeled oligonucleotides [32]. SERS provides a fingerprint spectrum with sharp peaks which enhances its multiplexing ability and allows the detection of multiple analytes from a mixture [33]. PCR-based SERS approach was used for the detection of three prominent mutations of melanoma (BRAF V600E, c-Kit L57P and NRAS Q61K) with a sensitivity of 0.1% (10 mutations from 10,000 wild-type alleles) [31].

UltraSEEK is a high-throughput, ultrasensitive method for the detection of the minor variants by enriching these variants by extension reactions following PCR using biotin labeled terminating nucleotide [31]. The extended products are then captured, washed and eluted followed by identification using matrix-assisted laser desorption/ionization time-of-flight mass spectrometry [34]. The advantage of UltraSEEK includes higher multiplexing ability, lesser time and smaller sample size (9 pg/μl to 4.2 ng/μl) [30].

13.3.4 Next-Generation Sequencing (NGS)-Based Methods

NGS employs parallel sequencing for identifying DNA sequences. NGS-based methods have gained prominence for ctDNA detection due to their high throughput and ability to detect both known and unknown mutations. NGS follows two approaches, targeted approach for known mutations and untargeted approach for unknown mutation. Targeted approach includes several subtypes such as CAncer Personalized Profiling by deep Sequencing (CAPP-Seq), Tagged Amplicon deep Sequencing (TAm-Seq), Safe-Sequencing System (Safe-SeqS) and Ion Torrent. Untargeted approach includes whole genome sequencing (WGS), whole exome sequencing (WES), personalized analysis of rearranged ends (PARE), digital karyotyping and Fast Aneuploidy Screening Test-Sequencing System (FAST-SeqS) [35]. Features and sensitivity of these techniques are briefly given in Table 13.1.

Jia et al. recently reported the detection of mutations in plasma ctDNA of metastatic colorectal cancer patients through NGS method (accuracy of 95.7%) [36]. Even though NGS has contributed immensely to the development of personalized treatment for cancer patients, it still has certain limitations such as high cost and requirement of proper infrastructure facility which has impeded its use in clinical settings. Also NGS generates extensive data, most of which is not required by the doctors who find it difficult to interpret.

Table 13.1 Targeted approach next-generation sequencing has various techniques which uses different parameters to obtain increased sensitivity

Technique	Unique feature	Sensitivity	Mutant allele frequency
TAm-Seq	Specially designed primers are used	~97%	~2%
eTAm-Seq	Single nucleotide variants	~98%	~1–2%
Safe-SeqS	Unique identifiers to each template	~100%	~0.25%
CAPP-Seq	Constructs library of recurrently mutated genomic regions from the population	~	~0.02%
Ion Torrent	Very less DNA input is required (1 ng)	Lesser sensitivity as compared to digital PCR	

13.3.5 Methylation Detection

ctDNA methylation profiling is an efficient tool for monitoring the prognosis in cancer. Methyl group is usually added to the CpG dinucleotide region in the DNA [37]. These epigenetic changes in the ctDNA have been very useful in the early diagnosis of colon cancer [38]. Three strategies are being used for methylation detection, namely, restriction enzyme (RE) digestion, affinity-based analysis and bisulphite modification [39]. RE method involves enzymes which digest only the unmethylated DNA [40]. Restriction landmark genomic scanning (RLGS) is one of the widely used RE methods which is useful in identifying regions of hypomethylation, tumour suppressor genes, hypermethylation and quantification of hypermethylation [41]. Affinity-based methylation analysis involves immunoprecipitation of methylated DNA fragments with anti-5-methylcytosine monoclonal antibodies following DNA denaturation [42]. The collected DNA is then analysed using microarray technologies to chalk out the methylation profile [43]. The bisulphite modification method is based on the conversion of unmethylated cytosines to uracil on DNA by sodium bisulphite (methylated cytosine remains unaffected) [44]. DeVos et al. (2009) developed an assay consisting of bisulphite-converted DNA for the measurement of hypermethylated SEPT9 DNA, a biomarker for colon cancer [45]. Detection of methylated SEPT9 is the first US FDA-approved blood-based screening test for colorectal cancer [35]. Other methylated genes in CC include VIM, ITGA4, OSM4, GATAF4 and NDRG4 [46]. The methods for ctDNA detection have seen a rapid progress in the past years. The translation of most of the techniques to the clinical setup requires further evaluation and standardization.

ctDNA isolated from plasma can be employed for detection of different stages of cancer depending mainly on the assay sensitivity. For example, next-generation sequencing techniques are resorted during the pre-neoplastic or non-metastatic stages, whereas standard NGS and dPCR are used to detect metastasis as they show approximately 100% sensitivity [47].

13.4 Release of ctDNA

DNA is often released into the bloodstream from the cells that have undergone either apoptosis or necrosis as part of various physiological processes. So there can be plenty of reasons why circulating DNA be misinterpreted as tumour DNA. Hence, to rule out the confusion existing amongst cell-free DNA and ctDNA genetic mutations and similar damages that are associated with that specific cancer has to be properly categorized. However, many challenges need to be addressed while monitoring liquid biopsy samples like mutation rate, fraction of ctDNA in the plasma sample, technique to be used, etc. [48]. Longitudinal studies are ongoing to bring ctDNA into clinical practice, but the outcome will be worth the effort due to the non-invasive nature [49]. Some studies suggest classification of plasma DNA according to their sizes as an easier method of screening [50]. Biologists working in various types of cancer enter into a debate on how exactly does ctDNA get released into the bloodstream. Another important question to be addressed is the presence of ctDNA in other physiological samples like urine and cerebrospinal fluid that may seemingly help more to find ways by which DNA is released into each of these. Lymphocytes can be one major source of ctDNA in serum samples, while very less of it will be in plasma samples. Plasma will contain DNA released from cells that have undergone either apoptosis or necrosis, and this can be understood based on the size of the DNA [51]. Radiation therapy is known to induce necrosis, and ctDNA analysis post-therapy will aid in analysing its efficacy.

Presence of ctDNA in urine samples is suggested to happen during the renal filtration system [52]. Some studies have shown positive correlation in the presence of mutated KRAS in urine samples of colon cancer-affected persons with respect to the progress of the treatment. This indicates possible use of urine samples for analysis purposes. Similarly, cerebrospinal fluid is another candidate for analysis which circulates in the central nervous system and is separated from the blood by the blood-brain barrier. As a result, it is more relevant for analysing solid tumours pertaining to the brain and other parts of the central nervous system. Nevertheless, these could be checked for analysis of extent of metastasis if any in case of advanced case of colon cancer [53].

13.5 Role of ctDNA as a Prognostic Biomarker in Colon Cancer

As stated earlier, treatment strategy for colon cancer involves surgical resection of the tumour and adjuvant chemotherapy (to eliminate tumour cells which may have remained) followed by steady patient monitoring to check for chemoresistance and response to therapy. Role of ctDNA as a potential prognostic biomarker has been evaluated by many researchers mainly because of its non-invasive nature and also its ability to detect the dynamic changes in the tumour which are of benefit in early clinical decision-making and improving the overall survival. Identifying the stage of the tumour is of importance in meeting out the necessary treatment. In their study, Wang et al. screened the serum ctDNA levels for APC, k-RAS and p53 mutations in 104 CRC patients at the time of the surgical resection [14]. They discovered a stage-dependent increase in the mutational changes (at least one marker) in the serum ctDNA samples, 0% in Dukes'A, 22.4% in Dukes'B, 48.7% in Dukes'C and 66.7% in Dukes'D stages. In another study by Yang et al. (2018), 47 early and late stage CRC patients were screened for 50 known oncogenes by targeted sequencing [54]. A correlation was observed between ctDNA concentration and stage of cancer (0.77 ng/μl for stage I and 1.52 ng/μl for stage IV). The ctDNA concentration was also found to increase with increased tumour size. They also compared the mutation detection rate of ctDNA with other known biomarkers (CEA, AFP, CA19-9, CA125, CA72-4); ctDNA was found to have a higher detection ability than the others. It is to be noted that detection of ctDNA at the early stages is limited by low abundance of tumour DNA in the bloodstream, around 1 to 10 ng/ml [55], and other confounding phenomenon such as clonal expansion of non-tumourous tissues [56]. Therefore, for detecting early stage cancer, technologies with high sensitivity should be employed. An account of such PCR-based, NGS-based methods has already been discussed in this chapter. Most of these techniques have only been demonstrated in the labs; bringing these technologies into the routine clinical diagnosis is a task (owing to the cost, infrastructure, etc.) which needs to be accomplished.

Another challenge associated with colon cancer treatment is the minimum residual disease (MRD) which occurs due to the incomplete tumour resection. Undetected MRD may lead to relapse or recurrence [8]. Post-operative ctDNA levels in colon cancer patients correspond to relapse [56]. Post-operative ctDNA measurement by both the methylation and somatic mutations contributes to selection of adjuvant therapy and identification of patients most prone to relapse [4]. Thamet et al. (2014) monitored the serum ctDNA from 150 CRC patients who underwent surgical resection [57]. Methylation of TAC1 (after 6-month follow-up) and Sept9 (after 1-year follow-up) in ctDNA corresponded to increased recurrence [58]. Reinhert et al. (2019) quantified ctDNA from pre-operative and post-operative stages of 122 CRC patients (stages I to III) [59]. 88.5% (108/122) patients had detectable pre-operative ctDNA. Post-resection, 89.4% (84 out of 94) patients were ctDNA negative, while 10.6% (10 out of 94) were ctDNA positive. ctDNA-positive group had a higher chance of relapse (70%) compared to the ctDNA-negative group (11.9%). Ng et al. (2017) designed a patient-specific ctDNA detection assay to monitor the disease progression after resection in CRC patients [60]. Recurrence was seen only in patients with post-operative plasma ctDNA. Thus, ctDNA plays an important role in the early detection of metastasis. From the above studies, it can be inferred that lower ctDNA levels post-resection correspond to better survival. On the basis of the ctDNA level, patients can be divided into high risk and low risk. These patients can then be provided with personalized treatment, thereby protecting low-risk patients from the potential hazards of overtreatment [61].

ctDNA can also be used to monitor response to treatment much earlier than imaging approaches [62]. In colon cancer, the mutational status of the tumour keeps on changing during the course of treatment through clonal evolution which may lead to a treatment resistance [63]. Inhibiting epidermal growth factor using monoclonal antibodies (cetuximab, bevacizumab, panitumumab) is a prominent treatment strategy in metastatic colorectal cancer [64]. Mutations in RAS pathway genes (KRAS and NRAS) and also BRAF are responsible for anti-EGFR resistance [65, 66]. ctDNA is most suited to check acquired resistance as it can monitor the tumour heterogeneity and tumour dynamics due to its non-invasive nature which enables drawing of multiple samples, thereby helping the oncologists in selecting the most ideal treatment strategy [63]. Thus, it can be concluded that ctDNA is indeed a promising prognostic tool in colon cancer.

13.6 Advantages and Disadvantages

Non-invasive nature is the prime advantage of ctDNA analysis. If this can be used as a diagnostic tool for predictive and tailored treatment strategy, the pain and suffering associated with obtaining the tissue biopsy will be greatly reduced. Several numbers of assessments, specificity, status of tumour metastasis and disease progression can be computed with ease in a short period of time. As described in the test, many high-throughput techniques can be used assuring precision and also amplification of specific tumour gene even if is obtained in small quantity which makes it more reliable. Also these modern molecular biology techniques employ use of very little amount of reagents which allows multiple tests to be carried out, thus making it a cost-effective venture. Such a screening method can be brought to practice to detect colon cancer (or any other type of cancer whose genetic biomarker profile is known) in a population, prediction of occurrence of the same and early diagnosis.

Many studies have tried to prove the potentiality of ctDNA as biomarker, but literature survey shows a lack in standard operating protocol. Another main drawback is associated with the mechanism of release of DNA from the cells; as a result, there are often chances of false-positive results to be obtained. A specific approved valid method has to be followed for a given type of cancer so as to obtain same set of results and avoid discrepancies.

13.7 Conclusion

To conclude, this chapter throws light into the significance of the use of ctDNA in the prediction and prognosis of colon cancer by highlighting the various high-throughput and cost-effective mechanisms. We have tried to analyse various reports based on use of ctDNA in colon cancer. However, most of it is limited by small number of subjects and longitudinal studies are required. What hinders the path of use of ctDNA into clinical setup is the inability to understand the mechanism of

DNA release that will generate unreliable results. But taken together ctDNA-based approach has more pros than cons, and more research in this area will definitely help in translating its purpose into a clinically relevant one. Moreover, use of ctDNA to monitor treatment efficacy and relapses is better suited as of now, and tailored treatment strategy can also be an added relief for cancer patients and possibly may aid in increasing survival rates.

References

1. Bray F, Ferlay J, Soerjomataram I, Siegel RL, Torre LA, Jemal A. Global cancer statistics 2018: GLOBOCAN estimates of incidence and mortality worldwide for 36 cancers in 185 countries. CA Cancer J Clin. 2018;68(6):394–424.
2. Vymetalkova V, Cervena K, Bartu L, Vodicka P. Circulating cell-free DNA and colorectal cancer: a systematic review. Int J Mol Sci. 2018;19(11):3356.
3. Dekker E, Tanis PJ, Vleugels JLA, Kasi PM, Wallace MB. Colorectal cancer. Lancet. 2019;394(10207):1467–80.
4. Reece M, Saluja H, Hollington P, Karapetis CS, Vatandoust S, Young GP, Symonds EL. The use of circulating tumour DNA to monitor and predict response to treatment in colorectal cancer. Front Genet. 2019;10:1118.
5. Berger AW, Schwerdel D, Welz H, Marienfeld R, Schmidt SA, Kleger A, Ettrich TJ, Seufferlein T. Treatment monitoring in metastatic colorectal cancer patients by quantification and KRAS genotyping of circulating cell-free DNA. PLoS One. 2017;12(3):e0174308.
6. Tanaka T, Tanaka M, Tanaka T, Ishigamori R. Biomarkers for colorectal cancer. Int J Mol Sci. 2010;11(9):3209–25.
7. Kim YW, Kim YH, Song Y, Kim HS, Sim HW, Poojan S, Eom BW, Kook MC, Joo J, Hong KM. Monitoring circulating tumour DNA by analyzing personalized cancer-specific rearrangements to detect recurrence in gastric cancer. Exp Mol Med. 2019;51(8):1–0.
8. Gorgannezhad L, Umer M, Islam MN, Nguyen NT, Shiddiky MJ. Circulating tumour DNA and liquid biopsy: opportunities, challenges, and recent advances in detection technologies. Lab Chip. 2018;18(8):1174–96.
9. Leon SA, Shapiro B, Sklaroff DM, Yaros MJ. Free DNA in the serum of cancer patients and the effect of therapy. Cancer Res. 1977;37(3):646–50.
10. Huang ZH, Li LH, Hua D. Quantitative analysis of plasma circulating DNA at diagnosis and during follow-up of breast cancer patients. Cancer Lett. 2006;243(1):64–70.
11. Fujiwara K, Fujimoto N, Tabata M, Nishii K, Matsuo K, Hotta K, Kozuki T, Aoe M, Kiura K, Ueoka H, Tanimoto M. Identification of epigenetic aberrant promoter methylation in serum DNA is useful for early detection of lung cancer. Clin Cancer Res. 2005;11(3):1219–25.
12. Shaw JA, Smith BM, Walsh T, Johnson S, Primrose L, Slade MJ, Walker RA, Coombes RC. Microsatellite alterations in plasma DNA of primary breast cancer patients. Clin Cancer Res. 2000;6(3):1119–24.
13. Brychta N, Krahn T, von Ahsen O. Detection of KRAS mutations in circulating tumour DNA by digital PCR in early stages of pancreatic cancer. Clin Chem. 2016;62(11):1482–91.
14. Wang JY, Hsieh JS, Chang MY, Huang TJ, Chen FM, Cheng TL, Alexandersen K, Huang YS, Tzou WS, Lin SR. Molecular detection of APC, K-ras, and p53 mutations in the serum of colorectal cancer patients as circulating biomarkers. World J Surg. 2004;28(7):721–6.
15. Lee JS, Kim M, Seong MW, Kim HS, Lee YK, Kang HJ. Plasma vs. serum in circulating tumour DNA measurement: characterization by DNA fragment sizing and digital droplet polymerase chain reaction. Clin Chem Lab Med (CCLM). 2020;58(4):527–32.

16. Busser B, Lupo J, Sancey L, Mouret S, Faure P, Plumas J, Chaperot L, Leccia MT, Coll JL, Hurbin A, Hainaut P. Plasma circulating tumour DNA levels for the monitoring of melanoma patients: landscape of available technologies and clinical applications. Biomed Res Int. 2017;2017:Article ID 5986129.
17. Taly V, Pekin D, Benhaim L, Kotsopoulos SK, Le Corre D, Li X, Atochin I, Link DR, Griffiths AD, Pallier K, Blons H. Multiplex picodroplet digital PCR to detect KRAS mutations in circulating DNA from the plasma of colorectal cancer patients. Clin Chem. 2013;59(12):1722–31.
18. Huggett JF, Whale A. Digital PCR as a novel technology and its potential implications for molecular diagnostics. Clin Chem. 2013;59:1691.
19. Quan PL, Sauzade M, Brouzes E. dPCR: a technology review. Sensors. 2018;18(4):1271.
20. Nakano M, Komatsu J, Matsuura SI, Takashima K, Katsura S, Mizuno A. Single-molecule PCR using water-in-oil emulsion. J Biotechnol. 2003;102(2):117–24.
21. Milbury CA, Zhong Q, Lin J, Williams M, Olson J, Link DR, Hutchison B. Determining lower limits of detection of digital PCR assays for cancer-related gene mutations. Biomol Detect Quantif. 2014;1(1):8–22.
22. Dressman D, Yan H, Traverso G, Kinzler KW, Vogelstein B. Transforming single DNA molecules into fluorescent magnetic particles for detection and enumeration of genetic variations. Proc Natl Acad Sci. 2003;100(15):8817–22.
23. Little S. Amplification-refractory mutation system (ARMS) analysis of point mutations. Curr Protoc Hum Genet. 1995;7(1):9–8.
24. Newton CR, Graham A, Heptinstall LE, Powell SJ, Summers C, Kalsheker N, Smith JC, Markham AF. Analysis of any point mutation in DNA. The amplification refractory mutation system (ARMS). Nucleic Acids Res. 1989;17(7):2503–16.
25. Chen Q, Lu P, Jones AV, Cross NC, Silver RT, Wang YL. Amplification refractory mutation system, a highly sensitive and simple polymerase chain reaction assay, for the detection of JAK2 V617F mutation in chronic myeloproliferative disorders. J Mol Diagn. 2007;9(2):272–6.
26. Spindler KL, Pallisgaard N, Andersen RF, Jakobsen A. Changes in mutational status during third-line treatment for metastatic colorectal cancer—results of consecutive measurement of cell free DNA, KRAS and BRAF in the plasma. Int J Cancer. 2014;135(9):2215–22.
27. Shu Y, Dhillon S, Ke X, Collins AR, Day NM. An efficient procedure for genotyping single nucleotide polymorphism. Nucleic Acids Res. 2001;29(17):e88.
28. Ahlawat S, Sharma R, Maitra A, Roy M, Tantia MS. Designing, optimization and validation of tetra-primer ARMS PCR protocol for genotyping mutations in caprine Fec genes. Meta Gene. 2014;2:439–49.
29. Mesrian Tanha H, Mojtabavi Naeini M, Rahgozar S, Rasa SM, Vallian S. Modified tetra-primer ARMS PCR as a single-nucleotide polymorphism genotyping tool. Genet Test Mol Biomarkers. 2015;19(3):156–61.
30. Elazezy M, Joosse SA. Techniques of using circulating tumour DNA as a liquid biopsy component in cancer management. Comput Struct Biotechnol J. 2018;16:370–8.
31. Wee EJ, Wang Y, Tsao SC, Trau M. Simple, sensitive and accurate multiplex detection of clinically important melanoma DNA mutations in circulating tumour DNA with SERS nanotags. Theranostics. 2016;6(10):1506.
32. Faulds K, Barbagallo RP, Keer JT, Smith WE, Graham D. SERRS as a more sensitive technique for the detection of labelled oligonucleotides compared to fluorescence. Analyst. 2004;129(7):567–8.
33. Dougan JA, Faulds K. Surface enhanced Raman scattering for multiplexed detection. Analyst. 2012;137(3):545–54.
34. Mosko MJ, Nakorchevsky AA, Flores E, Metzler H, Ehrich M, van den Boom DJ, Sherwood JL, Nygren AO. Ultrasensitive detection of multiplexed somatic mutations using MALDI-TOF mass spectrometry. J Mol Diagn. 2016;18(1):23–31.
35. Chen M, Zhao H. Next-generation sequencing in liquid biopsy: cancer screening and early detection. Hum Genomics. 2019;13(1):34.

36. Jia N, Sun Z, Gao X, Cheng Y, Zhou Y, Shen C, Chen W, Wang X, RONG S, Li N, Zhou J. Serial monitoring of circulating tumour DNA in patients with metastatic colorectal cancer to predict the therapeutic response. Front Genet. 2019;10:470.
37. Jeziorska DM, Murray RJ, De Gobbi M, Gaentzsch R, Garrick D, Ayyub H, Chen T, Li E, Telenius J, Lynch M, Graham B. DNA methylation of intragenic CpG islands depends on their transcriptional activity during differentiation and disease. Proc Natl Acad Sci. 2017;114(36):E7526–35.
38. Ma M, Zhu H, Zhang C, Sun X, Gao X, Chen G. "Liquid biopsy"—ctDNA detection with great potential and challenges. Ann Transl Med. 2015;3(16):235.
39. Olkhov-Mitsel E, Bapat B. Strategies for discovery and validation of methylated and hydroxymethylated DNA biomarkers. Cancer Med. 2012;1(2):237–60.
40. Singer J, Roberts-Ems J, Riggs AD. Methylation of mouse liver DNA studied by means of the restriction enzymes msp I and hpa II. Science. 1979;203(4384):1019–21.
41. Smiraglia DJ, Plass C. The study of aberrant methylation in cancer via restriction landmark genomic scanning. Oncogene. 2002;21(35):5414–26.
42. Weber M, Davies JJ, Wittig D, Oakeley EJ, Haase M, Lam WL, Schuebeler D. Chromosome-wide and promoter-specific analyses identify sites of differential DNA methylation in normal and transformed human cells. Nat Genet. 2005;37(8):853–62.
43. Down TA, Rakyan VK, Turner DJ, Flicek P, Li H, Kulesha E, Graef S, Johnson N, Herrero J, Tomazou EM, Thorne NP. A Bayesian deconvolution strategy for immunoprecipitation-based DNA methylome analysis. Nat Biotechnol. 2008;26(7):779–85.
44. Frommer M, McDonald LE, Millar DS, Collis CM, Watt F, Grigg GW, Molloy PL, Paul CL. A genomic sequencing protocol that yields a positive display of 5-methylcytosine residues in individual DNA strands. Proc Natl Acad Sci. 1992;89(5):1827–31.
45. Devos T, Tetzner R, Model F, Weiss G, Schuster M, Distler J, Steiger KV, Grützmann R, Pilarsky C, Habermann JK, Fleshner PR. Circulating methylated SEPT9 DNA in plasma is a biomarker for colorectal cancer. Clin Chem. 2009;55(7):1337–46.
46. Lam K, Pan K, Linnekamp JF, Medema JP, Kandimalla R. DNA methylation based biomarkers in colorectal cancer: a systematic review. Biochim Biophys Acta Rev Cancer. 2016;1866(1):106–20.
47. Pantel K, Alix-panabières C. Liquid biopsy and minimal residual disease — latest advances and implications for cure. Nat Rev Clin Oncol. 2019;16(July):409–24.
48. Ulz P, Heitzer E, Geigl JB, Speicher MR. Patient monitoring through liquid biopsies using circulating tumour DNA. Int J Cancer. 2017;141(5):887–96.
49. Bettegowda C, Sausen M, Leary RJ, Kinde I, Wang Y, Agrawal N, Bartlett BR, Wang H, Luber B, Alani RM, Antonarakis ES. Detection of circulating tumour DNA in early-and late-stage human malignancies. Sci Transl Med. 2014;6(224):224ra24.
50. Heitzer E, Auer M, Hoffmann EM, Pichler M, Gasch C, Ulz P, Lax S, Waldispuehl-Geigl J, Mauermann O, Mohan S, Pristauz G. Establishment of tumour-specific copy number alterations from plasma DNA of patients with cancer. Int J Cancer. 2013;133(2):346–56.
51. Haber DA, Velculescu VE. Blood-based analyses of cancer: circulating tumour cells and circulating tumour DNA. Cancer Discov. 2014;4:650–61.
52. Stewart CM, Kothari PD, Mouliere F, Mair R, Somnay S, Benayed R, Zehir A, Weigelt B, Dawson SJ, Arcila ME, Berger MF. The value of cell-free DNA for molecular pathology. J Pathol. 2018;244(5):616–27.
53. De Mattos-Arruda L, Mayor R, Ng CK, Weigelt B, Martínez-Ricarte F, Torrejon D, Oliveira M, Arias A, Raventos C, Tang J, Guerini-Rocco E. Cerebrospinal fluid-derived circulating tumour DNA better represents the genomic alterations of brain tumours than plasma. Nat Commun. 2015;6:8839.
54. Yang, Ying-Chi, et al. Circulating tumour DNA detectable in early-and late-stage colorectal cancer patients. Biosci Rep. 2018;38:4.

55. Wan JC, Massie C, Garcia-Corbacho J, Mouliere F, Brenton JD, Caldas C, Pacey S, Baird R, Rosenfeld N. Liquid biopsies come of age: towards implementation of circulating tumour DNA. Nat Rev Cancer. 2017;17(4):223.
56. Marcuello M, Vymetalkova V, Neves RP, Duran-Sanchon S, Vedeld HM, Tham E, van Dalum G, Flügen G, Garcia-Barberan V, Fijneman RJ, Castells A. Circulating biomarkers for early detection and clinical management of colorectal cancer. Mol Asp Med. 2019;69:107.
57. Ryan BM, Lefort F, McManus R, Daly J, Keeling PW, Weir DG, Kelleher D. A prospective study of circulating mutant KRAS2 in the serum of patients with colorectal neoplasia: strong prognostic indicator in postoperative follow up. Gut. 2003;52(1):101–8.
58. Tham C, Chew M, Soong R, Lim J, Ang M, Tang C, Zhao Y, Ong SY, Liu Y. Postoperative serum methylation levels of TAC1 and SEPT9 are independent predictors of recurrence and survival of patients with colorectal cancer. Cancer. 2014;120(20):3131–41.
59. Reinert T, Henriksen TV, Christensen E, Sharma S, Salari R, Sethi H, Knudsen M, Nordentoft I, Wu HT, Tin AS, Rasmussen MH. Analysis of plasma cell-free DNA by ultradeep sequencing in patients with stages I to III colorectal cancer. JAMA Oncol. 2019;5(8):1124–31.
60. Ng SB, Chua C, Ng M, Gan A, Poon PS, Teo M, Fu C, Leow WQ, Lim KH, Chung A, Koo SL. Individualised multiplexed circulating tumour DNA assays for monitoring of tumour presence in patients after colorectal cancer surgery. Sci Rep. 2017;7(1):1–1.
61. Marshall JL. Risk assessment in stage II colorectal cancer. Oncology. 2010;24(1_Suppl_1):9.
62. Bi F, Wang Q, Dong Q, Wang Y, Zhang L, Zhang J. Circulating tumour DNA in colorectal cancer: opportunities and challenges. Am J Transl Res. 2020;12(3):1044.
63. Siravegna G, Lazzari L, Crisafulli G, Sartore-Bianchi A, Mussolin B, Cassingena A, Martino C, Lanman RB, Nagy RJ, Fairclough S, Rospo G. Radiologic and genomic evolution of individual metastases during HER2 blockade in colorectal cancer. Cancer Cell. 2018;34(1):148–62.
64. Tsang AHF, Cheng KH, Wong ASP, Ng SSM, Ma BBY, Chan CML, et al. Current and future molecular diagnostics in colorectal cancer and colorectal adenoma. World J Gastroenterol. 2014;20(14):3847–57.
65. Di Nicolantonio F, Martini M, Molinari F, Sartore-Bianchi A, Arena S, Saletti P, et al. Wild-type BRAF is required for response to panitumumab or cetuximab in metastatic colorectal cancer. J Clin Oncol. 2008;26(35):5705–12.
66. Douillard JY, Oliner KS, Siena S, Tabernero J, Burkes R, Barugel M, Humblet Y, Bodoky G, Cunningham D, Jassem J, Rivera F. Panitumumab–FOLFOX4 treatment and RAS mutations in colorectal cancer. N Engl J Med. 2013;369(11):1023–34.

Chapter 14
Immuno-modulating Mediators of Colon Cancer as Immuno-therapeutic: Mechanism and Potential

Chanchal Kumar, Rajat Pratap Singh, Mrigendra Kumar Dwiwedi, and Ajay Amit

Abstract Colorectal cancer is responsible for more than half of all intestinal malignancies with very high metastatic rate. Although there are vast improvement and advancement made in recent time, surgery still remains the only potentially curative treatment choice. The success of colon cancer surgery depends upon early diagnosis, and it is not an effective choice in patients with advance stage or metastatic stage. Other traditional pharmaceutical therapeutic approaches including chemo-radiotherapy are associated with non-specificity and toxicity. These treatment regimens at best reduce the death rate depending upon time of diagnosis and in metastatic stage have moderate effect on survival time. Alternative therapeutic strategies are clearly needed, and the current thrust is to explore immunotherapy. Immunotherapy in a way is a treatment regimen against a disease in which augmentation of immune response takes place. As with various different classes of advanced-stage cancer, anti-tumour immunotherapy has a broad potential against colon cancer due to its capacity to elicit long-lasting and effective responses across a wide range of tumour. The basis of success of any immunotherapy regimens is the ability of the host immune system to differentiate between "self" and "non-self" and to respond accordingly. This can be either monoclonal antibody (mAb)-mediated-specific immune cell activation therapy or adoptive immune cell-mediated therapy (ACT). This can be achieved by the identification of cancer-associated antigens and development of therapeutic vaccination strategies. These cancer-associated antigens are also referred to as tumour-associated antigens (TAAs) and are mostly the proteins which modulate the host immune response in favour of tumour in the particular tumour microenvironment. These TAAs can be normal proteins which are expressed

C. Kumar · A. Amit (✉)
Department of Forensic Science, Guru Ghasidas Vishwavidyalaya, Bilaspur, India

R. P. Singh
Department of Biotechnology, Guru Ghasidas Vishwavidyalaya, Bilaspur, India

M. K. Dwiwedi
Department of Biochemistry, Government Nagarjuna PG College of Science, Raipur, India

G. P. Nagaraju et al. (eds.), *Colon Cancer Diagnosis and Therapy*,
https://doi.org/10.1007/978-3-030-63369-1_14

in normal cells too albeit at low level or "neo-antigens" which originate due to mutation-induced alteration in normal protein, subsequently making these otherwise self-proteins immunogenic. The current chapter deals with the advancement made on the use of these various immuno-modulators as an immuno-therapeutic with special emphasis on the treatment of colon and colorectal cancer.

Keywords Colorectal cancer · Monoclonal antibody · Chemotherapy · VEGF

14.1 Introduction

Colorectal cancer is the abnormal growth of the inner lining of the rectum or colon known as polyp, and subsequent angiogenesis escalates the metastasis resulting in tumour development at other sites. Mucous making gland of the inner lining of the colon and rectum constitutes over 95% of colorectal cancer known as adenocarcinomas [1]. Other less frequent colorectal cancers include cancers which initiate in hormone-producing intestinal cells (carcinoid tumours) and specialized colonic cells or interstitial cells of Cajal (gastrointestinal stromal tumours), immune system cancer (lymphomas) and tumours which start in the blood vessel of the colon (sarcomas). Once very rare, nowadays colorectal cancer-related mortality has increased, and population ageing, change in food preference, smoking and more sedentary lifestyle with obesity are the more cited reasons behind this upsurge [2, 3].

The intervention of chemotherapeutics like oxaliplatin and irinotecan has helped to achieve a 30-month median overall survival with metastatic disease, but the development of such therapeutics which is cancer specific is essential for effective cancer treatment [4]. Immuno-therapeutic is one such approach. The basis of immuno-therapeutics in cancer is an old knowing fact that the immune system is capable of supressing development of tumours as postulated by Paul Ehrlich in 1909 [5]. Although immuno-therapeutic-based treatment models have been evaluated and trialled in different disease models, research on the development of immuno-therapeutics for tumour are few. This scenario of negligence has been changing as many cancer immuno-therapeutic agents are at various stages of their clinical trial. The results were and are very promising which generated a huge interest in exploring the potential of immuno-therapeutics in cancer. The basis of success of any immunotherapy treatment regimens depends upon the understanding of particular basic cancer immunology and exploitation of two characteristics of particular immune response, i.e. memory and specificity.

When the immature peripheral immune cells like dendritic cells recognize pathogen through DAMP (damage-associated molecular pattern) or PAMP (pathogen-associated molecular pattern) interaction by its pathogen recognition receptors (PRRs), phagocytosis takes place followed by maturation of immune cells [6]. Subsequently the antigen-presenting cells (APCs) like macrophages and dendritic cells activate both CD8+ and CD4+ T cell via major histocompatibility complex

(MHC) class I and II molecules [7]. Dendritic cell (DC) is the most potent APC, and it exerts its effect on T cells by various signals. Interaction between MHC of DC and T-cell receptors (TCR) initiates the activation which is getting strengthened through co-stimulatory interaction between CD28 on T cells and CD80 or CD86 on APCs [8, 9]. Activation of CD8+ cells required additional signal for optimal effector functions which is provided by cytokines. This fine-tuned balance of suppressive and activating cytokines decides the directionality of particular immune response. A tumour cell exploits this balance and modulates the host immune response in their favours resulting in their immune escape.

14.2 Immunotherapy in Colon Cancer

Identification of specific tumour-associated antigens (TAAs) is the first step for the success of immunotherapy of a particular cancer. TAAs are immunogenic and can be associated with a particular cancer type or with a broad range of cancers [10]. These TAAs are capable of activating and inducing almost all types of immune effector cells. Melanoma antigen family A1 (MAGE-A1) was identified as a first TAA associated with melanoma [11]. MAGE-A1 belongs to big cancer-germline genes consisting of 25 related genes [12]. Initially discovered TAAs were normal tissue differentiation antigens with a certain role in target tissue but are very important to the expression of tumour characteristic. On the other hand, there are other constitutive proteins like p53 and human telomerase reverse transcriptase (hTERT) whose overexpression leads to malignancy, and we can't simply target them for immunotherapy [11]. This problem is solved to some extent by the identification of tumour- and patient-specific antigens arising due to somatic mutation in tumour cells. These antigens are known as neo-antigens and generated due to alteration in normal gene sequence identified by deep sequencing technology. Ideally, TAAs selected for immunotherapy should be tumour specific and recognized by APCs to trigger the adaptive arm of immune response. Similar to other cancer, colon cancer modulates host immune response towards Th2 and down-regulates MHC-I-mediated processing of cancer-specific antigen by altering the normal functioning of APCs like dendritic cells [13, 14]. This results in the escape from immunosurveillance of tumour cells further escalated by immunosuppressive agent, like arginase, present in the microenvironment of colon cancer which inhibits anti-tumour T-cell function through NO production [15]. This is evident when down-regulation in protective cytokines such as IFN-γ and tumour necrosis factor α (TNFα) and overall decrease in the number of circulatory CD8+ T cell were reported [16].

Table 14.1 enlists some recently concluded or on-going immuno-therapeutic clinical trials in colon cancer. Like any immunotherapy regimens, immunotherapy targeted against colon cancer is either active or passive in nature. Passive immunotherapy uses in vitro-produced effector mediators of immunity like monoclonal antibodies (mAbs) and adaptive transfer of antigen-specific effector cells which in turn inhibits the tumour progression and growth.

Table 14.1 Some important recent biological clinical trials on colon cancer

Serial number	Sponsor	Intervention/ treatment (Biological)	Phase	Status	References (*ClinicalTrials.gov*, US National Library of Science)
1	Eli Lilly and Company	Biological: ramucirumab	Phase 3	On-going	NCT01183780
2	Joanne Jeter	Nivolumab	Phase 2	On-going	*NCT03631641*
3	Thomas Jefferson University	Ad5-hGCC-PADRE vaccine	Phase 1	Completed	*NCT01972737*
4	University of Medicine and Dentistry of New Jersey	Therapeutic allogeneic lymphocytes	Phase 1	Completed	*NCT00161187*
5	University of Birmingham	Panitumumab	Phase 2 Phase 3	On-going	NCT00647530
6	National Cancer Institute (NCI)	Bevacizumab	Phase 1	Completed	*NCT00060411*
7	National Institutes of Health Clinical Center (CC)	Ipilimumab	Phase 1	Completed	*NCT00047164*
8	National Cancer Institute (NCI)	Bevacizumab	Phage 3	On-going	*NCT00217737*
9	Sabz Biomedicals	Cytokine-induced killer cell	Phase 1 Phase 2	On-going	*NCT03329664*
10	Vaccinogen Inc.	OncoVAX	Phase 3	On-going	*NCT02448173*
11	National Cancer Institute (NCI)	Edrecolomab	Phase 3	Completed	*NCT00002968*
12	Mansoura University	Panitumumab	Phase 3	Completed	*NCT04342676*
13	National Cancer Institute (NCI)	Cetuximab	Phase 3	Completed	*NCT00079274*
14	Duke University	AVX701	Phase 1	Completed	*NCT01890213*
15	National Cancer Institute (NCI)	Cetuximab	Phase 1	Completed	*NCT00134069*
16	National Cancer Institute (NCI)	Cetuximab	Phase 1	Completed	*NCT00397384*
17	National Cancer Institute (NCI)	Bevacizumab, cetuximab	Phase 1 Phase 2	Completed	*NCT00101348*
18	George E. Peoples	PalloV-CC	Phase 1	On-going	*NCT03827967*
19	Etubics Corporation	AD5 CEA vaccine	Phase 1 Phase 2	Completed	*NCT01147965*
20	Sidney Kimmel Comprehensive Cancer Center at Johns Hopkins	GVAX vaccine	Phase 1	On-going	*NCT01966289*
21	Epimmune	EP2101 vaccine	Phase 1	Completed	*NCT00054912*

(continued)

Table 14.1 (continued)

Serial number	Sponsor	Intervention/ treatment (Biological)	Phase	Status	References (*ClinicalTrials.gov*, US National Library of Science)
22	INTRAcel	BCG vaccine, autologous tumour cell vaccine	Phase 1 Phase 2	Completed	*NCT00016133*
23	M.D. Anderson Cancer Center	Anti-PD-L1/ TGFbetaRII *Fusion Protein* M7824	Phase 1 Phase 2	On-going	*NCT03436563*
24	Altor BioScience	Fusion protein ALT-801	Phase 1	Completed	*NCT00496860*

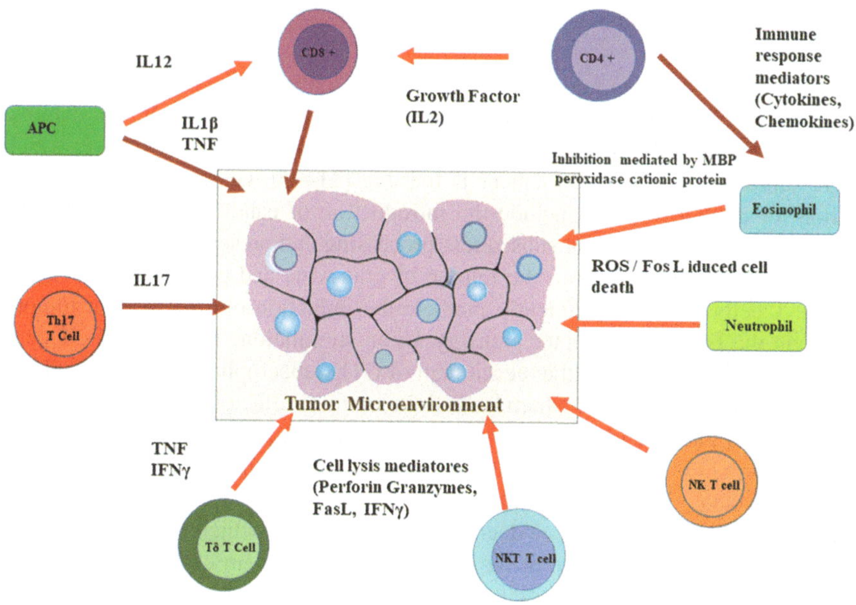

Fig. 14.1 Different white blood cells (WBC) and their respective anti-tumour mediators

14.2.1 Active Immunotherapy in Colon Cancer

Active immunotherapy involves boosting of individuals' immune capacity, and vaccination is one of its examples. So, basic understanding of colon cancer immunology is of utmost importance in designing immunotherapy regimens against it. The white blood cell (WBC)-mediated immune response is very important in checking the tumour initiation and proliferation (Fig. 14.1). In the following sections, we will discuss some active immuno-therapeutic approaches such as vaccination, adoptive immunotherapy, cytokine-based therapy and fusion protein-based therapy.

14.2.1.1 Vaccine as a Prophylactic and Curative Immuno-therapeutic

Vaccination against cancer is an active immuno-therapeutic regimen which targets to activate and induce proliferation of tumour-specific T cells. Traditionally, vaccines are preventive in nature, but in the case of cancer, vaccines are implemented as a curative measure to destroy tumours once present by triggering the patient's immune system. The vaccines targeting TAAs have been developed in various forms and formats. TAA vaccines can be epitope based, DNA based, carbohydrate based (against glycosylated protein and lipid of TME), viral vector based or in the form of peptide conjugate vaccine [17–20]. Like any other vaccine, an ideal preventive tumour vaccine would be cost-effective, durable and safe. It is desired that these vaccines should be able to give long-time protection with the need of fewer booster doses.

Theoretically, all immunogenic proteins expressed in the course of colon cancer development can be a good target for the activation of T-cell-mediated adaptive immune responses. Studies have shown that restoration of immune responses which were supressed due to colon cancer is feasible [21–25]. General mechanisms of action for peptide vaccine include the introduction of candidate peptide into the colon cancer patients and its subsequent processing and presentation to the T cells by APCs [26]. This results in the release of granzyme and perforins by CTLs or CD8+ T cells which subsequently mediate the induction of apoptosis in tumour cells via the Fas death receptor pathway. Upon stimulation, Type 1 CD4+ T cells and T-helper cells facilitate the recruitment of CTLs, macrophages and NK cells by secreting specific cytokines which leads these immune effector cells to release their own set of cytokines and effectively induce the cytotoxic pathways [27]. Nowadays, with the help of bioinformatics tools, it is possible to alter the amino acid sequence of target protein resulting in its stronger interaction with the T-cell receptor (TCR), improve biostability and reduce degradation by proteases which could increase the effectiveness of vaccine. One of the various immune system evasion mechanisms used by tumour cells is the expression of FasL [28]. The FasL is a ligand for Fas receptor present on CTL, and its binding with this receptor leads to the induced apoptosis of CTL, imparting resistance to tumour cells from Fas-induced apoptosis. Immunogenic peptide analogues known as altered peptide ligands (APLs) are ligands for T-cell receptor, and its binding to TCRs does not result in the destruction of tumour cells [29, 30]. Regulatory T cells can induce the expression of cell membrane molecules that lead to the inhibition of effector T-cell activation and function, resulting in the suppression of antitumor immunity. The defective antigen presentation of TAAs by MHC leads to further fall in anti-tumour immune responses. Generally, vaccines are used as a prophylactic measure, but against cancer, in situ *vaccine* gives an alternative means to vaccination by showing curative effects. In this type of vaccination model, identification of such target antigen which is responsible for immuno-inhibitory tumour microenvironment (TME) is a must [31]. By targeting these antigens, in situ vaccine enables host effector immune cells to enter TME and mount anti-tumour activity resulting in tumour clearance.

The main objective of this section is to discuss progress made in the development of colon cancer vaccine. It will highlight the safety, side effects and efficacy associated with vaccines that are currently in use and vaccines still undergoing clinical trials. For better understanding, we have classified vaccine as (A) tumour-associated antigen (TAA)-based vaccine, (B) oncolytic virus-based vaccine and (C) heat shock protein-based vaccine.

A. *Tumour-Associated Antigen (TAA)-Based Vaccine*

The earliest example of the therapeutic use of tumour antigens was in the form of crude tumour extract being introduced to tumour patients [32], but identification and characterization of well-defined TAAs are of uttermost importance in the development of vaccine. When the peptide fragments of TAAs are introduced into the patients, these fragments get processed and presented by MHC-I and MHC-II to the TCR which leads to immune cells including CTLs priming against these antigens. Now these activated CTLs primed by peptide vaccine recognize the respective TAAs on the surface of tumour cells resulting in the CTL-mediated destruction of tumour cells [33]. Uses of suitable adjuvants can significantly and positively influence the uptake and presentation of the antigens by APCs. DNA vaccinations based upon TAAs are another mode of vaccination [17]. In this mode, DNA sequences coding for TAAs get inserted into virus-based vector and get transcribed and translated by host machinery, but the problem arises when the host immune system initiates responses against the viral antigens rather than the target peptide which may further attenuate the antitumor immune response (Fig. 14.2).

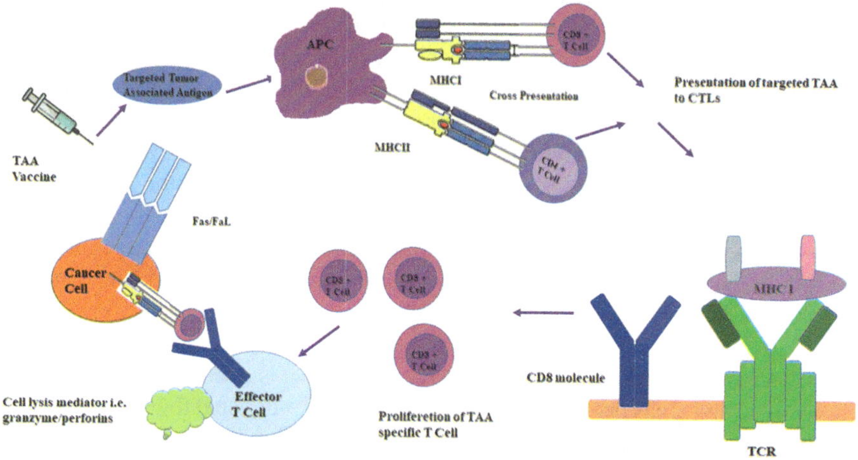

Fig. 14.2 A graphical representation of mode of action of tumour-associated antigen (TAA)-based vaccine

Vaccination through TAAs' primed DCs has been reported too [18]. The crude tumour lysates were used to prime the DCs because the ideal source of TAAs is the tumour itself. After introduction into the host, these TAAs' primed DCs presented TAAs to immune cells via MHC receptors resulting in the activation of various arms of immune cells against TAAs expressing tumour cells. DC-based immunization strategy lacks control over subsequent development which has been overcome by the use of synthetic peptides. Synthetic peptides are analogue to TAAs which allow modification in the target protein to enhance immune response along with viable monitoring and evaluation. It has been observed that anti-tumour immunological function restores after tumour resection which suggests the immunosuppressive effects of colon tumour and it is at both cellular and molecular levels [34, 35]. This immune evasion is multifactorial. There are many TAAs, and MHC-restricted epitopes for T-cell-mediated immune response in colon-specific tumour have been reported [36, 37] (Table 14.1). It has been also shown that there is a small population of antigen-specific memory T cell which exists and their number is linked to metastasis progression [11, 38]. These all findings are clearly suggestive of an immunological basis of disease control as evident by best survival of patient with high levels of infiltrating CD8+ T cells and T cells with elevated granzyme B expression [39]. The following are some TAAs and their mode of actions in detail.

(a) *Inhibition of beta human chorionic gonadotropin (βhCG) by in situ vaccination:* Human chorionic gonadotropin (hCG) is made up of two non-covalently joined polypeptide subunits, α and β, and belongs to a class of glycoprotein hormone [40]. Normal colorectal cells do not produce hCG, but tumour cells of the colon do. Further hCG level is associated with aggressiveness of the cancer and patients' survival [41]. It can promote metastasis in autocrine/paracrine fashion with promotion of neo-vascularization [42]. The immuno-inhibitory and pro-tumour activities of hCG are mainly due to a cysteine-rich structural motif. Such structural patterns are also present in other factors (TGF-β2, platelet-derived growth factor-β) [43]. Studies have shown that in the case of colorectal cancer, immunization against hCG leads to humoral or cellular effector responses resulting in the lysis of tumour cells which expressed hCG [44, 45]. It has been also shown that neutralization of soluble hCG with antibody abrogates hCG-mediated tumour progression.
(b) *Carcinoembryonic antigen (CEA) as a target for in situ vaccination:* Carcinoembryonic antigen (CEA) of 180 kDa is an oncofoetal glycoprotein and well-known TAA [35, 46]. Normally, they are expressed in the large intestine, but in the case of cancer, its overexpression takes place in colon cancer and in other gastrointestinal malignancies [47]. Since it is easy to detect circulating CEA in CEA-positive tumours, it is used to monitor therapy response [48]. CEAs are an attractive vaccine candidate because it is a self-tumour-associated antigen and it has been shown that in patients CTLs directed towards CEAs can be induced [49]. The main hindrance in its use in vaccine development is that this CEA is a usual member of foetus proteome and hence well tolerated by the adult immune system. To overcome this problem, an engineered CEA known as

CeaVac has been developed which is an anti-idiotypic antibody and has the same functionality as that of CEAs [50]. Another important TAA is 5T4 (leucine-rich membrane glycoprotein) which is associated with patient's survival and belongs to an oncofoetal class of protein, very limited in normal cells but overtly expressed in colon cancer cells ([51, 52]). A 5T4-based drug, TroVax, whose clinical trials showed very significant reduction in cancer load is in use with a pox virus vector and a modified vaccinia virus [53, 54].

(c) *Onyvax-105:* It is an anti-idiotypic antibody. It mimics the role of CD55, a GPI (glycosylphosphatidylinositol)-anchored protein. CD55 is an important complement regulator protein which protects the tumour cells from complement-mediated immune attack [35, 55].

(d) *Gastrin (gastric acid-stimulating hormone):* The precursor of gastrin is overexpressed in colon cancer causing metastasis by promoting angiogenesis and cell proliferation. Bulk of the peptide of gastrin (sometimes 100%) are formed from these precursors in early colon cancer cells which are normally absent from normal cells. Vaccination regimen by targeting this protein has shown promise which actually inhibits the tumour cell growth, division and translocation or metastasis [35, 46, 55, 56].

(e) *MET proto-oncogene:* Onartuzumab is another good candidate for in situ vaccination. It is a monoclonal antibody against human growth factor receptor (HGFR). It showed benefit in patients who overexpressed HGFR. It exerts its anti-tumour activity by blocking MET proto-oncogene, a cancer-specific receptor tyrosine kinase [55, 57].

(f) *The FANG TM, a novel vaccine*: This is a vaccine developed by combining patient's tumour cells with granulocyte-macrophage colony-stimulating factor (GM-CSF) small bi-functional RNA segment which is a kind of hairpin loop known as RNA furin [47]. This vaccine controls colon cancer progression by inhibition of synthesis of precursor protein of targeted cancer-specific active protein, whereas GM-CSF induce growth and proliferation of DCs. This approach of vaccination mainly targets the TGF β1 and 2 (TGFβ) which are responsible and linked with immunosuppression by interfering in the development of APCs mainly through blocking GM-CSF. For the development of this vaccine, GM-CSF and IL-13 are used to develop mDCs (myeloid DCs) from monocytes and subsequently for the priming of these mDCs with 6HLA-A*0201-binding peptide derivative of CEA, MAGE-2 (melanoma antigen over-expressed in gastrointestinal cancer) and HER2/neu [35, 55, 58].

B. *Oncolytic Virus-Based Vaccine*

It has been a well-established fact that when viruses infect any animal including human, it results in antigen expression which can be recognized by the host immune system, and subsequently vaccination against various viral diseases has been designed. Generally, vaccination is a prophylactic measure, but in the case of cancer, vaccination is more or less a means of cure and control of existing tumour. It has been observed that when viral infection occurred in cancer patients, their immune systems get boosted [35, 59, 60]. This increase in antitumor activity is evident by

Lindeman and Klein work of 1967 in which they have shown that antigenicity of tumour antigen became stronger after influenza infection [61]. The understanding of basic cancer biology and mechanisms of its immune escape change the direction of cancer immunotherapy. Now, instead of targeting individual tumour causing gene antigen, researchers are targeting such genes which have the potential of blocking cancer supporting pathways. In light of this, the vaccines against cancer are now being designed to trigger the more potent effector immune response by host to combat carcinogenesis. A therapeutic vaccine, Provenge, has been approved by FDA in 2010 which aims to inhibit the progression of prostate cancer. Also known as Sipuleucel-T, Provenge is the first vaccine which triggers the patient's own immune system to recognize and combat his cancer [62, 63].

In recent years, oncolytic viruses (OVs) have emerged as an effective tool of inhibiting cancer progression as evident in clinical trials [64–67]. The OVs are the class of viruses which attack tumour cells and kill them. OVs can be RNA- or DNA-based virus derived from human or animals. The reasons behind this specific infectivity of OVs to tumour cell include impaired antiviral defence mechanism of cancer cell. Further, these OVs can be genetically engineered so their infectivity capacity to normal cells decreases and gives these viruses the ability to deliver immunotherapeutic molecules into tumour cells [66, 68]. Ultimately, these viruses cause the bursting of the cancer cells and subsequent release of tumour antigen which can result in the triggering of effector immune cells (Fig. 14.3). Now, these activated immune cells clear the remaining tumours from the host. Toda and his team have shown that HSV G207, a genetically modified OV, can induce antitumor activity in CT26 colon cancer cells [69–71]. The OV therapy has direct effects on various signal transduction pathways important for cancer progression. OVs can interfere with Ras, Wnt, anti-apoptosis and EGFR signal transduction pathway, and this

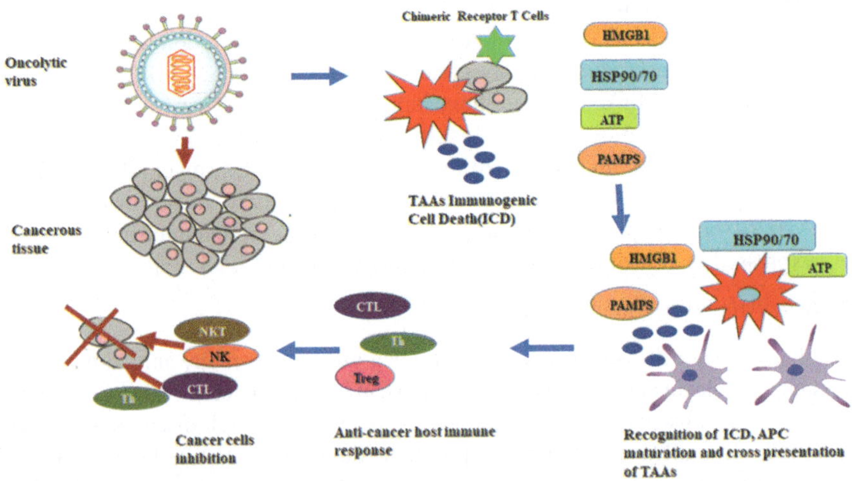

Fig. 14.3 Diagrammatic representation of immuno-therapeutic strategy based upon cancer-specific oncolytic viruses

alternation resulted in the inhibition of tumour development [64, 72–75]. As mentioned earlier in this section, genetic alternation in OVs makes them safe, specific and highly selective [64, 73, 76]. OV-based vaccination regimen is very effective because there is no issue of drug resistance since OVs' attack on tumour is multidirectional and, most importantly, virus dose in a tumour increases with time due to in situ virus replication [64, 68, 71–73].

The side effects associated with OV vaccination include the development of anti-OV antibodies and problem associated with the delivery of OVs to cancerous target cells. The anti-OV antibodies can neutralize or kill OV, and to avoid this, some specific cell carriers are used which can nullify the effect of these antibodies. The neural stem cells and myeloid-derived suppressor cells are example of frequently used carrier cells for OVs [47]. If we talk about OV-based colon cancer immunotherapy, then ONYX-015, a OV-based vaccine, is in phase 2 clinical trials along with chemotherapy. *TroVax* is another vaccine which has shown promise against colon cancer. It is actually an attenuated vaccinia virus-based vaccine which contains the gene for expression of 5T4, an oncofoetal protein as discussed above. The vaccination resulted in the induction of effector immune response as evident by antibody formation against 5T4 [53, 54]. Since technology is developing at a rapid pace, there are more reasons to hope that OV-based vaccination will be available against colon cancer or any other cancer sooner than expected.

C. *Heat Shock Protein-Based Vaccine*

HSPs and its role in cancer progression are well documented [77,78–81]. Specially, in the case of colon cancer, overexpression of HSP72 and glucose-regulated protein 96 (gp96) occur which are considered to be very important for cancer metastasis as they have important roles in tumour cell growth and tumour-associated signalling [82]. Study revealed that although their expression is not linked to patient's survival, as a diagnostic and prognostic marker, they are very important [78, 80]. It is a well-established fact that HSPs have a role in MHC-I-mediated antigen presentation where they work as chaperons and assist in the transportation of peptides to the heterodimeric transporters associated with antigen processing [78, 83–85]. Glucose-regulated protein 96 (gp96) has a major role in the assembly of the MHC-Iβ-2 macroglobulin-peptide complexes which takes place in the lumen of ER [82]. Various studies in animal models have reported the effectiveness of HSP-based vaccines in cancer treatment [78, 80, 81]. Since HSPs are responsible for the presentation of peptides on the surface of APCs, it has been proposed to develop a fusion protein of HSP with target protein as an immuno-therapeutic means against cancer [85–87]. This will promote presentation of target antigen to T cells and by so doing more potent immune response generation against target protein. In colon cancer scenario, CD44 is coupled with HSPs to improve the targeted immune response [82].

14.2.1.2 Adoptive Immunity-Based Immuno-therapeutics

The effectiveness of any cancer treatment regimen based on approaches like chemotherapy, immunotherapy or radiotherapy is marred by treatment-associated side effects, development of tolerance in tumour and toxicity [88–91]. In recent times, a novel approach known as adoptive immunotherapy has been explored which involves the ex vivo transfer of activated anti-cancer CD8+ T cell into cancer patients [92–96]. Almost six decades ago, in their classical experiment, Delorme and Alexander showed that the transfer of activated immune cells particularly T cells was able to inhibit the development of carcinogen-induced sarcoma [97]. Since then, there are many advances which have been made in the field of adoptive T-cell therapy with the aim of triggering the anti-cancer response through the ex vivo manipulation of T cells involving host immune cells [88–91]. The various ways to achieve this goal have been designed including the characterization of tumour-infiltrating lymphocytes (TILs), transfer of genetically engineered synthetic TCR (sTCR) and addition of chimeric antigen receptor (CAR) to T cells [98]. The main objective of this therapy module is to activate host's (cancer patient in this case) immune system and subsequently inhibition of tumour growth and development by effector immune cells (Fig. 14.4).

It is a well-known fact that each and every immune cell have a defined role in inhibiting tumour growth and the main purpose of adoptive immunotherapy is to trigger and involve these all cells in tumour control. Studies performed in animal model highlight the anti-tumour potential of adaptive transfer of T cells with requisition of only a small number of ex vivo activated T cells [93–95]. With advancement in technology now, it is possible to add different TAA-specific TCRs to T cells or attach co-stimulatory receptors to T cells [92]. This has opened up the field for the development of T-cell immuno-therapeutics targeting novel TAA. As reports suggested, these modified T cells are able to inhibit the immune escape pathway of tumour cells [94]. The natural killer cells (NK cells) are other attractive immune cells to use in adoptive immunotherapy, and its immuno-therapeutic potential was explored by Rosenberg and his team [99]. An NK cell induces cell death mainly through perforins and granzyme. On the basis of every day growing information regarding adoptive immunotherapy, it has been postulated that combining both T and NK cells will have greater success in combating cancer since these two potent immune cells are capable of attacking tumour cells from multi-direction [100, 101]. In spite of so many advances made, still we have not been able to fully explore this very attractive immunotherapy mode till now.

14.2.1.3 Cytokines as an Immuno-therapeutic Against Colon Cancer

Growth of immune cells and co-ordination within immuno effector cells are controlled by cytokines, a small protein produced by WBC. Cytokine as a therapeutic has a broad-based anti-tumour activity, independent of tumour types [102–104]. Two major cytokine classes which are in use for cancer treatment are interferon

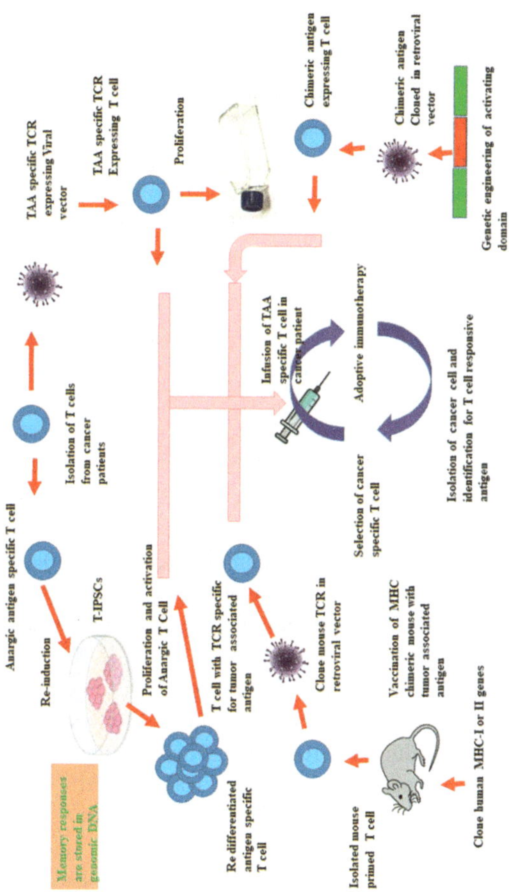

Fig. 14.4 A pictorial representation of the mechanism of action of various anti-tumour activities mediated by the host's adaptive immune system

(IFN) and interleukins (IL). Many inflammatory cells migrate at the site of tumour under the influence of tumour-secreted factors like cytokines, and chemokine promotes tumour progression. Some important cytokines which promote anti-tumour activities are GM-CSF, IL-15, IL-2, TNFα and IL-12 [102–105]. These cytokines have the potential to be explored as immuno-therapeutics either in single or in combination with other immuno-therapeutic agents. The anti-tumour activity of NK cells is inhibited by IL-10 secreted by tumour cells through activation of Stat3 and Braf [101]. The Wnt/β-catenin signalling is a major oncogene activation pathway in colon cancer, and this pathway is induced by TNFα, hepatocyte growth factor, PDGF, FGF19 and IL-1β [106, 107]. After activation of this pathway, β-catenin gets accumulated in the cytoplasm of cell which promotes cell growth and differentiation in colon cancer. The NF-kB pathway is another oncogene-inducing pathway which activates through TNFα [76, 108] as evident by antitumor activity shown by neutralizing TNFα antibodies (Enbrel or Remicade) in colon cancer [107]. Continuous overexpression of TNFα in tumour cells protects the cell from induced cell death by initiating NF-kB signalling. The etanercept, a TNFα antagonist, reduced the level of active β-catenin in the cytoplasm of tumour cells by inhibiting Wnt/β-catenin signalling pathway [47].

(a) *Interleukins as inducer of active immunity:* Interleukins are growth and differentiation causing cytokines which play very important roles in immune cell trafficking and immuno-modulation. The role of inflammation in colon cancer may be dual; it can either promote or suppress colon cancer pathogenesis. The interleukins are very important factor which determine the fate of tumour by controlling the tumour microenvironment (TME). There is no dearth of researches which explored several interleukins for its potential immuno-therapeutic value in cancer treatment. In this section of the chapter, we will discuss some interleukins important in colon cancer treatment.

    IL-1β is a well-defined pro-inflammatory cytokine released by activated macrophages. It promotes the TNFα, IL-6, IL-8, IL-17, Cox-2 and PGE2 expression [107, 109]. It helps in the development of tumour supporting microenvironment as evident by the increase in number of cancer in mice animal model by IL-1β gene induction [109–111]. The two main receptors present on target cells are IL-1RI and IL-1RII which transduce the signal through two cytoplasmic adaptor molecules MyD88 and IRAK after activation by IL-1β binding. The release of IL-1β by macrophages is STAT1 dependent, and blocking of STAT1 has shown to prevent the tumour formation [107]. It has been shown that IL-1β causes the overexpression of mitogenic, proto-oncogene HGF-cMET in colon cancer cells [107, 109]. A phase 1B clinical trial in colon cancer patients is undergoing for canakinumab (ACZ885) in combination with PDR001, a checkpoint inhibitor [107]. This canakinumab is very specific for IL-1β and developed as a human IgG1/j mAbI [112,113].

    IL-6 is another important interleukin released by a variety of immune cells like monocytes, fibroblasts and endothelial cells, macrophages, T cells and B lymphocytes after activation. In colon cancer, macrophages are activated to release IL-6 and induce STAT3 pathway in cancer cells. Blockage of IL-6 pathway inhibits the tumour cell growth and saves them from apoptosis as evident by studies which revealed that the inhibition of STAT3 has a negative impact on tumour progression [114, 115]. It has been reported that simultaneous expression of STAT3 and β-catenin is linked to the poor survival of colon cancer patients [76, 108]. Several therapeutics' mode has been proposed and developed by targeting IL-6/STAT-3 pathway by anti-IL-6 (siltuximab) or anti-IL-6R (tocilizumab) antibodies, soluble gp130Fc (sgp130Fc is a designer cytokine that blocks trans-signalling of IL-6/sIL-6R-mediated pathway by binding to this complex) and selective small molecule JAK inhibitors (ruxolitinib and CEP-33779) [116, 117]. Th17 cell is a subset of T-helper cell whose role in immuno-modulation during protozoan infection like leishmaniasis has been reported [118]. These cells are the producers of IL-17, IL-22 and TNFα, and release of these cytokines by Th17 cells is induced by IL-6, TGFβ, IL-1β and IL-23, while IFN-γ and IL-4 inhibit the differentiation of these cells [119]. Paneth cells residing at the bottom of the intestinal crypts are a major source of IL-17 in the colon [120]. The role of IL-17 is ambiguous in colon cancer or in any other cancer. Some have reported an anti-tumour role, while other reports are indicative of their pro-tumour activity [119, 120]. Evaluation of three mAbs (secukinumab, ixekizumab and brodalumab) targeting the IL-17/IL-17RA axis (for their anti-tumour potential) are in progress [121]. It has been observed in the mice model that targeting the IL-17/IL-17RA axis in colon cancer simultaneously with the VEGF pathway will be a viable and suitable alternative to explore in future clinical trials [122].

(b) *Tumour necrosis factor-related apoptosis-inducing ligand (TRAIL) as a target to induce active immunity:* TNF-related apoptosis-inducing ligand (TRAIL) belongs to death receptor (DR) ligand family (TNF family) [123]. This TRAIL protein has soluble and immune cell membrane bounded versions. Although five receptors are reported for TRAIL, only DR4 (TRAIL receptor 1) and DR5 (TRAIL receptor 2) are able to induce apoptosis since they are trans-membrane receptor containing cytoplasmic death domain [124]. The other two receptors (DcR1 and DcR2) are decoy receptors which lack cytoplasmic death domain, and the fifth receptor osteoprotegerin is a weak receptor [123, 125]. Various agonistic antibodies and recombinant human TRAIL ligand have been designed to induce TRAIL-mediated pathway mainly through DR4 and DR5 to induce apoptosis in cancer cell with better safety profile in vivo [126]. It has been reported that TRAIL-targeted therapies enhanced the effectiveness of conventional chemotherapy regime in colon cancer. It has been also reported that in a TRAIL unresponsive colon cancer cell line, *sorafenib*, a Raf kinase inhibitor, can trigger TRAIL-induced apoptosis by preventing the NF-kB-dependent expression of the anti-apoptotic genes, IAP2 and MCl-1 [107, 124–126].

14.2.1.4 Bispecific Antibodies (BsAbs) as a Connective Link to Induce Active Immunity

By understanding the potential of mAbs, 13 different monoclonal antibodies have been approved for tumour therapy, while more than 100 mAbs that are undergoing different phases of clinical trial with 33 mAbs for cancer treatment are in advance development stage to evaluate their clinical value including 11 immune checkpoints and 8 antibody-drug conjugates (ADC) [107, 127].

The specificity and toxicity associated with the use of antibodies as a therapeutic have been evaluated by phase display and hybridoma technology [128]. Generally antibodies are antigen specific with a binding capacity of two, but with the advent of new technology now, it is possible to induce manipulation in antibody structure and function [129]. It is possible to produce unnatural antibodies by fusion of two different hybridomas known as dual antibodies, fusion antibodies or bispecific antibodies. These dual antibodies are formed by random pairing of two different heavy and light chains with the ability to bind to two different antigens. The whole antibodies are big in size (150 kDa) so it is very difficult to deliver it at the tumour site. To fine-tune the antibody therapeutic value, the antibody has been cleaved by enzyme-based digestion, and instead of the whole antibody-only Fab, the antigen-binding domain of the antibody has been used [130]. But since these Fabs are very small, they have a real short stay in the system due to their clearance by the excretory system. Bispecific antibodies (BsAbs) were developed to overcome these hindrances for their effective therapeutic use as an immuno-therapeutic [131]. These laboratory-developed BsAbs can bind two different antigens or two different epitopes on the same region. Due to this bivalency, BsAbs have a greater therapeutic potential than monospecific mAbs [130–133]. There is a cross-talk between different transduction pathways like MET, VEGFR and IGFR-IR which exists, and interactions between them play a crucial role in tumour development and immune escape. It has been reported that the effectiveness of anti-EGFR mAbs decreased in colon cancer after some time due to the triggering of new pathway [134]. The complexity of tumour signalling became evident when Engelman et al. showed that gefitinib resistance starts when ERBB3 pathway is activated by mesenchymal-epithelial transition factor (MET) amplification [135, 136]. These findings are suggestive to design such therapeutic regimen which can be able to hit at multiple targets.

In the cancer immunotherapy based upon BsAbs, the obvious target is the T cell because it is the single most potent immune effector cell against cancer. The main mechanism by which tumour escapes the immune system is to interfere in the effective presentation of tumour antigen by APCs [130, 132]. This results in defective T-cell activation and proliferation. In tumour immunotherapy based on BsAbs, targeted antigens are differentiation antigens and are overexpressed in tumour cells [131]. The target antigens include CD19, CD33, CEA, EpCAM (epithelial cell adhesion molecule), PMSA (prostate-specific membrane antigen) and EGF receptors. The expression of these target antigens of BsAb is up-regulated in tumour cells [129–133].

Blinatumomab was developed by fusing two single chain antibodies (anti-CD19 and anti-CD3) [137]. This duobody or bispecific antibody is of 55 kDa. The joining of two single chain antibodies was performed so that these chains come into close proximity. For this purpose, the linker used was non-immunogenic short peptide containing five non-glycosylated amino acids [138]. This fusion antibody binds with CD19 expressed on malignant B cells and CD3 expressed on T cells simultaneously. This simultaneous binding brings the two cells, i.e. malignant B cell and T cell, very close to each other resulting in the activation of T cells and subsequent destruction of malignant B cells as evident by the increased expression of T-cell-inducing markers (CD2, CD69, IL-10, TNFα, CD25, IL-6, IFN-γ) [139–141]. This T-cell-mediated killing does not require antigen presentation or TCR involvement. There is no drug resistance with the use of blinatumomab because its working mechanism is independent of MHC expression pattern [141]. It has been also observed that blinatumomab binding with CD3 and CD19 induces cell lysis mediated by perforin and granzymes released by cytotoxic T cells [142].

Antibody-cytokine fusion proteins termed as immunocytokines give a new dimension in cancer immunotherapy. These engineered biopharmaceuticals are able to increase the therapeutic index of cytokine payloads and have the potential to preferentially target the tumour cells and trigger the trafficking of effector immune cells at the site of tumour. It has been reported in animal model that IL-2-based immunocytokines have an anti-tumour potential against colon cancer. There are various IL-2-based immunocytokines in combination with other therapeutic targets (L19-IL2 plus RT, L19-IL2 plus CTLA-4, L19-IL2 plus AAZ+-ValCit-MMAE) that are in the preclinical stage for the evaluation of their anti-tumour activity in colon cancer [143, 144].

14.2.2 Passive Immunotherapy or Monoclonal Antibody (mAb)-Based Immuno-therapeutics

Passive immunotherapy uses in vitro-produced monoclonal antibodies (mAbs) which, after introduction into the patient, inhibit the tumour progression and growth. Monoclonal antibodies which block a specific pathway important for tumour survival by binding to the ligand or the extracellular domain of a receptor are a very attractive way to control cancer [47]. Immuno-modulatory mAbs are specific antibodies which exert their anti-tumour activity by inducing immune cells and do not target cancer cells, and hence it is not cancer specific. It works by activating or blocking the regulatory receptors of immune cells. Even a single molecule blockade like programmed cell death protein 1 (PD-1) has shown an effective anti-tumour activity and was approved to be used in melanoma and non-small cell lung cancer (NSCLC) by the FDA [53, 56]. PD-1 is an immune checkpoint signalling receptor responsible for lymphocyte maintenance of self-tolerance. mAbs can work either by blocking the inhibitory receptors or by activating T-cell stimulatory receptors.

However, checkpoint blocking is generally tumour specific, whereas T-cell stimulatory mAbs may be independent of cancer type with tumour-specific variation in route of administration as therapeutic [47, 99].

For an effective cancer therapy, the development of continuous immunological memory response is a critical factor [36, 39, 145]. It is still not clear how this immunological memory generates but its role in tumour reduction and eradication is proven. The finding that T-cell stimulation alone is sufficient for anti-tumour T-cell-mediated response without any external intervention clearly suggested that these responsive patients were immunologically primed and had an immunological memory which directs this anti-cancer response [39]. So, for the success of mAb-based immunotherapy, exploitation of this latent potential of the immune system is needed [126, 128, 133]. Identification of T-cell stimulatory therapy responsive patient is important to save them from undue treatment and associated toxicity. There are several predictive biomarkers like C-reactive protein (CRP) and absolute lymphocyte count that have identified which level is correlated with T-cell stimulatory therapy response [146, 147]. Other such markers can be the number of circulating myeloid-derived suppressor cell (MDSC) and baseline levels of soluble CD25. Whole exome-sequencing in patients with melanoma and NSCLC and treated with mAbs were performed to identify a genetic basis of response to immuno-therapeutics. The successes in the identification of genetic altered neoepitopes are of paramount importance as this can allow selectivity of immunotherapy [146–148]. There are various clinical trials that are on-going or recently concluded on mAb-mediated immunotherapy in colon cancer (Table 14.2).

For better clearance, we classified mAb-based immuno-therapeutics on the basis of their target which may be overlapping since some antibodies have effect on more than one pathway. The broad classification will be as follows.

14.2.2.1 The mAbs Against a Target Pathway for Immunotherapy

In this segment, we will have an emphasis on such mAbs whose target is a pathway which is essential for tumour survival and progression. These antibodies are either analogues to the ligands of these receptors or antagonist. Following are some important examples of such antibodies used in cancer immunotherapy.

A. *Vascular Endothelial Growth Factor (VEGF)-Targeted mAbs*

   VEGF is very important for cancer progression since it is involved in angiogenesis and vascular permeability. Further, VEGF mediates many tumour cell signalling pathways which are important for cancer initiation and development [149]. The neuropilins, trans-membrane glycoproteins and co-receptors for class 3 semaphorins, play an important role in VEGF-mediated signalling of tumour cells. These neuropilins have the ability to impart regulation on the function and migration of various growth factor receptors and integrins [150]. There are three VEGF receptors present on endothelial cells and angioblasts, and it has been observed that the VEGF receptor 2 is overtly expressed in colorectal

Table 14.2 List of novel monoclonal antibody-based colorectal cancer immuno-therapeutics undergoing clinical trials for their efficacy and safety

Name of the mAbs	Format	Target in host	Proposed mode of action	References
RG7212	Fully humanized IgG1 kappa	Fn14	Supress TweAK; inhibit proliferation, survival and NF-κB	[220]
Tigatuzumab	Humanized IgG	DR5 (TNFRSF10B or TRAIL-R2)	Agonist of DR5, apoptosis induction and cytotoxic activity	[221]
Nimotuzumab	Humanized IgG1	Extracellular domain of eGFR	Inhibits EGFR	[222]
Figitumumab	Fully humanized IgG2	IGF-1R	Reduces the activation of IGF-1R	[223]
Drozitumab	Fully humanized IgG1	DR5	Agonist of DR5, apoptosis induction, cytotoxic activity	[224]
I-huA33	Fully humanized IgG1	A33 glycoprotein	Stimulates CTL response against A33-positive colorectal cancer	[225]
Dalotuzumab	Fully humanized IgG1 isotype	IGF-1R	Antagonist of iGF-1R; inhibits IGF-1- and IGF-2-mediated tumour cell proliferation, IGF-1R autophosphorylation and Akt phosphorylation	[226]
Robatumumab	Fully humanized IgG1 kappa isotype	IGF-1R	Antagonist of IGF-1R; inhibits VEGF and angiogenesis	[227]
MNRP1685A	Fully humanized IgG1	NRP1	Targets the VEGF binding domain of NRP1; reduces angiogenesis, cell survival, migration and invasion	[228]
KRN330	Fully humanized IgG	A33 glycoprotein	Stimulates CTL response against A33-positive colorectal cancer	[229]

cancer. The angiogenesis-promoting factors like VEGF-A, VEGF-B, VEGF-C, VEGF-D and VEGF-E help in the proliferation and migration of endothelial cells by degrading the extracellular matrix by binding to the receptors VEGFR-1, R-2 and R-3 [149–151]. In the case of colon cancer, VEGF-A along with its receptor VEGFR-2 is in abundance [151]. These informations have a great value for interpreting the cancer developmental biology and by virtue of so in developing new immuno-therapeutic regimen for cancer treatment by targeted blockage of new blood vessel formation for nutrient supply to tumour. Studies have revealed that the monoclonal antibody-based anti-VEGF therapies have a positive effect on the survival of colon cancer patients.

(i) *Bevacizumab:* Bevacizumab is a classic example of a mAb-based anti-VEGF immuno-therapeutic [151]. It interferes in VEGFR binding with its respective ligand and hence blocks the downstream signalling through VEGFR. It has been reported that there is no relation with the efficacy of bevacizumab with VEGF expression pattern and microvessel number. Microvessel density (MVD) assessment is a very good technique to predict metastasis in which by the help of specific antibodies like endoglin, one can differentiate between cancer-associated vascularization from normal vessels [152]. Endoglin (CD105) expression significantly increases on endothelial cells during tumour-associated vascularization which is further enhanced once the blockage of VEGF pathway occurs [151]. The role of endoglin as a possible prognostic marker in colon cancer has been evaluated, and it was concluded that endoglin is a more precise and sensitive marker than the other pan-endothelial markers and its positive staining is directly linked to lymphatic invasion and metastases to lymph nodes and liver in colon cancer [153]. Although it can be used alone, bevacizumab is generally used in combination with chemotherapy which enhances the efficacy of chemotherapy. This combination therapy leads to a decrease in raised interstitial pressure in tumours and improves the patient's survival [151, 153].

(ii) *Ramucirumab:* By using phage display library of big size, a fully humanized IgG1 mAb known as ramucirumab has been developed [47]. Ramucirumab blocks VEGFR-2 by targeting outer extracellular domain of VEGFR-2 [154]. It has shown a very positive anti-cancer activity during a large-scale clinical trial as evident by the increased VEGF expression accompanied with down-regulation in VEGFR-1/2, and more significantly it is well tolerated by patients [154]. These effects of ramucirumab were assessed by the level of VEGF-A and soluble VEGFR-1/2 during phase 1 trials. This clearly indicates about saturation of receptors as suggested by its dose independency. After very positive phase 1 and subsequent phase 2 trials of these antibodies which resulted in 6-month survival without any further tumour progression, a phase 3 trial of ramucirumab has been started. Phase 3 trials have very promising results as evident by the positive change in overall patient survival [154]. Administration of this antibody is associated with hypertension, vascular thrombotic events and proteinuria in patients [155].

(iii) *Aflibercept:* By combining human IgG1 with VEGFR-1 and VEGFR-2, a fusion protein has been developed. This therapeutic fusion protein is known as aflibercept [149]. It is basically developed by fusing the second Ig domain of VEGFR-1 and the third immunoglobulin domain of VEGFR-2 with IgG1. It has a high degree of tolerability in patients with high binding affinity for VEGF-A, VEGF-B and PIGF [149–151]. Studies have been revealed that this antibody is very promising for colon cancer treatment because it blocks VEGFR-1-mediated signalling. IMC-18F1 is a human VEGFR-1-neutralizing antibody which has shown great promise by exhibiting anti-angiogenic and anti-proliferative activity [155].

B. *Epidermal Growth Factor Receptor (EGFR)-Targeted mAbs*
EGFR belongs to erbB class of tyrosine kinase (TK) receptor. As all TK receptors, EGFR has three segments, extracellular, trans-membrane and cytoplasmic, and as usual cytoplasmic domain possesses the kinase activity. The signals mediated by EGFR pathway are crucial for many cellular functions like growth, proliferation and communications. These receptors (EGFRs) use various downstream transduction pathways like STAT, MAPK and AKT [156] (Fig. 14.5). It has been reported that many abnormalities in colon cancer are associated with the overexpression of EGFR [157].

Panitumumab and cetuximab are the two monoclonal antibodies which have been used as therapeutics against colon cancer [157]. These antibodies prevent metastasis by targeting the epidermal growth factor receptor (EGFR). Panitumumab is a fully human IgG2 mAb which blocks EGFR tyrosine phosphorylation-mediated signalling along with the initiation of carcinogenesis and cancer cell proliferation. This antibody has a high affinity for the EGFR extracellular domain and binds strongly with it. Panitumumab along with cetuximab (a chimeric human-mouse IgG1 mAb) has been cleared for the treatment of advanced colorectal cancer. This combinational antibody-based therapy has shown positive effects on colon-associated tumour in most of the patients with the exception of KRAS-mutated patients at codons 12 and 13 [158]. The KRAS is a type of oncogene belonging to the rat sarcoma virus (Ras) gene family which interferes with the EGFR-mediated

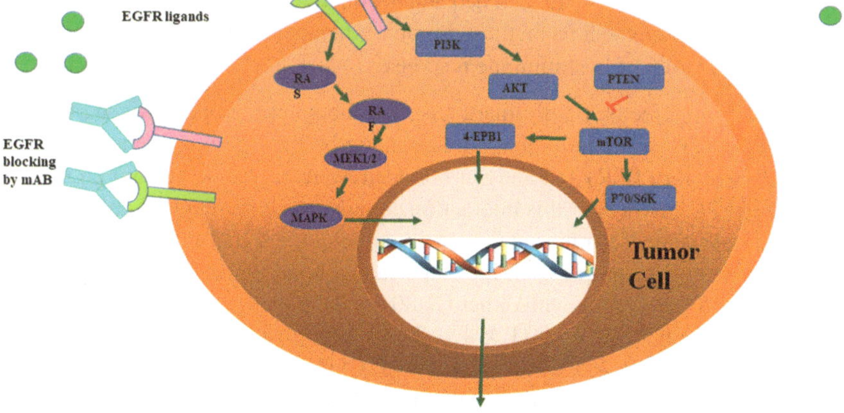

Fig. 14.5 Epidermal growth factor receptor (EGFR)-mediated signalling pathway and its blockade through anti-EGFR monoclonal antibodies in tumour cells

downstream signalling and subsequently controls the gene transcription pattern [157]. Both cetuximab and panitumumab have a greater affinity for EGFR than its natural ligands like EGF and TGFα, and by so doing, they outcompete these ligands. Due to the antibodies binding with EGFR, progression of cell cycle gets blocked and arrested at G1 phase which in effect inhibits angiogenesis along with metastasis [159]. Reduced level of matrix metalloproteinase formation is one of the mechanisms by which angiogenesis and metastasis are inhibited and effectiveness of chemotherapy and radiotherapy increases. Since panitumumab is an IgG2 antibody, it does not exert antibody-dependent cell cytotoxicity in chemotherapy-refractory colon cancer. These two antibodies (cetuximab and panitumumab) are used in combination since blocking of only one transduction pathway through one mAb has a limited effect because generally for any signalling receptor, alternative pathways exist and so inhibiting two transduction pathways is always better [157–159]. Other benefits of combinational therapy are limitation of overlapping toxicity with almost no pharmacokinetic interactions between antibodies [159]. However, deciding the combination of mAbs for immunotherapy needs fine-tuning because any random combination may result in disaster as evident in the case of combinations such as bevacizumab with cetuximab or panitumumab which resulted in the reduction in survival time along with increased toxicity in the case of colon cancer [159]. Sometimes mild side effects can be associated with better outcome in cancer patients as in the case with panitumumab where skin toxicity was observed to be linked with positive treatment response [157, 159].

14.2.2.2 Immuno-therapeutic mAbs Targeting Immune Checkpoint

Effective immune cell activation is of uttermost importance in the inhibition of tumour progression. The added advantage for targeting immune checkpoint through mAbs is that it is not limited to a certain type of cancer. The effectiveness of these immuno-therapeutics is broad, and hence it is effective in colon cancer too [160]. In this section, our focus will be on those immuno-therapeutic mAbs which have influence over activation of host immune response.

A. *CTLA-4*: An effector T-cell function is dependent upon proper antigen presentation and subsequent initiation signal generation through the interaction of the T-cell receptor (TCR) and antigen-bounded MHC molecule present on the surface of APCs. However, this interaction alone is not sufficient to mount an effective T-cell response; rather, another co-stimulatory signal is required to avoid T-cell anergy or apoptosis. This important second signal comes from T-cell receptor CD28 binding with either CD80 or CD86 on the APC which eventually leads to the shuttling of CTLA-4, a T-cell inhibitory receptor, to cell surface. Once on cell surface, CTLA-4 binds with CD80 or CD86 with higher affinity than CD28 and subsequently restricts T-cell stimulation by competing for its ligand with CD28 receptor [99].

Study on knock-out mice for CTLA-4 leads to the development of lethal autoimmune condition which clearly suggests that CTLA-4 plays an important role in the suppression of T-cell activation and, thus, inhibiting its anti-tumour activity [161]. It has been shown that regulatory T cells (Tregs) express a higher level of CTLA-4 than normal T cell which in turn helps Treg cells to exert a maximal immunosuppressive function [162]. Studies in mice model revealed that use of anti-CTLA-4 mAbs decreases intramural TREGs and reduces its interaction time with normal T cell and this leads to a more proper interaction between APC and conventional T cell [162, 163]. Due to this, CTLA-4 blockade has been regarded as a potent immuno-therapeutic against a broad spectrum of cancer [164].

As it became clear that CTLA-4 interferes with T-cell activity, its blocking agent emerged as a promising "adjuvant" candidate to use along with therapeutic cancer vaccination. This approach has shown good results with DNA vaccine [165]. *Ipilimumab* is an anti-CTLA-4 human mAb included in phase 3 trial alone or with gp100 peptide vaccine, and results showed that the survival of ipilimumab-receiving patients was better than peptide vaccine where their combination had not exerted any extra benefits [166]. This was a milestone in cancer immunotherapy because no other treatment had shown a significant difference in survival before ipilimumab, but it also revealed that immunotherapy targeting immune checkpoint has a significant effect on patient survival. These reports clearly suggest that once immune checkpoint is blocked, the anti-tumour immune response can last long and these agents do not target tumour but instead of that they modulate the patient's immune system to control tumour development. The use of ipilimumab introduced a new type of side effects known as immune-related adverse events (irAEs), and they arise due to uninhibited immune response [167]. This irAE can occur in any organ, but some particular organs like the spleen are more susceptible; however, the good thing is that it is manageable without altering the anti-tumour effects of the treatment and most of the irAEs are reversible. Endocrinopathies like hypophysitis and thyroiditis caused by irAEs are managed by chronic hormone replacement. It is of uttermost importance to develop unique response kinetics of ipilimumab for every patient and design immune-related response criteria (irRC) accordingly [168]. This irRC is important to decide the duration of the therapy. In 2011, the Food and Drug Administration (FDA) approved ipilimumab or its combination with nivolumab (discussed later) as an immunotherapy drug in metastatic colorectal cancer patients who have gone through standard chemotherapy regimens previously. This immunotherapy is allowed in patients over 12 years of age whose tumours have any one from two genetic markers either mismatch repair deficiency (dMMR) or high microsatellite instability (MSI-H) because their presence is associated with high rates of DNA mutation which subsequently leads to the generation of various tumour-related neo-antigens that can be targeted by immune cells [169].

B. *PD-1 axis targeting mAbs as cancer immuno-therapeutics:* PD-1 is another inhibitory receptor expressed on T cells with its ligands; PD-L1 and PD-L2 are expressed in response to IFN-γ on the surface of APCs and tumour cells. It has been proven that PD-1 ligation inhibits downstream signalling of the TCR and its ligand present on malignant cells has the potential to induce T-cell suppression [170, 171]. Two anti-PD-1 mAbs, *pembrolizumab* and *nivolumab*, have shown a 40% positive response in advanced-stage melanoma patients and are subsequently approved by FDA in 2014, and its combination was approved in 2015 on the basis of phase 3 data [99]. Since PDL-1 can bind both PD-1 and CD80 present on T cell, the effect of anti-PD-1- or anti-PDL-1-based immunotherapeutics may differ. It is evident that anti-PDL-1-based therapy has an advantage over anti-PD-1-based immuno-therapeutic because use of anti-PDL-1 will block both PD-1- and CD80-mediated pathway, while anti-PD-1 treatment can only block PD-1-mediated signal transduction [172, 173]. Simultaneous use of CTLA-4 and anti-PD-1 as a combination therapy has shown great promises. This combination treatment regimen has an overall 58% response rate with 11.5% complete response rate in phase 3 trial with late-stage melanoma [174]. Although toxicity is associated with PD-1-based immunotherapies too, it is less serious than CTLA-4-associated toxicity, and it can be managed through corticosteroid intervention and by stopping anti-PD-1 treatment at the appropriate time [174] (Fig. 14.6).

C. *Lymphocyte-activation gene 3 (LAG-3), an immunosuppressive receptor as a target for immunotherapy:* LAG-3 present on activated conventional T cells, Treg cells, B cells and plasmacytoid dendritic cells transmits an inhibitory signal which binds with MHC-II of APCs and supports Treg cells in their suppressive functions [99, 175]. It has been observed that simultaneous expression of LAG-3 and PD-1 on the surface of T cells is associated with T-cell anergy [99, 176]. Due to this exact reason, anti-PD-1 and anti-LAG-3 in combination have shown additive anti-tumour activity [177]. Various studies funded by the National Cancer Institute of NIH on the effect of anti-LAG-3 mAb relatlimab (BMS-986016) alone or in combination with nivolumab on cancer and especially on colon cancer are in advance stage with lots of promise [178].

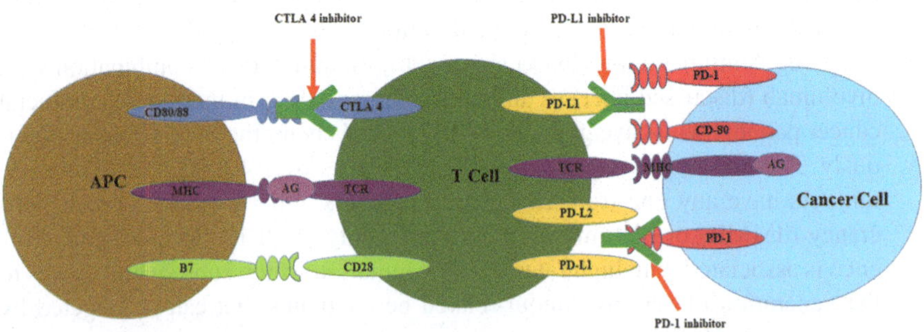

Fig. 14.6 A diagrammatic representation of various immune checkpoint interactions and their blockade through specific monoclonal antibody

D. *T-cell membrane protein 3 (TIM-3) as a target for cancer immunotherapy:* Another T-cell exhaustion-associated inhibitory receptor is T-cell membrane protein-3 (TIM-3) which induces apoptosis in T cells. TIM-3 is generally expressed on Th1 subset of T cells and not expressed on Th2 cells [179]. There are four natural ligands, galectin-9, CEACAM-1, phosphatidylserine and HMGB1, for the TIM-3 receptor which have been reported [99]. Studies have highlighted the various critical roles played by TIM-3-mediated pathway in colon cancer development. Colon cancer development is related with overexpression of TIM-3. It has been observed in the colon cancer mouse model that TIM-3 blockage results in anti-tumour activity. These reports also suggested that tumour volume and stage are associated with the number of Tim-3+ γδ T cell in colon cancer patients. These Tim-3+ γδ T cells (Vγ9Vδ2 T cells) are important for tumour control as they kill tumour cells by releasing perforin/granzyme B. This anti-tumour activity is mediated through ERK1/2 pathway. These activities of Vγ9Vδ2 T cells were reported to be inhibited by TIM-3 overexpression [180]. It has been also reported that immuno-therapeutics targeting TIM-3 enhance CD8+ T-cell-mediated anti-melanoma activity.
E. *T-cell immuno-receptor with immunoglobulin and ITIM domains (TIGIT):* TIGIT is expressed on CD4+ T cells and is a marker of exhausted cytotoxic cells. Anti-tumour activity has been observed with TIGIT blockade in animal in combination with anti-TIM-3 or anti-PD-1 mAbs, and this had not shown any addition in toxicity associated with these drugs which clearly suggests its potential role in anti-tumour immunotherapy. It has been reported that aspirin has exerted its protective effect through TIGIT-CD155 pathway [181–183].

14.2.2.3 Monoclonal Antibodies for T-Cell Co-stimulation in Colon Cancer Immunotherapy

After substantial proof for anti-tumour response generation by inhibitory T-cell receptor blockage, now the emphasis has been given to explore the anti-cancer potential of co-stimulatory T-cell receptor activation. After the binding of TCR with peptide containing MHC of APCs, these co-stimulatory receptors bind their respective ligands present on the surface of APC which generates the secondary signal that subsequently activates T cell. Following are some important co-stimulatory proteins which have an immuno-therapeutic potential for colon cancer.

A. *T-cell antigen 4-1BB homologue (4-1BB) targeting:* It has been well documented that T-cell activation needs two signals, one through TCR and another through co-stimulatory signal. The CD28:B7-mediated co-stimulatory pathway is the principal pathway responsible for T-cell activation, but a number of other pathways have been also studied and reported which actually amplifies the primary signal [99]. Recently described 4-1BB and its ligands are involved in such amplification mechanism. The 4-1BB (CD137) belongs to the TNF receptor family expressed on various effector immune cells and has a role in immune response persistence along with the generation of immunological memory [184, 185]. 4-1BB binding with its ligand 4-1BBL supports T-cell division and avoids T-cell anergy [185]. This 4-1BB-mediated binding induces apoptosis inhibitory proteins like CASP8, Bcl-2-like protein 1, Bcl-2-related protein A1 (Bfl-1) and FADD-like apoptosis regulator. The immuno-therapeutics designed on the basis of 4-1-BB-mediated pathway have shown anti-tumour activity [186–188]. The CTLs specific against tumour get activated by the introduction of urelumab, a fully human agonist of anti-4-1BB [184]. Although solo use of urelumab had been suspended due to an instance of severe hepatotoxicity, combination therapy with other anti-tumour mAbs like rituximab or cetuximab has been reported to boost the anti-tumour activity. This combination therapy also induces NK cells for increased anti-tumour activities [189, 190].

B. *Glucocorticoid-induced TNFR-related protein (GITR):* Another important T-cell activation co-stimulatory signal comes from glucocorticoid-induced TNFR-related protein (GITR)-mediated signal transduction [191]. T-regulatory cells constitutively expressed this receptor, and its up-regulation occurs during the activation of T cells [191]. GITR activation results in the inhibition of Tregs-mediated immunosuppression, release of pro-inflammatory cytokines and T-cell proliferation [192–194]. In the case of colorectal cancer, fibrosarcoma and melanoma, treatment with anti-GITR resulted in tumour-specific immuno-memory development in syngeneic mouse models [195–197]. GITR ligation does not allow Treg cells' lineage to be established and by so doing blocks Treg-mediated inhibition of T-cell effector functions [198]. Many different treatment regimen bases on anti-GITR approaches are at various stages of the clinical trials covering a wide cancer spectrum [199].

C. *CD40:* CD40 is a class of TNF receptor which is mainly expressed on B cells, dendritic cells, monocytes and macrophages [200]. In addition to these immune cells, tumour cells also express these receptors. The ligand for CD40 is CD40L which has been expressed by CD4+ T cells, and subsequent binding of CD40 of APCs with its ligand induces T-cell activation [201]. This binding induces APCs to increase the expression of MHC class II and to secrete pro-inflammatory cytokines like IL-12. This CD40-mediated signalling is important for antibody class switching in B cells. Although mAbs that target CD40 on tumour cells have therapeutic values, the mAb which is CD40 agonist can induce anti-tumour activity in normal B cells and so have wider applications [202–205]. It has been shown that in colon cancer CD40 expression gets uplifting and SW48 colon cancer cell apoptosis can be achieved by the transfection of CD40L-expressing gene [206].

D. *CD134:* CD134 or OX40 is a tumour necrosis factor ligand superfamily member 4 expressed on T cells', NK cells' and neutrophils' surface with various immune cells, viz. APCs express its ligand, OX40L [207]. When the OX40 present on T cells' surface interacts with its ligand, it induces proliferation and Th1/Th2-associated cytokine release [208, 209]. The effect of CD40-mediated pathways is also evident in blocking the suppressive effect of Tregs by inducing activation-associated cell death [210]. Recent study has shown that the activation of CD40 by binding with its ligand resulted in an anti-malignant activity through CD4+ and CD8+ T cells and the generation of immunological memory which prevents the re-emergence of tumour [211]. The correlation between the survival of colon cancer patients and the number of OX-40-positive lymphocytes is reported which strongly suggests that there is an immuno-therapeutic potential in OX40 [212]. Observation of various phase 1 trials clearly indicated that an agonist mAb targeting OX40 introduced as a monotherapy induces anti-tumour activity in melanoma and colon cancer [213, 214]. Currently, many clinical trials are in progress to explore the anti-tumour potential of OX40 agonists in combination with other mAbs against a broad range of cancer type [215, 216].

Checkpoint blockade plus co-stimulation of effector T-cell function is an appealing anti-tumour approach in which enhancing the T-cell activity by mAbs and simultaneous blocking of PD-1 or PD-L1 result in tumour cell lysis [99]. Several anti-cancer investigations with this bi-factorial approach are on-going with the anticipation of developing a new therapeutic or improving the current immuno-therapeutic effectiveness [216–219].

14.3 Conclusion

The designing of colon cancer immuno-therapeutics has been based upon the identification of colon tumour-specific antigens in addition to general TAAs. The immuno-therapeutic approach against colon cancer is and should be flexible to be used in conjunction with standard chemotherapies with little side effects. For sustained anti-tumour activity in colon cancer, it is important to develop and evaluate various combinations of different antibodies and OV-based immuno-therapeutics with no or little side effects. Although immuno-therapeutic-based treatment regimens have tremendous potential, there is a need of caution. If one is targeting checkpoint inhibitors as his or her target for immuno-therapeutic, then he/she should be aware of the exact level of inhibition required by each individual patient. As immuno-therapeutics involve the host immune system in one way or another for cancer cures, patient-specific customization of dose and duration of treatment will be essential. The other major important factor important for the success of any immuno-therapeutics is the identification of a biomarker associated with the response of a particular therapy in patient. It will help in the identification of tumour patients who are responsive to certain immuno-therapeutics but non-responding to another. Although lots of progress have been made in cancer immuno-therapeutic and many of such therapeutic agent are in clinical or preclinical phase of their testing, still studies and researches are needed to fine-tune this wonderful treatment modality for cancer.

References

1. Fleming M, Ravula S, Tatishchev SF, Wang HL. Colorectal carcinoma: pathologic aspects. J Gastrointest Oncol. 2012;3(3):153.
2. Colditz GA, Wolin KY, Gehlert S. Applying what we know to accelerate cancer prevention. Sci Transl Med. 2012;4(127):127rv4.
3. Chu, K. M. (2011). Epidemiology and risk factors of colorectal cancer. Early Diagnosis and Treatment of Cancer Series: Colorectal Cancer, 1–11.
4. Parsyan, A., Robichaud, N., & Meterissian, S. (2014). Colorectal Cancers. In Translation and Its Regulation in Cancer Biology and Medicine (pp. 593-610). Springer, Dordrecht.
5. Souglakos J, Androulakis N, Syrigos K, Polyzos A, Ziras N, Athanasiadis A, et al. FOLFOXIRI (folinic acid, 5-fluorouracil, oxaliplatin and irinotecan) vs FOLFIRI (folinic acid, 5-fluorouracil and irinotecan) as first-line treatment in metastatic colorectal cancer (MCC): a multicentre randomised phase III trial from the Hellenic Oncology Research Group (HORG). Br J Cancer. 2006;94(6):798–805.
6. Smyth MJ, Dunn GP, Schreiber RD. Cancer immunosurveillance and immunoediting: the roles of immunity in suppressing tumor development and shaping tumor immunogenicity. Adv Immunol. 2006;90:1–50.
7. Zipfel C. Early molecular events in PAMP-triggered immunity. Curr Opin Plant Biol. 2009;12(4):414–20.
8. Fodde R, Smits R, Clevers H. APC, signal transduction and genetic instability in colorectal cancer. Nat Rev Cancer. 2001;1(1):55–67.
9. Tseng SY, Dustin ML. T-cell activation: a multidimensional signaling network. Curr Opin Cell Biol. 2002;14(5):575–80.
10. Vasilevko V, Ghochikyan A, Holterman MJ, Agadjanyan MG. CD80 (B7-1) and CD86 (B7-2) are functionally equivalent in the initiation and maintenance of CD4+ T-cell proliferation after activation with suboptimal doses of PHA. DNA Cell Biol. 2002;21(3):137–49.
11. Line A, Slucka Z, Stengrevics A, Silina K, Li G, Rees RC. Characterisation of tumour-associated antigens in colon cancer. Cancer Immunol Immunother. 2002;51(10):574–82.
12. Minev BR. Melanoma vaccines. In: Seminars in oncology, vol. 29, No. 5: WB Saunders; 2002. p. 479–93. Philadelphia, USA.
13. Schooten E, Di Maggio A, en Henegouwen PMVB, Kijanka MM. MAGE-A antigens as targets for cancer immunotherapy. Cancer Treat Rev. 2018;67:54–62.
14. Djaldetti M, Bessler H. Modulators affecting the immune dialogue between human immune and colon cancer cells. World J Gastrointest Oncol. 2014;6(5):129.
15. Atkins D, Breuckmann A, Schmahl GE, Binner P, Ferrone S, Krummenauer F, Störkel S, Seliger B. MHC class I antigen processing pathway defects, ras mutations and disease stage in colorectal carcinoma. Int J Cancer. 2004;109(2):265–73.
16. Mielczarek M, Chrzanowska A, Ścibior D, Skwarek A, Ashamiss F, Lewandowska K, Barańczyk-Kuźma A. Arginase as a useful factor for the diagnosis of colorectal cancer liver metastases. Int J Biol Markers. 2006;21:40.
17. Rao CV. Nitric oxide signaling in colon cancer chemoprevention. Mut Res/Fundamental and Molecular Mechanisms of Mutagenesis. 2004;555(1-2):107–19.
18. Bei R, Scardino A. TAA polyepitope DNA-based vaccines: a potential tool for cancer therapy. Biomed Res Int. 2010;2010:Article ID 102758.
19. Brody JD, Engleman EG. DC-based cancer vaccines: lessons from clinical trials. Cytotherapy. 2004;6(2):122–7.
20. Chen X, Chang CH, Goldenberg DM. Novel strategies for improved cancer vaccines. Expert Rev Vaccines. 2009;8(5):567–76.
21. Vergati M, Intrivici C, Huen NY, Schlom J, Tsang KY. Strategies for cancer vaccine development. Biomed Res Int. 2010;2010:Article ID 596432.

22. Ferri M, Del Monte SR, Salerno G, Bocchetti T, Angeletti S, Malisan F, et al. Recovery of immunological homeostasis positively correlates both with early stages of right-colorectal cancer and laparoscopic surgery. PLoS One. 2013;8(9):e74455.
23. Hong S, Hwang I, Lee YS, Park S, Lee WK, Fernandes-Alnemri T, et al. Restoration of ASC expression sensitizes colorectal cancer cells to genotoxic stress-induced caspase-independent cell death. Cancer Lett. 2013;331(2):183–91.
24. Terzić J, Grivennikov S, Karin E, Karin M. Inflammation and colon cancer. Gastroenterology. 2010;138(6):2101–14.
25. Maeda K, Hazama S, Tokuno K, Kan S, Maeda Y, Watanabe Y, et al. Impact of chemotherapy for colorectal cancer on regulatory T-cells and tumor immunity. Anticancer Res. 2011;31(12):4569–74.
26. Galon J, Fridman WH, Pagès F. The adaptive immunologic microenvironment in colorectal cancer: a novel perspective. Cancer Res. 2007;67(5):1883–6.
27. Arens R, van Hall T, van der Burg SH, Ossendorp F, Melief CJ. Prospects of combinatorial synthetic peptide vaccine-based immunotherapy against cancer. In: Seminars in immunology, vol. 25, No. 2: Academic Press; 2013. p. 182–90. Philadelphia, USA.
28. Noguchi M, Sasada T, Itoh K. Personalized peptide vaccination: a new approach for advanced cancer as therapeutic cancer vaccine. Cancer Immunol Immunother. 2013;62(5):919–29.
29. Villa-Morales M, Fernández-Piqueras J. Targeting the Fas/FasL signaling pathway in cancer therapy. Expert Opin Ther Targets. 2012;16(1):85–101.
30. Fong L, Hou Y, Rivas A, Benike C, Yuen A, Fisher GA, et al. Altered peptide ligand vaccination with Flt3 ligand expanded dendritic cells for tumor immunotherapy. Proc Natl Acad Sci. 2001;98(15):8809–14.
31. Katsara M, Minigo G, Plebanski M, Apostolopoulos V. The good, the bad and the ugly: how altered peptide ligands modulate immunity. Expert Opin Biol Ther. 2008;8(12):1873–84.
32. Locy H, De Mey S, De Mey W, De Ridder M, Thielemans K, Maenhout SK. Immunomodulation of the tumor microenvironment: turn foe into friend. Front Immunol. 2018;9:2909.
33. Nair SK, Snyder D, Rouse BT, Gilboa E. Regression of tumors in mice vaccinated with professional antigen-presenting cells pulsed with tumor extracts. Int J Cancer. 1997;70(6):706–18.
34. Seliger B, Maeurer MJ, Ferrone S. Antigen-processing machinery breakdown and tumor growth. Immunol Today. 2000;21(9):455–64.
35. Evans C, Dalgleish AG, Kumar D. Immune suppression and colorectal cancer. Aliment Pharmacol Ther. 2006;24(8):1163–77.
36. Merika E, Saif MW, Katz A, Syrigos C, Morse M. Colon cancer vaccines: an update. In Vivo. 2010;24(5):607–28.
37. Roovers RC, Van der Linden E, de Bruïne AP, Arends JW, Hoogenboom HR. Identification of colon tumour-associated antigens by phage antibody selections on primary colorectal carcinoma. Eur J Cancer. 2001;37(4):542–9.
38. Bonertz A, Weitz J, Pietsch DHK, Rahbari NN, Schlude C, Ge Y, et al. Antigen-specific Tregs control T cell responses against a limited repertoire of tumor antigens in patients with colorectal carcinoma. J Clin Invest. 2009;119(11):3311–21.
39. Jameson SC, Masopust D. Understanding subset diversity in T cell memory. Immunity. 2018;48(2):214–26.
40. Durgeau A, Virk Y, Corgnac S, Mami-Chouaib F. Recent advances in targeting CD8 T-cell immunity for more effective cancer immunotherapy. Front Immunol. 2018;9:14.
41. Hotakainen K, Ljungberg B, Paju A, Rasmuson T, Alfthan H, Stenman UH. The free β-subunit of human chorionic gonadotropin as a prognostic factor in renal cell carcinoma. Br J Cancer. 2002;86(2):185–9.
42. Li J, Yin M, Song W, Cui F, Wang W, Wang S, Zhu H. B subunit of human chorionic gonadotropin promotes tumor invasion and predicts poor prognosis of early-stage colorectal cancer. Cell Physiol Biochem. 2018;45(1):237–49.
43. Arora SP, Mahalingam D. Immunotherapy in colorectal cancer: for the select few or all? J Gastroint Oncol. 2018;9(1):170.

44. Galat A. Common structural traits for cystine knot domain of the TGFβ superfamily of proteins and three-fingered ectodomain of their cellular receptors. Cell Mol Life Sci. 2011;68(20):3437–51.
45. Moulton HM, Yoshihara PH, Mason DH, Iversen PL, Triozzi PL. Active specific immunotherapy with a β-human chorionic gonadotropin peptide vaccine in patients with metastatic colorectal cancer: antibody response is associated with improved survival. Clin Cancer Res. 2002;8(7):2044–51.
46. Tsuruma T, Hata F, Furuhata T, Ohmura T, Katsuramaki T, Yamaguchi K, et al. Peptide-based vaccination for colorectal cancer. Expert Opin Biol Ther. 2005;5(6):799–807.
47. Dlamini Z, Khoza T, Hull R, Choene M, Mkhize-Kwitshana Z. Current immunotherapeutic treatments in colon cancer. Colorectal cancer: from pathogenesis to treatment. Colorectal Cancer. 2016:211.
48. Margalit O, Mamtani R, Yang YX, Reiss KA, Golan T, Halpern N, et al. Assessing the prognostic value of carcinoembryonic antigen levels in stage I and II colon cancer. Eur J Cancer. 2018;94:1–5.
49. Campos-da-Paz M, Dórea JG, Galdino AS, Lacava ZG, de Fatima Menezes Almeida Santos M. Carcinoembryonic antigen (CEA) and hepatic metastasis in colorectal cancer: update on biomarker for clinical and biotechnological approaches. Recent Pat Biotechnol. 2018;12(4):269–79.
50. Ojima T, Iwahashi M, Nakamura M, Matsuda K, Nakamori M, Ueda K, et al. Successful cancer vaccine therapy for carcinoembryonic antigen (CEA)-expressing colon cancer using genetically modified dendritic cells that express CEA and T helper-type 1 cytokines in CEA transgenic mice. Int J Cancer. 2007;120(3):585–93.
51. Naveed A, Rahman SU, Arshad MI, Aslam B. Recapitulation of the anti-idiotype antibodies as vaccine candidate. Transl Med Commun. 2018;3(1):1.
52. Codd AS, Kanaseki T, Torigo T, Tabi Z. Cancer stem cells as targets for immunotherapy. Immunology. 2018;153(3):304–14.
53. Bashir B, Snook AE. Immunotherapy regimens for metastatic colorectal carcinomas. Hum Vaccin Immunother. 2018;14(2):250–4.
54. Harrop R, Connolly N, Redchenko I, Valle J, Saunders M, Ryan MG, et al. Vaccination of colorectal cancer patients with modified vaccinia Ankara delivering the tumor antigen 5T4 (TroVax) induces immune responses which correlate with disease control: a phase I/II trial. Clin Cancer Res. 2006;12(11):3416–24.
55. Zhang RT, Bines SD, Ruby C, Kaufman HL. TroVax® vaccine therapy for renal cell carcinoma. Immunotherapy. 2012;4(1):27–42.
56. Comeau JM, Labruzzo MB. From bench to bedside: promising colon cancer clinical trials. Am J Manag Care. 2013;19(1 Spec No):SP32.
57. Song LJ, Liu RJ, Zeng Z, Alper SL, Cui HJ, Lu Y, et al. Gastrin inhibits a novel, pathological colon cancer signaling pathway involving EGR1, AE2, and P-ERK. J Mol Med. 2012;90(6):707–18.
58. Raghav K, Bailey AM, Loree JM, Kopetz S, Holla V, Yap TA, et al. Untying the gordion knot of targeting MET in cancer. Cancer Treat Rev. 2018;66:95–103.
59. Senzer N, Barve M, Kuhn J, Melnyk A, Beitsch P, Lazar M, et al. Phase I trial of "bi-shRNAifurin/GMCSF DNA/autologous tumor cell" vaccine (FANG) in advanced cancer. Mol Ther. 2012;20(3):679–86.
60. Kelly E, Russell SJ. History of oncolytic viruses: genesis to genetic engineering. Mol Ther. 2007;15(4):651–9.
61. Xiang B, Snook AE, Magee MS, Waldman SA. Colorectal cancer immunotherapy. Discov Med. 2013;15(84):301.
62. Lindenmann J, Klein PA. Viral oncolysis: increased immunogenicity of host cell antigen associated with influenza virus. J Exp Med. 1967;126(1):93–108.
63. Winter H, Fox BA, Rüttinger D. Future of cancer vaccines. In: Cancer Vaccines. New York: Humana Press; 2014. p. 555–64.

64. Cheever MA, Higano CS. PROVENGE (Sipuleucel-T) in prostate cancer: the first FDA-approved therapeutic cancer vaccine. Clin Cancer Res. 2011;17(11):3520–6.
65. Raja J, Ludwig JM, Gettinger SN, Schalper KA, Kim HS. Oncolytic virus immunotherapy: future prospects for oncology. J Immunother Cancer. 2018;6(1):140.
66. Tang J, Pearce L, O'Donnell-Tormey J, Hubbard-Lucey VM. Trends in the global immuno-oncology landscape. Nat Rev Drug Discov. 2018;17:783.
67. Rosewell Shaw A, Suzuki M. Oncolytic viruses partner with T-cell therapy for solid tumor treatment. Front Immunol. 2018;9:2103.
68. Jing Y, Chavez V, Khatwani NK, Merchan J. Antitumor efficacy of a dual stromal and tumor targeted oncolytic measles virus in breast and colon cancer models. Cancer Res. 2018;78:5920.
69. Twumasi-Boateng K, Pettigrew JL, Kwok YE, Bell JC, Nelson BH. Oncolytic viruses as engineering platforms for combination immunotherapy. Nat Rev Cancer. 2018;18(7):419–32.
70. Toda M, Martuza RL, Kojima H, Rabkin SD. In situ cancer vaccination: an IL-12 defective vector/replication-competent herpes simplex virus combination induces local and systemic antitumor activity. J Immunol. 1998;160(9):4457–64.
71. Toda M, Rabkin SD, Kojima H, Martuza RL. Herpes simplex virus as an in situ cancer vaccine for the induction of specific anti-tumor immunity. Hum Gene Ther. 1999;10(3):385–93.
72. Bauzon M, Hermiston T. Armed therapeutic viruses–a disruptive therapy on the horizon of cancer immunotherapy. Front Immunol. 2014;5:74.
73. Chiocca EA. Oncolytic viruses. Nat Rev Cancer. 2002;2(12):938–50.
74. Bommareddy PK, Shettigar M, Kaufman HL. Integrating oncolytic viruses in combination cancer immunotherapy. Nat Rev Immunol. 2018;18(8):498–513.
75. Marelli G, Howells A, Lemoine NR, Wang Y. Oncolytic viral therapy and the immune system: a double-edged sword against cancer. Front Immunol. 2018;9:866.
76. Struzik J, Szulc-Dąbrowska L. NF-κB signaling in targeting tumor cells by oncolytic viruses—therapeutic perspectives. Cancers. 2018;10(11):426.
77. Jamal M, Oglu A. Review of the basis for oncolytic virotherapy and development of the genetically modified tumor-specific viruses. MedBioTech J. 2018;2(03):95–102.
78. Yamaguchi T, Uchida E. Oncolytic virus: regulatory aspects from quality control to clinical studies. Curr Cancer Drug Targets. 2018;18(2):202–8.
79. Saini J, Sharma PK. Clinical, prognostic and therapeutic significance of heat shock proteins in cancer. Curr Drug Targets. 2018;19(13):1478–90.
80. Nylandsted J, Brand K, Jäättelä M. Heat shock protein 70 is required for the survival of cancer cells. Ann N Y Acad Sci. 2000;926(1):122–5.
81. Olotu F, Adeniji E, Agoni C, Bjij I, Khan S, Elrashedy A, Soliman M. An update on the discovery and development of selective heat shock protein inhibitors as anti-cancer therapy. Expert Opin Drug Discovery. 2018;13(10):903–18.
82. Kelly M, McNeel D, Fisch P, Malkóvsky M. Immunological considerations underlying heat shock protein-mediated cancer vaccine strategies. Immunol Lett. 2018;193:1–10.
83. Wang X, Wang Q, Lin H, Li S, Sun L, Yang Y. HSP72 and gp96 in gastroenterological cancers. Clin Chim Acta. 2013;417:73–9.
84. Li Z, Menoret A, Srivastava P. Roles of heat-shock proteins in antigen presentation and cross-presentation. Curr Opin Immunol. 2002;14(1):45–51.
85. Murshid A, Gong J, Calderwood SK. The role of heat shock proteins in antigen cross presentation. Front Immunol. 2012;3:63.
86. Shevtsov M, Multhoff G. Heat shock protein–peptide and HSP-based immunotherapies for the treatment of cancer. Front Immunol. 2016;7:171.
87. Huang C, Zhao J, Li Z, Li D, Xia D, Wang Q, Jin H. Multi-chaperone-peptide-rich mixture from colo-carcinoma cells elicits potent anticancer immunity. Cancer Epidemiol. 2010;34(4):494–500.
88. Liu B, Ye D, Song X, Zhao X, Yi L, Song J, et al. A novel therapeutic fusion protein vaccine by two different families of heat shock proteins linked with HPV16 E7 generates potent antitumor immunity and antiangiogenesis. Vaccine. 2008;26(10):1387–96.

89. Jensen-Jarolim E, Bax HJ, Bianchini R, Crescioli S, Daniels-Wells TR, Dombrowicz D, et al. AllergoOncology: opposite outcomes of immune tolerance in allergy and cancer. Allergy. 2018;73(2):328–40.
90. Nurgali K, Jagoe RT, Abalo R. Adverse effects of cancer chemotherapy: anything new to improve tolerance and reduce sequelae? Front Pharmacol. 2018;9:245.
91. Kroschinsky F, Stölzel F, von Bonin S, Beutel G, Kochanek M, Kiehl M, Schellongowski P. New drugs, new toxicities: severe side effects of modern targeted and immunotherapy of cancer and their management. Crit Care. 2017;21(1):89.
92. Graham K, Unger E. Overcoming tumor hypoxia as a barrier to radiotherapy, chemotherapy and immunotherapy in cancer treatment. Int J Nanomedicine. 2018;13:6049.
93. Zhang H, Chen J. Current status and future directions of cancer immunotherapy. J Cancer. 2018;9(10):1773.
94. June CH, O'Connor RS, Kawalekar OU, Ghassemi S, Milone MC. CAR T cell immunotherapy for human cancer. Science. 2018;359(6382):1361–5.
95. Ruella M, Kalos M. Adoptive immunotherapy for cancer. Immunol Rev. 2014;257(1):14–38.
96. Dalerba P, Maccalli C, Casati C, Castelli C, Parmiani G. Immunology and immunotherapy of colorectal cancer. Crit Rev Oncol Hematol. 2003;46(1):33–57.
97. Kang CW, Dutta A, Chang LY, Mahalingam J, Lin YC, Chiang JM, et al. Apoptosis of tumor infiltrating effector TIM-3+ CD8+ T cells in colon cancer. Sci Rep. 2015;5(1):1–12.
98. Delorme EJ, Alexander P. Treatment of primary fibrosarcoma in the rat with immune lymphocytes. Lancet. 1964;284(7351):117–20.
99. Khalil DN, Smith EL, Brentjens RJ, Wolchok JD. The future of cancer treatment: immunomodulation, CARs and combination immunotherapy. Nat Rev Clin Oncol. 2016;13(5):273.
100. Rosenberg SA, Lotze MT, Muul LM, Leitman S, Chang AE, Ettinghausen SE, et al. Observations on the systemic administration of autologous lymphokine-activated killer cells and recombinant interleukin-2 to patients with metastatic cancer. N Engl J Med. 1985;313(23):1485–92.
101. Restifo NP, Dudley ME, Rosenberg SA. Adoptive immunotherapy for cancer: harnessing the T cell response. Nat Rev Immunol. 2012;12(4):269–81.
102. Baggio L, Laureano ÁM, da Rocha Silla LM, Lee DA. Natural killer cell adoptive immunotherapy: coming of age. Clin Immunol. 2017;177:3–11.
103. Shimabukuro-Vornhagen A, Gödel P, Subklewe M, Stemmler HJ, Schlößer HA, Schlaak M, et al. Cytokine release syndrome. J Immunother Cancer. 2018;6(1):56.
104. Waldmann TA. Cytokines in cancer immunotherapy. Cold Spring Harb Perspect Biol. 2018;10(12):a028472.
105. Berraondo P, Sanmamed MF, Ochoa MC, Etxeberria I, Aznar MA, Pérez-Gracia JL, et al. Cytokines in clinical cancer immunotherapy. Br J Cancer. 2019;120(1):6–15.
106. Wagner S, Mullins CS, Linnebacher M. Colorectal cancer vaccines: tumor-associated antigens vs neoantigens. World J Gastroenterol. 2018;24(48):5418.
107. Klampfer L. Cytokines, inflammation and colon cancer. Curr Cancer Drug Targets. 2011;11(4):451–64.
108. Han SY, Choung SY, Paik IS, Kang HJ, Choi YH, KIM SJ, Lee MO. Activation of NF-κB determines the sensitivity of human colon cancer cells to TNFα-induced apoptosis. Biol Pharm Bull. 2000;23(4):420–6.
109. Kaler P, Augenlicht L, Klampfer L. Macrophage-derived IL-1β stimulates Wnt signaling and growth of colon cancer cells: a crosstalk interrupted by vitamin D 3. Oncogene. 2009;28(44):3892–902.
110. Voronov E, Dotan S, Krelin Y, Song X, Elkabets M, Carmi Y, et al. Unique versus redundant functions of IL-1α and IL-1β in the tumor microenvironment. Front Immunol. 2013;4:177.
111. Li Y, Wang L, Pappan L, Galliher-Beckley A, Shi J. IL-1β promotes stemness and invasiveness of colon cancer cells through Zeb1 activation. Mol Cancer. 2012;11(1):87.
112. Myint ZW, Goel G. Role of modern immunotherapy in gastrointestinal malignancies: a review of current clinical progress. J Hematol Oncol. 2017;10(1):86.

113. Kurzrock R, Hickish T, Wyrwicz L, Saunders M, Wu Q, Stecher M, et al. Interleukin-1 receptor antagonist levels predict favorable outcome after bermekimab, a first-in-class true human interleukin-1α antibody, in a phase III randomized study of advanced colorectal cancer. Onco Targets Ther. 2019;8(3):1551651.
114. Bromberg J, Wang TC. Inflammation and cancer: IL-6 and STAT3 complete the link. Cancer Cell. 2009;15(2):79–80.
115. Li YY, Hsieh LL, Tang RP, Liao SK, Yeh KY. Interleukin-6 (IL-6) released by macrophages induces IL-6 secretion in the human colon cancer HT-29 cell line. Hum Immunol. 2009;70(3):151–8.
116. Jones SA, Scheller J, Rose-John S. Therapeutic strategies for the clinical blockade of IL-6/gp130 signaling. J Clin Invest. 2011;121(9):3375–83.
117. Waldner MJ, Foersch S, Neurath MF. Interleukin-6-a key regulator of colorectal cancer development. Int J Biol Sci. 2012;8(9):1248.
118. Amit A, Dikhit MR, Singh AK, Kumar V, Suman SS, Singh A, et al. Immunization with Leishmania donovani protein disulfide isomerase DNA construct induces Th1 and Th17 dependent immune response and protection against experimental visceral leishmaniasis in Balb/c mice. Mol Immunol. 2017;82:104–13.
119. Knochelmann HM, Dwyer CJ, Bailey SR, Amaya SM, Elston DM, Mazza-McCrann JM, Paulos CM. When worlds collide: Th17 and Treg cells in cancer and autoimmunity. Cell Mol Immunol. 2018;15(5):458–69.
120. Doulabi H, Rastin M, Shabahangh H, Maddah G, Abdollahi A, Nosratabadi R, et al. Analysis of Th22, Th17 and CD4+ cells co-producing IL-17/IL-22 at different stages of human colon cancer. Biomed Pharmacother. 2018;103:1101–6.
121. Ibrahim S, Girault A, Ohresser M, Lereclus E, Paintaud G, Lecomte T, Raoul W. Monoclonal antibodies targeting the IL-17/IL-17RA axis: an opportunity to improve the efficiency of anti-VEGF therapy in fighting metastatic colorectal cancer? Clin Colorectal Cancer. 2018;17(1):e109–13.
122. Mésange P, Poindessous V, Sabbah M, Escargueil AE, de Gramont A, Larsen AK. Intrinsic bevacizumab resistance is associated with prolonged activation of autocrine VEGF signaling and hypoxia tolerance in colorectal cancer cells and can be overcome by nintedanib, a small molecule angiokinase inhibitor. Oncotarget. 2014;5(13):4709.
123. Zhang L, Fang B. Mechanisms of resistance to TRAIL-induced apoptosis in cancer. Cancer Gene Ther. 2005;12(3):228–37.
124. Stuckey DW, Shah K. TRAIL on trial: preclinical advances in cancer therapy. Trends Mol Med. 2013;19(11):685–94.
125. von Karstedt S, Montinaro A, Walczak H. Exploring the TRAILs less travelled: TRAIL in cancer biology and therapy. Nat Rev Cancer. 2017;17(6):352.
126. Françoso A, Simioni PU. Immunotherapy for the treatment of colorectal tumors: focus on approved and in-clinical-trial monoclonal antibodies. Drug Des Devel Ther. 2017;11:177.
127. Kaplon H, Reichert JM. Antibodies to watch in 2019. In: MAbs, vol. 11, No. 2: Taylor & Francis; 2019. p. 219–38. Oxfordshire,UK.
128. Nelson AL, Dhimolea E, Reichert JM. Development trends for human monoclonal antibody therapeutics. Nat Rev Drug Discov. 2010;9(10):767–74.
129. Frenzel A, Schirrmann T, Hust M. Phage display-derived human antibodies in clinical development and therapy. In: MAbs, vol. 8, No. 7: Taylor & Francis; 2016. p. 1177–94. Oxfordshire,UK.
130. Kontermann RE, Brinkmann U. Bispecific antibodies. Drug Discov Today. 2015;20(7):838–47.
131. Krishnamurthy A, Jimeno A. Bispecific antibodies for cancer therapy: a review. Pharmacol Ther. 2018;185:122–34.
132. Sedykh SE, Prinz VV, Buneva VN, Nevinsky GA. Bispecific antibodies: design, therapy, perspectives. Drug Des Devel Ther. 2018;12:195.
133. Chames P, Baty D. Bispecific antibodies for cancer therapy: the light at the end of the tunnel? In: MAbs, vol. 1, No. 6: Taylor & Francis; 2009. p. 539–47. Oxfordshire,UK.

134. Dienstmann R, De Dosso S, Felip E, Tabernero J. Drug development to overcome resistance to EGFR inhibitors in lung and colorectal cancer. Mol Oncol. 2012;6(1):15–26.
135. Nahta R, Esteva FJ. HER2 therapy: molecular mechanisms of trastuzumab resistance. Breast Cancer Res. 2006;8(6):215.
136. Engelman JA, Zejnullahu K, Mitsudomi T, Song Y, Hyland C, Park JO, et al. MET amplification leads to gefitinib resistance in lung cancer by activating ERBB3 signaling. Science. 2007;316(5827):1039–43.
137. Nagorsen D, Kufer P, Baeuerle PA, Bargou R. Blinatumomab: a historical perspective. Pharmacol Ther. 2012;136(3):334–42.
138. Hoffman L, Gore L. Blinatumomab, a bi-specific anti-CD19/CD3 BiTE® antibody for the treatment of acute lymphoblastic leukemia: perspectives and current pediatric applications. Front Oncol. 2014;4:63.
139. Hoffmann P, Hofmeister R, Brischwein K, Brandl C, Crommer S, Bargou R, et al. Serial killing of tumor cells by cytotoxic T cells redirected with a CD19-/CD3-bispecific single-chain antibody construct. Int J Cancer. 2005;115(1):98–104.
140. Fujimoto M, Poe JC, Inaoki M, Tedder TF. CD19 regulates B lymphocyte responses to transmembrane signals. In: Seminars in immunology, vol. 10, No. 4: Academic Press; 1998. p. 267–77. Cambridge,UK.
141. Brandl C, Haas C, d'Argouges S, Fisch T, Kufer P, Brischwein K, et al. The effect of dexamethasone on polyclonal T cell activation and redirected target cell lysis as induced by a CD19/CD3-bispecific single-chain antibody construct. Cancer Immunol Immunother. 2007;56(10):1551–63.
142. Haas C, Krinner E, Brischwein K, Hoffmann P, Lutterbüse R, Schlereth B, et al. Mode of cytotoxic action of T cell-engaging BiTE antibody MT110. Immunobiology. 2009;214(6):441–53.
143. Vilgelm AE, Johnson DB, Richmond A. Combinatorial approach to cancer immunotherapy: strength in numbers. J Leukoc Biol. 2016;100(2):275–90.
144. Bootz F, Neri D. Immunocytokines: a novel class of products for the treatment of chronic inflammation and autoimmune conditions. Drug Discov Today. 2016;21(1):180–9.
145. Sahin U, Türeci Ö. Personalized vaccines for cancer immunotherapy. Science. 2018;359(6382):1355–60.
146. Sproston NR, Ashworth JJ. Role of C-reactive protein at sites of inflammation and infection. Front Immunol. 2018;9:754.
147. Darvin P, Toor SM, Nair VS, Elkord E. Immune checkpoint inhibitors: recent progress and potential biomarkers. Exp Mol Med. 2018;50(12):1–11.
148. Bailey AM, Mao Y, Zeng J, Holla V, Johnson A, Brusco L, et al. Implementation of biomarker-driven cancer therapy: existing tools and remaining gaps. Discov Med. 2014;17(92):101.
149. Goel HL, AM M. Mercurio AM VEGF targets the tumour cell. Nat Rev Cancer. 2013;13(12):871–82.
150. Ellis LM, Hicklin DJ. VEGF-targeted therapy: mechanisms of anti-tumour activity. Nat Rev Cancer. 2008;8(8):579–91.
151. Martins SF, Reis RM, Rodrigues AM, Baltazar F, Longatto Filho A. Role of endoglin and VEGF family expression in colorectal cancer prognosis and anti-angiogenic therapies. World J Clin Oncol. 2011;2(6):272.
152. Tol J, Punt CJ. Monoclonal antibodies in the treatment of metastatic colorectal cancer: a review. Clin Ther. 2010;32(3):437–53.
153. Saad RS, Liu YL, Nathan G, Celebrezze J, Medich D, Silverman JF. Endoglin (CD105) and vascular endothelial growth factor as prognostic markers in colorectal cancer. Mod Pathol. 2004;17(2):197–203.
154. Clarke JM, Hurwitz HI. Targeted inhibition of VEGF receptor 2: an update on ramucirumab. Expert Opin Biol Ther. 2013;13(8):1187–96.
155. Saif MW. Anti-VEGF agents in metastatic colorectal cancer (mCRC): are they all alike? Cancer Manag Res. 2013;5:103.

156. Herbst RS. Review of epidermal growth factor receptor biology. Int J Radiat Oncol Biol Phys. 2004;59(2):S21–6.
157. Peeters M, Cohn A, Köhne CH, Douillard JY. Panitumumab in combination with cytotoxic chemotherapy for the treatment of metastatic colorectal carcinoma. Clin Colorectal Cancer. 2012;11(1):14–23.
158. Vale CL, Tierney JF, Fisher D, Adams RA, Kaplan R, Maughan TS, et al. Does anti-EGFR therapy improve outcome in advanced colorectal cancer? A systematic review and meta-analysis. Cancer Treat Rev. 2012;38(6):618–25.
159. You B, Chen EX. Anti-EGFR monoclonal antibodies for treatment of colorectal cancers: development of cetuximab and panitumumab. J Clin Pharmacol. 2012;52(2):128–55.
160. Son CH, Bae JH, Shin DY, Lee HR, Choi YJ, Jo WS, et al. CTLA-4 blockade enhances anti-tumor immunity of intratumoral injection of immature dendritic cells into irradiated tumor in a mouse colon cancer model. J Immunother. 2014;37(1):1–7.
161. Tivol EA, Borriello F, Schweitzer AN, Lynch WP, Bluestone JA, Sharpe AH. Loss of CTLA-4 leads to massive lymphoproliferation and fatal multiorgan tissue destruction, revealing a critical negative regulatory role of CTLA-4. Immunity. 1995;3(5):541–7.
162. Takahashi T, Tagami T, Yamazaki S, Uede T, Shimizu J, Sakaguchi N, et al. Immunologic self-tolerance maintained by CD25+ CD4+ regulatory T cells constitutively expressing cytotoxic T lymphocyte–associated antigen 4. J Exp Med. 2000;192(2):303–10.
163. Read S, Malmström V, Powrie F. Cytotoxic T lymphocyte–associated antigen 4 plays an essential role in the function of CD25+ CD4+ regulatory cells that control intestinal inflammation. J Exp Med. 2000;192(2):295–302.
164. Tanaka A, Sakaguchi S. Regulatory T cells in cancer immunotherapy. Cell Res. 2017;27(1):109–18.
165. Gregor PD, Wolchok JD, Ferrone CR, Buchinshky H, Guevara-Patiño JA, Perales MA, et al. CTLA-4 blockade in combination with xenogeneic DNA vaccines enhances T-cell responses, tumor immunity and autoimmunity to self antigens in animal and cellular model systems. Vaccine. 2004;22(13-14):1700–8.
166. Hodi FS, O'Day SJ, McDermott DF, Weber RW, Sosman JA, Haanen JB, et al. Improved survival with ipilimumab in patients with metastatic melanoma. N Engl J Med. 2010;363(8):711–23.
167. Weber JS, Kähler KC, Hauschild A. Management of immune-related adverse events and kinetics of response with ipilimumab. J Clin Oncol. 2012;30(21):2691–7.
168. Wolchok JD, Hoos A, O'Day S, Weber JS, Hamid O, Lebbé C, et al. Guidelines for the evaluation of immune therapy activity in solid tumors: immune-related response criteria. Clin Cancer Res. 2009;15(23):7412–20.
169. Andre T, Lonardi S, Wong KYM, Morse M, McDermott RS, Hill AG, et al. Combination of nivolumab (nivo)+ ipilimumab (ipi) in the treatment of patients (pts) with deficient DNA mismatch repair (dMMR)/high microsatellite instability (MSI-H) metastatic colorectal cancer (mCRC): CheckMate 142 study. J Clin Oncol. 2017;35(suppl 15):3531a.
170. Chemnitz JM, Parry RV, Nichols KE, June CH, Riley JL. SHP-1 and SHP-2 associate with immunoreceptor tyrosine-based switch motif of programmed death 1 upon primary human T cell stimulation, but only receptor ligation prevents T cell activation. J Immunol. 2004;173(2):945–54.
171. Parry RV, Chemnitz JM, Frauwirth KA, Lanfranco AR, Braunstein I, Kobayashi SV, et al. CTLA-4 and PD-1 receptors inhibit T-cell activation by distinct mechanisms. Mol Cell Biol. 2005;25(21):9543–53.
172. Park JJ, Omiya R, Matsumura Y, Sakoda Y, Kuramasu A, Augustine MM, et al. B7-H1/CD80 interaction is required for the induction and maintenance of peripheral T-cell tolerance. Blood J Am Soc Hematol. 2010;116(8):1291–8.
173. Paterson AM, Brown KE, Keir ME, Vanguri VK, Riella LV, Chandraker A, et al. The programmed death-1 ligand 1: B7-1 pathway restrains diabetogenic effector T cells in vivo. J Immunol. 2011;187(3):1097–105.

174. Larkin J, Chiarion-Sileni V, Gonzalez R, Grob JJ, Cowey CL, Lao CD, et al. Combined nivolumab and ipilimumab or monotherapy in untreated melanoma. N Engl J Med. 2015;373(1):23–34.
175. Huard B, Gaulard P, Faure F, Hercend T, Triebel F. Cellular expression and tissue distribution of the human LAG-3-encoded protein, an MHC class II ligand. Immunogenetics. 1994;39(3):213–7.
176. Blackburn SD, Shin H, Haining WN, Zou T, Workman CJ, Polley A, et al. Coregulation of CD8+ T cell exhaustion by multiple inhibitory receptors during chronic viral infection. Nat Immunol. 2009;10(1):29.
177. Woo SR, Turnis ME, Goldberg MV, Bankoti J, Selby M, Nirschl CJ, et al. Immune inhibitory molecules LAG-3 and PD-1 synergistically regulate T-cell function to promote tumoral immune escape. Cancer Res. 2012;72(4):917–27.
178. Zhou G, Noordam L, Sprengers D, Doukas M, Boor PP, van Beek AA, et al. Blockade of LAG3 enhances responses of tumor-infiltrating T cells in mismatch repair-proficient liver metastases of colorectal cancer. Onco Targets Ther. 2018;7(7):e1448332.
179. He Y, Cao J, Zhao C, Li X, Zhou C, Hirsch FR. TIM-3, a promising target for cancer immunotherapy. Onco Targets Ther. 2018;11:7005.
180. Li X, Lu H, Gu Y, Zhang X, Zhang G, Shi T, Chen W. Tim-3 suppresses the killing effect of Vγ9Vδ2 T cells on colon cancer cells by reducing perforin and granzyme B expression. Exp Cell Res. 2020;386(1):111719.
181. Lozano E, Dominguez-Villar M, Kuchroo V, Hafler DA. The TIGIT/CD226 axis regulates human T cell function. J Immunol. 2012;188(8):3869–75.
182. Kurtulus S, Sakuishi K, Zhang H, Joller N, Tan D, Smyth M, et al. Mechanisms of TIGIT-driven immune suppression in cancer. J Immunother Cancer. 2014;2(S3):O13.
183. Ma B, Duan X, Zhou Q, Liu J, Yang X, Zhang D, et al. Use of aspirin in the prevention of colorectal cancer through TIGIT-CD155 pathway. J Cell Mol Med. 2019;23(7):4514–22.
184. Bartkowiak T, Curran MA. 4-1BB agonists: multi-potent potentiators of tumor immunity. Front Oncol. 2015;5:117.
185. Cheuk AT, Mufti GJ, Guinn BA. Role of 4-1BB: 4-1BB ligand in cancer immunotherapy. Cancer Gene Ther. 2004;11(3):215–26.
186. Lee HW, Park SJ, Choi BK, Kim HH, Nam KO, Kwon BS. 4-1BB promotes the survival of CD8+ T lymphocytes by increasing expression of Bcl-xL and Bfl-1. J Immunol. 2002;169(9):4882–8.
187. Stärck L, Scholz C, Dörken B, Daniel PT. Costimulation by CD137/4–1BB inhibits T cell apoptosis and induces Bcl-xL and c-FLIPshort via phosphatidylinositol 3-kinase and AKT/protein kinase B. Eur J Immunol. 2005;35(4):1257–66.
188. Chester C, Sanmamed MF, Wang J, Melero I. Immunotherapy targeting 4-1BB: mechanistic rationale, clinical results, and future strategies. Blood J Am Soc Hematol. 2018;131(1):49–57.
189. James AM, Cohen AD, Campbell KS. Combination immune therapies to enhance anti-tumor responses by NK cells. Front Immunol. 2013;4:481.
190. Kohrt HE, Colevas AD, Houot R, Weiskopf K, Goldstein MJ, Lund P, et al. Targeting CD137 enhances the efficacy of cetuximab. J Clin Invest. 2014;124(6):2668–82.
191. Schaer DA, Cohen AD, Wolchok JD. Anti-GITR antibodies--potential clinical applications for tumor immunotherapy. Curr Opin Investig Drugs (London, England: 2000). 2010;11(12):1378–86.
192. Kanamaru F, Youngnak P, Hashiguchi M, Nishioka T, Takahashi T, Sakaguchi S, et al. Costimulation via glucocorticoid-induced TNF receptor in both conventional and CD25+ regulatory CD4+ T cells. J Immunol. 2004;172(12):7306–14.
193. Ronchetti S, Nocentini G, Bianchini R, Krausz LT, Migliorati G, Riccardi C. Glucocorticoid-induced TNFR-related protein lowers the threshold of CD28 costimulation in CD8+ T cells. J Immunol. 2007;179(9):5916–26.

194. Valzasina B, Guiducci C, Dislich H, Killeen N, Weinberg AD, Colombo MP. Triggering of OX40 (CD134) on CD4+ CD25+ T cells blocks their inhibitory activity: a novel regulatory role for OX40 and its comparison with GITR. Blood. 2005;105(7):2845–51.
195. Mitsui J, Nishikawa H, Muraoka D, Wang L, Noguchi T, Sato E, et al. Two distinct mechanisms of augmented antitumor activity by modulation of immunostimulatory/inhibitory signals. Clin Cancer Res. 2010;16(10):2781–91.
196. Bulliard Y, Jolicoeur R, Windman M, Rue SM, Ettenberg S, Knee DA, et al. Activating Fc γ receptors contribute to the antitumor activities of immunoregulatory receptor-targeting antibodies. J Exp Med. 2013;210(9):1685–93.
197. Cohen AD, Schaer DA, Liu C, Li Y, Hirschhorn-Cymmerman D, Kim SC, et al. Agonist anti-GITR monoclonal antibody induces melanoma tumor immunity in mice by altering regulatory T cell stability and intra-tumor accumulation. PLoS One. 2010;5(5):e10436.
198. Schaer DA, Budhu S, Liu C, Bryson C, Malandro N, Cohen A, et al. GITR pathway activation abrogates tumor immune suppression through loss of regulatory T-cell lineage stability. Cancer Immunol Res. 2013;1(5):320–31.
199. Zappasodi R, Sirard C, Li Y, Budhu S, Abu-Akeel M, Liu C, et al. Rational design of anti-GITR-based combination immunotherapy. Nat Med. 2019;25(5):759–66.
200. Eliopoulos AG, Young LS. The role of the CD40 pathway in the pathogenesis and treatment of cancer. Curr Opin Pharmacol. 2004;4(4):360–7.
201. van Kooten C, Banchereau J. CD40-CD40 ligand. J Leukoc Biol. 2000;67(1):2–17.
202. Kawabe T, Naka T, Yoshida K, Tanaka T, Fujiwara H, Suematsu S, et al. The immune responses in CD40-deficient mice: impaired immunoglobulin class switching and germinal center formation. Immunity. 1994;1(3):167–78.
203. Burington B, Yue P, Shi X, Advani R, Lau JT, Tan J, et al. CD40 pathway activation status predicts response to CD40 therapy in diffuse large B cell lymphoma. Sci Transl Med. 2011;3(74):74ra22.
204. Beatty GL, Chiorean EG, Fishman MP, Saboury B, Teitelbaum UR, Sun W, et al. CD40 agonists alter tumor stroma and show efficacy against pancreatic carcinoma in mice and humans. Science. 2011;331(6024):1612–6.
205. Vonderheide RH. CD40 agonist antibodies in cancer immunotherapy. Annu Rev Med. 2019;71:41.
206. Pang X, Zhang L, Wu J, Ma C, Mu C, Zhang G, Chen W. Expression of CD40/CD40L in colon cancer, and its effect on proliferation and apoptosis of SW48 colon cancer cells. J BUON. 2017;22(4):894–9.
207. Baumann R, Yousefi S, Simon D, Russmann S, Mueller C, Simon HU. Functional expression of CD134 by neutrophils. Eur J Immunol. 2004;34(8):2268–75.
208. Rogers PR, Song J, Gramaglia I, Killeen N, Croft M. OX40 promotes Bcl-xL and Bcl-2 expression and is essential for long-term survival of CD4 T cells. Immunity. 2001;15(3):445–55.
209. Arestides RS, He H, Westlake RM, Chen AI, Sharpe AH, Perkins DL, Finn PW. Costimulatory molecule OX40L is critical for both Th1 and Th2 responses in allergic inflammation. Eur J Immunol. 2002;32(10):2874–80.
210. Hirschhorn-Cymerman D, Rizzuto GA, Merghoub T, Cohen AD, Avogadri F, Lesokhin AM, et al. OX40 engagement and chemotherapy combination provides potent antitumor immunity with concomitant regulatory T cell apoptosis. J Exp Med. 2009;206(5):1103–16.
211. Pan PY, Zang Y, Weber K, Meseck ML, Chen SH. OX40 ligation enhances primary and memory cytotoxic T lymphocyte responses in an immunotherapy for hepatic colon metastases. Mol Ther. 2002;6(4):528–36.
212. Petty JK, He K, Corless CL, Vetto JT, Weinberg AD. Survival in human colorectal cancer correlates with expression of the T-cell costimulatory molecule OX-40 (CD134). Am J Surg. 2002;183(5):512–8.
213. Curti BD, Kovacsovics-Bankowski M, Morris N, Walker E, Chisholm L, Floyd K, et al. OX40 is a potent immune-stimulating target in late-stage cancer patients. Cancer Res. 2013;73(24):7189–98.

214. Weixler B, Cremonesi E, Sorge R, Muraro MG, Delko T, Nebiker CA, et al. OX40 expression enhances the prognostic significance of CD8 positive lymphocyte infiltration in colorectal cancer. Oncotarget. 2015;6(35):37588.
215. Buchan SL, Rogel A, Al-Shamkhani A. The immunobiology of CD27 and OX40 and their potential as targets for cancer immunotherapy. Blood J Am Soc Hematol. 2018;131(1):39–48.
216. Carter PJ, Lazar GA. Next generation antibody drugs: pursuit of the'high-hanging fruit'. Nat Rev Drug Discov. 2018;17(3):197.
217. Chae YK, Arya A, Iams W, Cruz MR, Chandra S, Choi J, Giles F. Current landscape and future of dual anti-CTLA4 and PD-1/PD-L1 blockade immunotherapy in cancer; lessons learned from clinical trials with melanoma and non-small cell lung cancer (NSCLC). J Immunother Cancer. 2018;6(1):39.
218. Park YJ, Kuen DS, Chung Y. Future prospects of immune checkpoint blockade in cancer: from response prediction to overcoming resistance. Exp Mol Med. 2018;50(8):1–13.
219. Marin-Acevedo JA, Soyano AE, Dholaria B, Knutson KL, Lou Y. Cancer immunotherapy beyond immune checkpoint inhibitors. J Hematol Oncol. 2018;11(1):8.
220. Lassen UN, Meulendijks D, Siu LL, Karanikas V, Mau-Sorensen M, Schellens JH, et al. A phase I monotherapy study of RG7212, a first-in-class monoclonal antibody targeting TWEAK signaling in patients with advanced cancers. Clin Cancer Res. 2015;21(2):258–66.
221. Ciprotti M, Tebbutt NC, Lee FT, Lee ST, Gan HK, McKee DC, et al. Phase I imaging and pharmacodynamic trial of CS-1008 in patients with metastatic colorectal cancer. J Clin Oncol. 2015;33(24):2609.
222. Takeda M, Okamoto I, Nishimura Y, Nakagawa K. Nimotuzumab, a novel monoclonal antibody to the epidermal growth factor receptor, in the treatment of non-small cell lung cancer. Lung Cancer Targets Ther. 2011;2:59.
223. Becerra CR, Salazar R, Garcia-Carbonero R, Thomas AL, Vázquez-Mazón FJ, Cassidy J, et al. Figitumumab in patients with refractory metastatic colorectal cancer previously treated with standard therapies: a nonrandomized, open-label, phase II trial. Cancer Chemother Pharmacol. 2014;73(4):695–702.
224. Rocha Lima CM, Bayraktar S, Flores AM, MacIntyre J, Montero A, Baranda JC, et al. Phase Ib study of drozitumab combined with first-line mFOLFOX6 plus bevacizumab in patients with metastatic colorectal cancer. Cancer Investig. 2012;30(10):727–31.
225. Herbertson RA, Tebbutt NC, Lee FT, Gill S, Chappell B, Cavicchiolo T, et al. Targeted chemoradiation in metastatic colorectal cancer: a phase I trial of 131I-huA33 with concurrent capecitabine. J Nucl Med. 2014;55(4):534–9.
226. Doi T, Muro K, Yoshino T, Fuse N, Ura T, Takahari D, et al. Phase 1 pharmacokinetic study of MK-0646 (dalotuzumab), an anti-insulin-like growth factor-1 receptor monoclonal antibody, in combination with cetuximab and irinotecan in Japanese patients with advanced colorectal cancer. Cancer Chemother Pharmacol. 2013;72(3):643–52.
227. Lin EH, Lenz HJ, Saleh MN, Mackenzie MJ, Knost JA, Pathiraja K, et al. A randomized, phase II study of the anti-insulin-like growth factor receptor type 1 (IGF-1R) monoclonal antibody robatumumab (SCH 717454) in patients with advanced colorectal cancer. Cancer Med. 2014;3(4):988–97.
228. Weekes CD, Beeram M, Tolcher AW, Papadopoulos KP, Gore L, Hegde P, et al. A phase I study of the human monoclonal anti-NRP1 antibody MNRP1685A in patients with advanced solid tumors. Investig New Drugs. 2014;32(4):653–60.
229. Bendell JC, Lenz HJ, Ryan T, El-Rayes BF, Marshall JL, Modiano MR, et al. Phase 1/2 study of KRN330, a fully human anti-A33 monoclonal antibody, plus irinotecan as second-line treatment for patients with metastatic colorectal cancer. Investig New Drugs. 2014;32(4):682–90.

Chapter 15
Immune Checkpoint Inhibitors as an Armor for Targeted Immunotherapy of Colorectal Cancer

Smita Kapoor and Yogendra S. Padwad

Abstract Recent progress in understanding the interplay between tumor cells and immune cells has given emergence to a new field called immunotherapy. Tumor cells are dependent upon signals called "immune checkpoints" to escape themselves from immune surveillance. Despite the substantial advances in chemotherapy and radiotherapy, life expectancy of CRC patients has not been achieved successfully. Immunotherapy has recently emerged as a newfangled armor for combating cancer. Several immune checkpoint inhibitors have received approval from FDA for colon cancer treatment in clinical settings. The blocking of these checkpoints such as PD-1 or PDL-1 and CTLA-4 can help the immune system to fight against the tumor cells. Treatment with selective anti-PD-1/PDL-1 and anti-CTLA-4 monoclonal antibodies (mAbs) has revolutionized the therapeutic scenario of different cancer types. Advancements in combination chemotherapy regimens for colorectal cancer have led to significant improvement in disease-free survival. This chapter summarizes the rationale for immune checkpoint inhibitor therapy in colon cancer.

Keywords Immunotherapy · Immune checkpoint inhibitors · Colon cancer · PD-1/PD-L1 · CTLA-4

Abbreviations

BTLA	Band T-lymphocyte attenuator
CRC	Colorectal cancer
CTLA-4	Cytotoxic T-lymphocyte-associated protein 4

S. Kapoor · Y. S. Padwad (✉)
Pharmacology and Toxicology Laboratory, CSIR-Institute of Himalayan Bioresource Technology (CSIR-IHBT), Palampur, HP, India

Academy of Scientific and Innovative Research (AcSIR), Ghaziabad, Uttar Pradesh, India
e-mail: yogendra@ihbt.res.in

G. P. Nagaraju et al. (eds.), *Colon Cancer Diagnosis and Therapy*,
https://doi.org/10.1007/978-3-030-63369-1_15

DCR	Disease control rate
dMMR	Mismatch repair-deficient
FDA	Food and Drug Administration
ICBs	Immune checkpoint blockades
ICIs	Immune checkpoint inhibitors
ICOS	Inducible co-stimulator
IRAEs	Immune-related adverse events
LAG-3	Lymphocyte-activation gene 3
MAbs	Monoclonal antibodies mCRC- Metastatic colorectal cancer
MCSCs	Mesenchymal stem cells
MHC	Major histocompatibility complex
MSI-H	Microsatellite instability-high MSS-Microsatellite stable
NSCLS	Non-small cell lung carcinoma
ORR	Objective response rate OS- Overall survival
PD-1	Programmed cell death protein 1
pDC	Plasmacytoid dendritic cells
PDL-1	Programmed death ligand 1
PDL-2	Programmed death ligand 2 POLE- Polymerase epsilon
pMMR	Proficient MMR
TATE	Trans-arterial tirapazamine embolization
TCR	T-cell receptor
TILs	Tumor-infiltrating lymphocytes
TIM-3	T-cell immunoglobulin mucin-3
TME	Tumor microenvironment
Tregs	T regulatory cells
VISTA	V-domain immunoglobulin suppressor of T-cell activation

15.1 Introduction

Colon cancer is the third major cancer related to mortality in the United States and the second major type in terms of mortality and has caused around 700,000 annual deaths worldwide [57]. As per 2018 reports, over 1.8 million of colorectal cancer cases and 881,000 CRC-related deaths were estimated to occur [84].

The calculated global burden of CRC is estimated to increase by 60 percent by the year 2030 [87]. The overall survival rate of patient with mCRC remains poor even after remarkable advancements in CRC treatment [73]; in the United States, the 5-year survival rate is 12.5% in between 5 months and 2 years [89]. The role of chronic inflammation in gastrointestinal cancers can be clearly used for immune-based approaches and also have role in utilizing our immune system to selectively destroy the tumor [2, 71]. The role of immune checkpoint inhibitor was first demonstrated in metastatic melanoma; ICI immunotherapy is an emerging and revolutionized oncology field. Immunotherapy is effective against cancer because it targets not only the cancer cells but also the microenvironment of cancer; this strategy of

ICI immunotherapy is capable of causing delayed responses of tumors irrespective of the initial increase in the metastases [7]. CRC patients having MSI-H/dMMR can be benefitted from ICI therapy; KEYNOTE-177 clinical trial in recent study has described that MSI-H/dMMR patients showed CRC progression-free survival. There is a need for developing an effective and potent treatment for different subgroups of CRC [18].

15.1.1 Immunotherapy

Cancer immune surveillance is the response of the immune system against tumor [77]. The immune system has the potential of recognizing and destroying transformant cells in early stages of cancer through its innate and adaptive effector mechanisms [47]. Tumor microenvironment has helped us in understanding the relationship between tumor cells and our immune cells. One of the independent hallmarks of cancer is its escaping power from immune surveillance [20]. The field of immunotherapy has made advancement because of good understanding of the emerging new sphere called immuno-oncology. The first attempt to utilize the immune system for curing cancer was done by William B. Coley (Father of Immunotherapy) in the late nineteenth century. The Nobel Prize in Physiology and Medicine 2018 (James P. Allison and Tasuku Honjo) for the discovery of CTLA-4 protein and PD-1/PD-L1 has given immense recognition to the field of immunotherapy [5]. Immune checkpoint inhibitors have shown remarkable efficacy in patients with hyper-mutated subtypes of colorectal cancer, i.e., MSI-H and dMMR, and also with POLE, a hereditary mutation, when compared with traditional chemotherapy [13]. The immune system plays a crucial part in the emerging field of immunotherapy and can distinguish between non-self and self with the help of TCR present on T cells along with the MHC-1 molecules which are possessed by the surface of various tumor cells [47, 78]. Co-stimulatory or co-inhibitory signals are modulated by TCR-MHC complex which is further employed by tumor cells to escape destruction [8, 9]. ICIs are a kind of immunotherapy which includes the role of antibodies; CTLA-4 and PD-1 are co-receptors present on T cells (targeted by ICIs) and cancer cells and also in other immune cells. ICI immunotherapy is an emerging oncology field and has transformed the existing clinical treatments available (Fig. 15.1).

15.2 Paving the Way for Immune Checkpoint Inhibitor Immunotherapy in CRC

The role of ICIs was preliminary announced in the year 2010 and 2012, and they have converted into OS advantage in contrast to already known treatments in metastatic melanomas and NSCLS [6]. Earlier immunotherapy particularly immune checkpoint inhibition was not regarded as a good method for treating

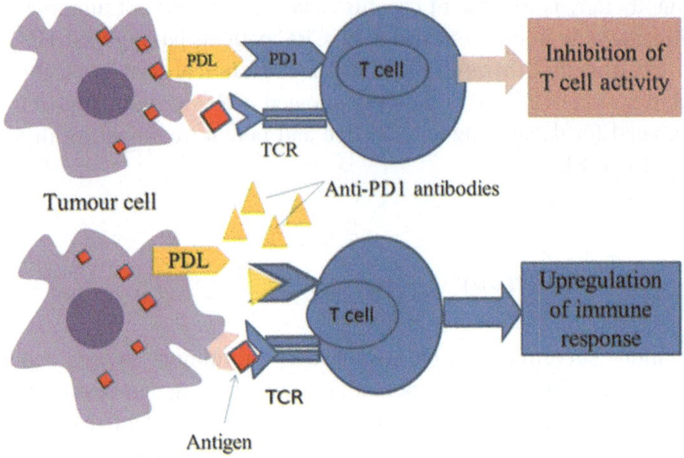

Fig. 15.1 Depicting immune checkpoint (immunotherapy) in tumor cell and T cell. It shows blockade of PD-1 which leads to the upregulation of immune response

CRC. Tremelimumab, a mAb against CTLA-4 during its initial phase II study, has depicted no improvement in the health of patient having recurrent CRC [46]. Another study of phase I anti-PD-1/PDL-1 antibodies showed no significant response among the previously treated CRC patients [49, 52]. Presently a large number of trials at the clinical levels to investigate the ICIs alone and in combination with other treatments of CRC have been conducted. Pembrolizumab and nivolumab are US FDA-approved drugs specifically for the patients with dMMR/MSI-H. Approval of different antibodies has appeared as a boon for the patients particularly dMMR/MSI-H CRC, as 31 percent ORR and 12 percent OSR have been observed in patients earlier having treatment resistance to dMMR/MSI-H. Thus the successful attempts of ICIs have paved the way for the study of FDA-approved drugs for combating the CRC [79].

15.2.1 Immune Checkpoints and Checkpoint Inhibitors

Immune checkpoints are important regulators of immune activation. They act as a signal for regulating antigen recognition receptors in the process of immune response. Whenever the immune system is attacked by a pathogen, co-stimulatory (CD28, ICOS, and CD137) and co-inhibitory (PD-1, CTLA-4, and VISTA) immune checkpoints are the two signals which play a vital role in protecting normal tissues from damage [3]. Cancer cells have property of escaping from immune attack by impairment of immune checkpoint proteins [97]. Checkpoint inhibitors have come out as a potent aid in the field of colorectal cancer immunotherapy; they have shown as promising target for treating colorectal cancer. These molecules which basically

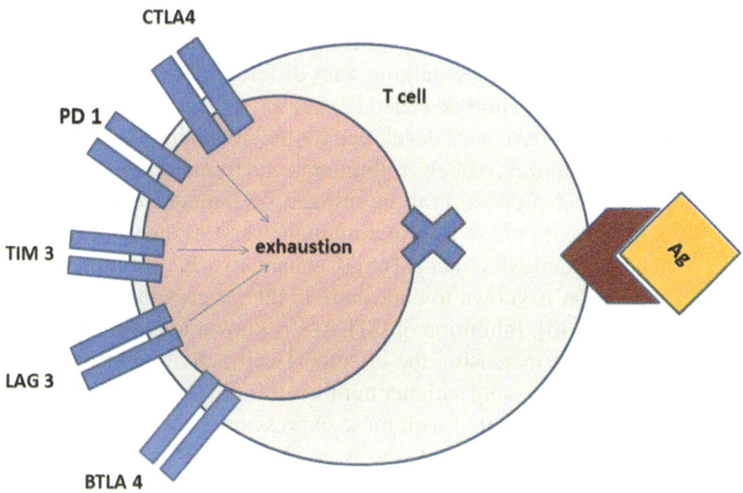

Fig. 15.2 Showing different immune checkpoints and immunosuppression in CRC tumor cells. Different immune checkpoints can activate inhibitory pathways in T cell which leads to T-cell-mediated immunosuppression. These immune checkpoints are opted by tumor cells and thus cause T-cell exhaustion and tumor immune tolerance [74]

function as blocking antibodies to various cell surface inhibitory molecules like PD-1/PDL-1 and CTLA-4 hinder the priming and regulator phases of adaptive T-cell immune response [52, 58]. TIM-3, BTLA, IDO, and LAG-3 are other important immune checkpoints and play a pivotal role in CRC. The major treatments for CRC have been surgery, chemotherapy, and radiotherapy. To improve the success rate of ICIs, the involvement of clinical trials and patients should be increased; also these should be combined with conventional therapies. In the last few decades, the cases of mCRC have shown the improved overall survival of patients; thus, checkpoint inhibitors have shown good outcomes [93] (Fig. 15.2).

15.2.1.1 CTLA-4

Cytotoxic T-lymphocyte-associated protein 4 also known as CD152, belongs to a membrane glycoprotein and is a molecular ligand. CTLA-4 is a surface receptor transiently present on effector T cells. The discovery of CTLA-4 occurred while performing differential screening of mouse cytolytic T-cell cDNA library [3, 21]. There lies the difference among the T cells for the expression of CTLA-4; T regulatory cells constitutively express CTLA-4 because of their high level of FoxP3 transcription factor, while some T cells need activation for possessing CTLA-4 expression [3, 24, 26]. During the initial studies of CTLA-4, it was considered to have structural similarities with CD28 and was believed to be a positive regulator of T cells. Later on, Professor Alison described the negative role associated with T-cell stimulation and CTLA-4, and his study explained the interaction of B7 ligands with CTLA-4 which removed IL-2 production and also proliferation of T cells and induced cell cycle arrest via cross-talking with different pathways whose roles are in the survival and proliferation of cells [17, 23, 25, 27, 28, 35, 42, 56]. Different anti-CTLA-4 antibodies have been developed for the treatment of colon cancer [25]. Currently CTLA-4 inhibitors, namely, ipilimumab and tremelimumab (anti-CTLA-4 IgG 2 mAb), are under production to be utilized by humans. Forty-seven mCRC patients were treated with phase II tremelimumab every 90 days after failure of all standard chemotherapeutic treatments [46]. Cancer cell which continuously exhibits CTLA-4 expression is known to contribute in the progression of hematological and solid tumors [33, 40]. Inhibition of CTLA-4 is known to reduce the colon cancer metastatic effect by increasing the effector T-cell activity and inhibiting Treg cells [3, 12]. Patients expressing a higher number of CTLA-4 are connected with the poorer prognosis when compared with those expressing low CTLA-4, thus making CTLA-4 a smarter and successful attempt in combating CRC.

15.2.1.2 PD-1 and PDL-1

Programmed cell death protein 1 (CD279), is one of the inhibitory receptors which is presented on the surface of T lymphocytes (T helper, T cytotoxic, NKT cells), B cells, and monocytes/macrophages [15, 36]. PD-1 has two ligands, namely, PD-L1 and PD-L2. PD-L1 is a transmembrane molecule belonging to B7-H1 family, and PD-L2 belongs to B7-DC family [15]. The main difference between the two ligands is their expression; for example, PD-L1 is possessed in a constitutive manner on different types of immune and non-immune cells, but the expression of PDL-2 is inducible which means it can be induced depending on the stimulus of microenvironment [51]. PD-1 and PD-L1 act via transduction route to inhibit and block the signals of different cytokines via acting on differentiation and multiplication of T cells and thus causing invasion and spreading of cancer cells [82]. Tumor's immune evasion causes T-cell exhaustion in cancer, and this has been linked to the increased expression of PD-1 on TILs and upregulation of its ligand on cancer-specific cytotoxic T cells [59]. The first evidence of importance of this pathway in CRC was shown among the Chinese population who exhibit correlation between SNP and PD-1 gene in CRC [67] and also in an Iranian population having colon cancer [50]. Droeser has showed the interlink of PD-L1 appearance with the better survival in colorectal cancer samples; also overexpression of PD-1 cytotoxic lymphocytes and IFN-γ gene was noticed in a sample of CRC patients [4, 54]. To control the suppression of the immune system, PD-1/PD-L1 mAbs have shown good reactions in metastatic solid tumors. PD-L1 is interlinked with tumor formation and development; still the expression of PD-L1 protein in colon cancer and its significance in clinical prognosis are yet to be elucidated [96].

15.2.1.3 TIM-3

The other immune checkpoint blocker targeted for treating CRC is TIM-3 which is abbreviated from T-cell immunoglobulin and mucin-containing protein 3. TIM-3 is known to be possessed by helper T cells and T cytotoxic cells. Galectin-9 is an important ligand presented by TIM-3 which is supposed to play an important role in decreasing TH1 responses and act as an inducer of cell death (apoptosis) of tumor-infiltrating CD8+ T cells [37, 69]. TIM-3 also plays a role in the depletion of CD8+ T cells by acting as co-inhibitory molecules in alignment to PD-1 and CTLA-4 [72]. Further, the role of TIM-3 in conjunction with PD-1 in T-cell depletion has been revealed in animal models in CD8+ T cells. In previous preclinical models, blockage of TIM-3 was capable of rejuvenating venture of anticancer, when compared to the outcome of PD-1 barricade with the considerable potency through merging of TIM-3 and PD-1 [68]. Normal tissues possess inflated expression of TIM-3 as compared to the CRC tissues and correspond to metastasis of lymphatic and TNM [72]. It has been revealed in the previous study that cytotoxic T cells express TIM-3 in the mice colon cancer model which leads to the enhancement of the secretion of effector cytokine and also causes programmed cell death in comparison to cells which do not possess TIM-3 [69]. Anti-TIM-3 antibodies fight against colorectal cancer by inhibiting cancer growth by disorganizing the galectin-9/TIM-3 signaling pathways and improve the healing potential of chemotherapy [69]. Many studies have been showing the link which supports the production of inhibitors of TIM-3 and have great value as an individual in colorectal cancer patients [16].

15.2.1.4 LAG-3

LAG-3 is lymphocyte-activation gene 3, also called CD223, basically a potential cancer immunotherapeutic target. This receptor is exhibited by activated CD4+ cells and CD8+ cells [31] and NK cells [94] and also on pDC [43, 95]. A crucial role of anti-regulation in the proliferation of T cells and its interlinkage with MHC-II is played by LAG-3; some studies have shown CD223 appearance to mitigate the Treg functions [11, 16]. The role of LAG-3 has been well established in the field of CRC progression [10]. The two forms of MSI differently express LAG-3 in CRC; it is dominantly present in microsatellite unstable when compared to the microsatellite stable [45, 65]. IL-10 and TGFβ1 increased level has been known to produce the activated form of CD223 Tregs which shows an immunosuppressive phenotype [45]. In previous studies, CD223 has been shown to target with PD-1 in a dual immunomodulator called MGD013 whose purpose was to produce additive effect on the tumor immunity [53]. Anti-LAG-3 antibody promotes effector T-cell activity and inhibits Treg-induced suppressive functions in the TME [55]. Currently most of the studies are undergoing in early phase of an anti-CD223 antibody or in amalgamation with nivolumab in metastatic colorectal cancer. LAG-3 is well investigated to take part in an exceptional inhibitory part in the maintenance of immune homeostasis in company with other immune checkpoints especially PD-1. Thus, LAG-3 is one of the promising therapeutic targets in colon cancer immunotherapy [85].

15.2.1.5 IDO

Indoleamine-2,3-dioxygenase is an enzyme present within the cells which results in tryptophan degradation known to have a suppressive effect on the immune system which further leads to the immune escape of tumors [1]. IDO1 and IDO2 are enzymes that catalyze the first and rate-limiting step involved in the conversion of essential amino acid L-tryptophan into L-kynurenine [32]. Depletion of tryptophan and accumulation of kynurenine leads to T-cell growth arrest in G1 phase and also induction of highly immunosuppressive T regulatory cells [29]. In colorectal cancer patient, IDO expression is linked to worse prognosis and lesser CD3+ infiltration of T cells [38]. Expression of IDO inhibition changes immune response in colon TME in mice by increasing expressions of proinflammatory cytokines and reducing Foxp3+ Tregs [70]. GDC-0919, an anti-IDO agent, is in phase I development along with epacadostat, and an IDO inhibitor is under investigation in combination with pembrolizumab and azacitidine.

15.3 Factors Influencing the Anti-tumor Benefits of Immune Checkpoint

Anti-tumor beneficial effects of immune checkpoint are influenced by different factors of immune checkpoint inhibitors. TILs' character, position, and solidness are strong predictors of survival of cancer patients [39, 41, 48]. ICBs need tumor-infiltrating CTLs and local expression of PDL-1 for its clinical efficacy; these ICB therapies are greatly potent in different forms of advanced cancer and show less potency in most forms of CRC and cancer of ovaries [49, 63, 66]. PD-1/PDL-1 blockers have exhibited to depend on the existence or absence of accumulation of CTL expression in TME [60-62]. Burden of mutations and presence of antigenic neoepitopes in tumor play important roles in the activity of ICIs; if CRC has low mutational load, then it is generally unresponsive to immune checkpoint inhibitors. Similarly, if CRC is MSI-H, having very high mutational burden, then it shows inhibition of PD-1 up to 50% ORR [64].

15.4 Biomarkers for Immune Checkpoint Inhibitors in Metastatic CRC

Around 20 percent of small subsets of patients have been served through cancer immunotherapy when assessed through clinical trials; the reason behind this is the IRAEs developed by some patients [14]. The role of biomarker prediction is very important in order to solve the problem, and the study of biomarkers is pivotal for both the current scenario of clinical care and further development of the field of ICIs. DNA repair pathways are operated by MMR genes including MLH-1, PMS-2, MSH-2, and MSH-6; loss of function of any of these genes and their products results in the change of the size of microsatellite called microsatellite instability (MSI) and also known as dMMR. Some of the pathological features like mutational load of tumor and TILs are believed to be linked with an enhanced risk of MSI-CRC [22, 30]. CRC with MSI have two different phenotypes: MSI-H and MSI-L [34]. It is clear that PD-1 blockade is having biomarker called MSI [75]. PD-L1 and PD-L2 are ligands present on cancer cells known to repress the response of the immune system by binding to PD-1 receptor present on T effector cells. Upregulation of PD-L1 on tumors will help them to escape the host immune response [64].

15.5 Drugs Available in the Market

Presently two drugs, pembrolizumab and nivolumab, have been accredited by FDA; both of these are immune checkpoint PD-1 blockers in metastatic CRC patients having dMMR/MSI-H [64, 79] US FDA, approval [88]. Ipilimumab (Yervoy), another fully humanized monoclonal antibody CTLA-4, has been approved by FDA to use in conjunction with nivolumab for treating the patients having dMMR/MSI-H colorectal cancer [83]. A summary of clinical trials for ongoing drugs involved in immune checkpoint inhibitors has been shown in Table 15.1.

15.6 Immune Checkpoint Blockades in Fusion with Chemotherapy

To improve the therapeutic efficacy of ICI treatment, a large number of trials at clinical and preclinical levels have been carried out to explore the effect of conventional therapies (chemotherapies, targeted therapies, radiation therapies) with combinatorial treatment (ICIs + conventional therapies) [90]. Chemotherapy has appeared as a favorable treatment to show additive immunomodulatory effects both in vitro and in vivo; further, ICIs can improve the treatment of MSS CRC. TILs, tumor antigens, and tumor PDl-1 expressions which are predictive biomarkers of ICI have appeared to enhance after 5-flourouracil plus oxaliplatin (FOLFOX)

Table 15.1 Summary of clinical trials for ongoing drugs involved in immune checkpoint inhibitors [80]

Identifier	Agent	Trial	Patient population	Phase
NCT02860546	Nivolumab	A study evaluating TAS-102 plus nivolumab in patients with MSS CRC	mCRC	2
NCT02291289	Atezolizumab	A multi-center study of biomarker-driven therapy in metastatic colorectal cancer	mCRC	2
NCT02227667	MEDI4736	Evaluation and efficacy of MEDI4736 in immunological subsets of advanced colorectal cancer	mCRC	2
NCT03050814	Avelumab	Standard of care alone or in combination with Ad-CEA vaccine and avelumab in patients with previously untreated metastatic CRC (QUILT-2.004)	mCRC	2
NCT029815524	Pembrolizumab	Phase II study of GVAX (with CY) and pembrolizumab in pMMR advanced CRC	MMR-p mCRC	2
NCT01844505	Nivolumab + ipilimumab	Phase II, open-label, multi-center single-arm efficacy and safety clinical study of ipilimumab in subjects with untreated or previously treated advanced/metastatic melanoma	MSI-H	2
NCT02060188	Nivolumab	An investigational immunotherapy study of nivolumab and nivolumab in combination with other anticancer drugs in colon cancer that returned or spread (CheckMate 142)	MSI/MSS mCRC	2
NCT02992912	Atezolizumab	Atezolizumab with stereotactic ablative radiotherapy in patients with metastatic tumors (SABR-PD-L1)	Metastatic tumor	2
NCT02437071	Pembrolizumab	Assessment of the efficacy of pembrolizumab + radiotherapy or ablation in mCRC patients	mCRC	2

treatment both in mice models of colon cancer and in human tumor samples [92]. Likewise, immunomodulatory effects of host which include upregulation of cellular major histocompatibility complex (MHC) class 1, recruitment and activation of dendritic cells (DC), and repression of Tregs and myeloid derived suppressor cells have been known post-chemotherapy and also function coadjuvantly in promoting immune TME [44]. In an earlier study, it was well established as a verification of concept that the application of oxaliplatin led to an enhancement in the reaction of the immune system in an in vivo pMMR colon cancer mice model to catch a PD-L1 fusion protein [91]. Presently different trials have been conducted to estimate the capability of current chemotherapy with ICBs. FOLFOX (phase II study) in combination with pembrolizumab has shown to improve the overall ORR of 53% at

Table 15.2 List of clinical trials of combinatorial therapy of immune checkpoint inhibitors (ICIs) and chemotherapy in colorectal cancer [19]

Combination treatment	ICI	Study population	Trial ID	Phase	Status
Trifluridine + tipiracil hydrochloride	Nivolumab	Refractory, metastatic MSS CRC	NCT02860546	II	Completed
FOLFOX	Tremelimumab + durvalumab	First-line, KRAS-mt CRC	NCT030202758	Ib/II	Recruiting
Azacitidine	Durvalumab	Refractory, metastatic MSS CRC	NCT02811497	II	Recruiting
Guadecitabine	Nivolumab	Refractory, metastatic MSS CRC	NCT03576963	Ib/II	Not yet recruiting
Nordic FLOX regimen	Nivolumab	Untreated, metastatic MSS CRC	NCT0338819	II	Recruiting
Pemetrexed ± oxaliplatin	Pembrolizumab	Refractory, metastatic MSS	NCT03626922	I	Not yet recruiting
Romidepsin ± 5-azacitidine	Pembrolizumab	Refractory, metastatic MSS CRC	NCT02512172	I	Recruiting
TATE	Nivolumab or pembrolizumab	Metastatic CRC to the liver	NCT03259867	II	Recruiting

24-week median follow-up with a DCR of 100% at 8 weeks in MSS CRC [81]. Chemotherapy treatment in combination with ICIs (PD-1 inhibitors nivolumab and pembrolizumab, PDL-1 inhibitor durvalumab, and CTLA-4 inhibitor tremelimumab) in MSS CRC have been utilizing different agents such as histone deacetylase inhibitor romidepsin and thymidine phosphorylase inhibitor tipiracil (TAS-102) in addition to cytotoxin trifluridine to treat the condition of colon cancer. Other locally based drugs like TATE, a hypoxic selective cytotoxin, have been used in condition of mCRC. A list mentioning trials of combinatorial therapy of immune checkpoint inhibitors (ICIs) and chemotherapy in colorectal cancer has been discussed in Table 15.2.

15.6.1 Immune Checkpoint Inhibitor and Radiotherapy

Radiotherapy uses high-energy rays to destroy cancer cells; it employs local radio-embolization to CRC metastasis and external beam radiation therapy. There are a small number of trials of pre-diagnostic data supporting the involvement of radiotherapy as a powerful way to increase the effectiveness of ICBs in the treatment of MSS CRC by contributing directly to the procedure of immunogenic cell demise.

Table 15.3 List of combinatorial (radiotherapy + ICIs) clinical trials employed for CRC [19]

Radiation regimen	ICI	Study population	Study ID	Phase	Status
Standard radiation therapy	Nivolumab + ipilimumab	MSS and MSI-H CRC	NCT03104439	II	Recruiting
Hypofractionated palliative radiation	Durvalumab and tremelimumab	Metastatic MSS CRC	NCT03007407	II	Recruiting
Chemo-radiation	Durvalumab	Stage II–IV, MSS rectal cancer	NCT03102047	II	Recruiting
SBRT to the liver	Pembrolizumab	Metastatic CRC to liver CRC	NCT02837263	I	Recruiting
Radioembolization	Durvalumab and tremelimumab	Metastatic MSS to the liver	NCT03005002	I	Active not recruiting
High- or low-dose radiation therapy	Durvalumab and tremelimumab	Refractory metastatic MSS CRC to the liver	NCT02888743	II	Recruiting

Radiotherapy has shown to cause direct demolition of cancer both in vitro and in vivo by releasing tumor antigens, increasing the cytokines of inflammation and cell surface molecule, and recruitment of immune cells into the TME [86]. Early clinical efforts showing the combinatorial effect of radiotherapy and ICI are less; phase II non-randomized study evaluating pembrolizumab in inclusion to radiotherapy of patients in cancer metastases having foster, obstinate pMMR colorectal cancer has shown ORR of 9% [76]. There is a need of more data to fully measure the true efficacy of the combination of radiotherapy and ICIs; Table 15.3 has discussed a list of combinatorial (radiotherapy + ICIs) clinical trials employed for CRC.

15.7 Negative Effects of Immune Checkpoint Inhibitors

The main objective behind the development of immune checkpoint inhibitors was to improve the activity of the immune system against the tumor cells; there are some patients who developed some negative effects related to the immune system against non-tumor tissues, termed as IRAEs (immune-related adverse events). It leads to death and other effects particularly comorbidities. The use of drugs of immune checkpoint inhibitors among patients has not resulted in any specific side effects other than the reported in clinical trials across solid tumors [79]. Previously, some studies have shown the negative impact related to immune checkpoint inhibitor; 13 percent of patients have stopped their immunotherapy due to IRAEs to the non-cancerous tissues. Single-agent anti-PD-1 therapy and combinatorial therapies have led to the problems related to autoimmune liver inflammation and acute injuries to the kidney, rashes, diarrhea, and thyroid and pancreatic inflammation [64, 79, 83].

15.7.1 *Future Perspective of Immune Checkpoint Blockers*

The field of immuno-oncology with respect to ICIs has become one of the most widely scrutinized; there are still important unanswered questions regarding the mechanism behind the therapy and why some patient population get benefited from the treatment and others develop IRAEs. MAbs targeting novel ICI molecules in conjunction with combination therapy may further improve the immunotherapy. Therapeutic efficacy further will be enhanced by better understanding the interaction between the immune system and cancer cells and realizing the importance of biomarker-based approaches and overcoming the mechanism of resistance developed by some patients.

15.8 Conclusion

Even after continuous advanced research and multifaceted treatment, colorectal cancer is still one of the major reasons behind a large number of deaths worldwide. Therapy targeting the immune system (immunotherapy) is an emerging field that can play an important role in treating CRC; an improved knowledge of the immune system and tumor interaction has led to the production of novel molecules called ICIs or ICBs. It is known that mCRC patients having increased mutational load and infiltration of immune cells due to MSI-H or dMMR are considered to be the suitable candidates for immune checkpoint inhibitory therapy. A clear involvement of MSI/dMMR in CRC has paved a way for immunotherapy for treating the advanced refractory patients. Targeting of PD-1 or PD-L1 in the patients having MSI-H malignancy using ICIs has shown good success, and thus, in MSI-H population, the immunotherapy can be employed beneficially to treat the MSS CRCs. Combinatorial therapy has shown promising effects involving ICBs with chemotherapy, radiotherapy, or some other small molecule inhibitors. There is a need of better mastery in dMMR and its genomic features to find more selective markers and to improve the efficacy of immune checkpoint inhibition. These selective molecules grant hope to treat not just selective CRC patients but all other patients. CRC patients who have failed the previous treatment, the combinatorial therapy helps in improving the curative and therapeutic effect and give new hope for the direction of improved treatments. The main key challenge is to identify the selective mCRC patients from diverging stretch who will likely to get beneficial effect either from ICBs alone or from combinatorial cancer treatments. Further, there is a need to interpret the immune system's detailed characteristics for better utilization of targeted and combinatorial immunotherapy for immune checkpoint inhibition in the field of colorectal cancer.

Acknowledgments Authors are highly thankful to the Director, CSIR-IHBT, Palampur, for his continuous support and inspiration. SK is highly thankful to the Indian Council of Medical

Research (ICMR) for the fellowship and the Academy of Scientific and Innovative Research (AcSIR), Ghaziabad, for the Ph.D. registration.

Funding ICMR Fellowship (No 3/1/3 JRF) and MLP0204.

Authors' Contribution SK and YSP: Conceptualization of the manuscript, writing of the manuscript.

YSP: Significant revisions and improvement.

References

1. Zou W. Immunosuppressive networks in the tumour environment and their therapeutic relevance. Nat Rev Cancer. 2005;5(4):263–74.
2. Trinchieri G. Cancer and inflammation: an old intuition with rapidly evolving new concepts. Annu Rev Immunol. 2012;30:677–706.
3. Pardoll DM. The blockade of immune checkpoints in cancer immunotherapy. Nat Rev Cancer. 2012;12(4):252–64.
4. Heinimann K. Toward a molecular classification of colorectal cancer: the role of microsatellite instability status. Front Oncol. 2013;3:272.
5. Altmann DM. A Nobel Prize-worthy pursuit: cancer immunology and harnessing immunity to tumour neoantigens. Immunology. 2018;155(3):283–4.
6. Sholl LM. Understanding patterns of pathologic response following neoadjuvant immunotherapy for solid tumours. Ann Oncol. 2018;29:1630–2.
7. Robert C. A decade of immune-checkpoint inhibitors in cancer therapy. Nat Commun. 2020;11:3801.
8. Townsend SE, Allison JP. Tumour rejection after direct costimulation of CD8+ T cells by B7-transfected melanoma cells. Science. 1993;15(5093):368–70.
9. Sharma P, Allison JP. The future of immune checkpoint therapy. Science. 2015;348:56–61.
10. Chen J, Chen Z. The effect of immune microenvironment on the progression and prognosis of colorectal cancer. Med Oncol. 2014;31(8):82.
11. Goldberg MV, Drake CG. LAG-3 in cancer immunotherapy. In: Cancer immunology and immunotherapy. Berlin, Heidelberg: Springer; 2010. p. 269–78.
12. Nishikawa H, Sakaguchi S. Regulatory T cells in tumor immunity. Int J Cancer. 2010;127(4):759–67.
13. Hermel DJ, Gruber SB. Hereditary colorectal cancer: immunotherapy approaches. In: Hereditary colorectal cancer. Cham: Springer; 2018. p. 385–99.
14. Kourie HR, Klastersky J. Immune checkpoint inhibitors side effects and management. Immunotherapy. 2016;8(7):799–807.
15. Berger KN, Pu JJ. PD-1 pathway and its clinical application: a 20 year journey after discovery of the complete human PD-1 gene. Gene. 2018;638:20–5.
16. Shin DS, Ribas A. The evolution of checkpoint blockade as a cancer therapy: what's here, what's next? Curr Opin Immunol. 2015;33:23–35.
17. Bhandaru M, Rotte A. Monoclonal antibodies for the treatment of melanoma: present and future strategies. In: Human monoclonal antibodies. New York: Humana Press; 2019. p. 83–108.
18. Wrobel P, Ahmed S. Current status of immunotherapy in metastatic colorectal cancer. Int J Color Dis. 2019;34(1):13–25.
19. Hermel DJ, Sigal D. The emerging role of checkpoint inhibition in microsatellite stable colorectal cancer. J Pers Med. 2019;9(1):5.

20. Hanahan D, Weinberg RA. Hallmarks of cancer: the next generation. Cell. 2011;144(5):646–74.
21. Brunet JF, Denizot F, Luciani MF, Roux-Dosseto M, Suzan M, Mattei MG, Golstein P. A new member of the immunoglobulin superfamily—CTLA-4. Nature. 1987;328(6127):267–70.
22. Liu B, Nicolaides NC, Markowitz S, Willson JK, Parsons RE, Jen J, Papadopolous N, Peltomäki P, de la Chapelle A, Hamilton SR, Kinzler KW. Mismatch repair gene defects in sporadic colorectal cancers with microsatellite instability. Nat Genet. 1995;9(1):48–55.
23. Krummel MF, Allison JP. CD28 and CTLA-4 have opposing effects on the response of T cells to stimulation. J Exp Med. 1995;182(2):459–65.
24. Alegre ML, Noel PJ, Eisfelder BJ, Chuang E, Clark MR, Reiner SL, Thompson CB. Regulation of surface and intracellular expression of CTLA4 on mouse T cells. J Immunol. 1996;157(11):4762–70.
25. Leach DR, Krummel MF, Allison JP. Enhancement of antitumour immunity by CTLA-4 blockade. Science. 1996;271(5256):1734–6.
26. Perkins D, Wang Z, Donovan C, He H, Mark D, Guan G, Wang Y, Walunas T, Bluestone J, Listman J, Finn PW. Regulation of CTLA-4 expression during T cell activation. J Immunol. 1996;156(11):4154–9.
27. Chambers CA, Sullivan TJ, Allison JP. Lymphoproliferation in CTLA-4–deficient mice is mediated by costimulation-dependent activation of CD4+ T cells. Immunity. 1997;7(6):885–95.
28. Fraser JH, Rincón M, McCoy KD, Le Gros G. CTLA4 ligation attenuates AP-1, NFAT and NF-κB activity in activated T cells. Eur J Immunol. 1999;29(3):838–44.
29. Munn DH, Shafizadeh E, Attwood JT, Bondarev I, Pashine A, Mellor AL. Inhibition of T cell proliferation by macrophage tryptophan catabolism. J Exp Med. 1999;189(9):1363–72.
30. Wood RD, Mitchell M, Sgouros J, Lindahl T. Human DNA repair genes. Science. 2001;291(5507):1284–9.
31. Workman CJ, Rice DS, Dugger KJ, Kurschner C, Vignali DA. Phenotypic analysis of the murine CD4-related glycoprotein, CD223 (LAG-3). Eur J Immunol. 2002;32(8):2255–63.
32. Moffett JR, Namboodiri MA. Tryptophan and the immune response. Immunol Cell Biol. 2003;81(4):247–65.
33. Pistillo MP, Tazzari PL, Palmisano GL, Pierri I, Bolognesi A, Ferlito F, Capanni P, Polito L, Ratta M, Pileri S, Piccioli M, Basso G, Rissotto L, Conte R, Gobbi M, Stirpe F, Ferrara GB. CTLA-4 is not restricted to the lymphoid cell lineage and can function as a target molecule for apoptosis induction of leukemic cells. Blood. 2003;101:202–9.
34. Pawlik TM, Raut CP, Rodriguez-Bigas MA. Colorectal carcinogenesis: MSI-H versus MSI-L. Dis Markers. 2004;20(4, 5):199–206.
35. Chikuma S, Abbas AK, Bluestone JA. B7-independent inhibition of T cells by CTLA-4. J Immunol. 2005;175(1):177–81.
36. Greenwald RJ, Freeman GJ, Sharpe AH. The B7 family revisited. Annu Rev Immunol. 2005;23:515–48.
37. Zhu C, Anderson AC, Schubart A, Xiong H, Imitola J, Khoury SJ, Zheng XX, Strom TB, Kuchroo VK. The Tim-3 ligand galectin-9 negatively regulates T helper type 1 immunity. Nat Immunol. 2005;6(12):1245–52.
38. Brandacher G, Perathoner A, Ladurner R, Schneeberger S, Obrist P, Winkler C, Werner ER, Werner-Felmayer G, Weiss HG, Georg G, Margreiter R. Prognostic value of indoleamine 2, 3-dioxygenase expression in colorectal cancer: effect on tumour-infiltrating T cells. Clin Cancer Res. 2006;12(4):1144–51.
39. Galon J, Costes A, Sanchez-Cabo F, Kirilovsky A, Mlecnik B, Lagorce-Pagès C, Tosolini M, Camus M, Berger A, Wind P, Zinzindohoué F. Type, density, and location of immune cells within human colorectal tumours predict clinical outcome. Science. 2006;313(5795):1960–4.
40. JZoshi AD, Hegde GV, Dickinson JD, Mittal AK, Lynch JC, Eudy JD, Armitage JO, Bierman PJ, Bociek RG, Devetten MP, Vose JM, Joshi SS. ATM, CTLA4, MNDA, and HEM1 in high versus low CD38 expressing B-cell chronic lymphocytic leukemia. Clin Cancer Res. 2007;13:5295–304.

41. Galon J, Fridman WH, Pagès F. The adaptive immunologic microenvironment in colorectal cancer: a novel perspective. Cancer Res. 2007;67(5):1883–6.
42. Schneider H, Valk E, Leung R, Rudd CE. CTLA-4 activation of phosphatidylinositol 3-kinase (PI 3-K) and protein kinase B (PKB/AKT) sustains T-cell anergy without cell death. PloS One. 2008;3(12):e3842.
43. Schneider CJ, Wang Y, El Kasmi KC, Pardoll DM, Murray PJ, Drake CG, Vignali DA. LAG-3 regulates plasmacytoid dendritic cell homeostasis. J Immunol. 2009;182(4):1885–91.
44. Liu WM, Fowler DW, Smith P, Dalgleish AG. Pre-treatment with chemotherapy can enhance the antigenicity and immunogenicity of tumours by promoting adaptive immune responses. Br J Cancer. 2010;102(1):115–23.
45. Camisaschi C, Casati C, Rini F, Perego M, De Filippo A, Triebel F, Parmiani G, Belli F, Rivoltini L, Castelli C. LAG-3 expression defines a subset of CD4+ CD25highFoxp3+ regulatory T cells that are expanded at tumour sites. J Immunol. 2010;184(11):6545–51.
46. Chung KY, Gore I, Fong L, Venook A, Beck SB, Dorazio P, Criscitiello PJ, Healey DI, Huang B, Gomez-Navarro J, Saltz LB. Phase II study of the anti-cytotoxic T-lymphocyte–associated antigen 4 monoclonal antibody, tremelimumab, in patients with refractory metastatic colorectal cancer. J Clin Oncol. 2010;28(21):3485–90.
47. Schreiber RD, Old LJ, Smyth MJ. Cancer immunoediting: integrating immunity's roles in cancer suppression and promotion. Science. 2011;331(6024):1565–70.
48. Fridman WH, Pagès F, Sautes-Fridman C, Galon J. The immune contexture in human tumours: impact on clinical outcome. Nat Rev Cancer. 2012;12(4):298–306.
49. Brahmer JR, Tykodi SS, Chow LQ, Hwu WJ, Topalian SL, Hwu P, Drake CG, Camacho LH, Kauh J, Odunsi K, Pitot HC. Safety and activity of anti–PD-L1 antibody in patients with advanced cancer. N Engl J Med. 2012;366(26):2455–65.
50. Mojtahedi Z, Mohmedi M, Rahimifar S, Erfani N, Hosseini SV, Ghaderi A. Programmed death-1 gene polymorphism (PD-1.5 C/T) is associated with colon cancer. Gene. 2012;508(2):229–32.
51. Rozali EN, Hato SV, Robinson BW, Lake RA, Lesterhuis WJ. Programmed death ligand 2 in cancer-induced immune suppression. Clin Dev Immunol. 2012;29:2012.
52. Topalian SL, Hodi FS, Brahmer JR, Gettinger SN, Smith DC, McDermott DF, Powderly JD, Carvajal RD, Sosman JA, Atkins MB, Leming PD. Safety, activity, and immune correlates of anti–PD-1 antibody in cancer. N Engl J Med. 2012;366(26):2443–54.
53. Woo SR, Turnis ME, Goldberg MV, Bankoti J, Selby M, Nirschl CJ, Bettini ML, Gravano DM, Vogel P, Liu CL, Tangsombatvisit S. Immune inhibitory molecules LAG-3 and PD-1 synergistically regulate T-cell function to promote tumoural immune escape. Cancer Res. 2012;72(4):917–27.
54. Droeser RA, Hirt C, Viehl CT, Frey DM, Nebiker C, Huber X, Zlobec I, Eppenberger-Castori S, Tzankov A, Rosso R, Zuber M. Clinical impact of programmed cell death ligand 1 expression in colorectal cancer. Eur J Cancer. 2013;49(9):2233–42.
55. Gagliani N, Magnani CF, Huber S, Gianolini ME, Pala M, Licona-Limon P, Guo B, De'Broski RH, Bulfone A, Trentini F, Di Serio C. Coexpression of CD49b and LAG-3 identifies human and mouse T regulatory type 1 cells. Nat Med. 2013;19(6):739.
56. Intlekofer AM, Thompson CB. At the bench: preclinical rationale for CTLA-4 and PD-1 blockade as cancer immunotherapy. J Leukoc Biol. 2013;94(1):25–39.
57. Siegel R, DeSantis C, Jemal A. Colorectal cancer statistics, 2014. CA Cancer J Clin. 2014;64(2):104–17.
58. Topalian SL, Sznol M, McDermott DF, Kluger HM, Carvajal RD, Sharfman WH, Brahmer JR, Lawrence DP, Atkins MB, Powderly JD, Leming PD. Survival, durable tumour remission, and long-term safety in patients with advanced melanoma receiving nivolumab. J Clin Oncol. 2014;32(10):1020.
59. Wu X, Zhang H, Xing Q, Cui J, Li J, Li Y, Tan Y, Wang S. PD-1+ CD8+ T cells are exhausted in tumours and functional in draining lymph nodes of colorectal cancer patients. Br J Cancer. 2014;111(7):1391–9.

60. Taube JM, Klein A, Brahmer JR, Xu H, Pan X, Kim JH, Chen L, Pardoll DM, Topalian SL, Anders RA. Association of PD-1, PD-1 ligands, and other features of the tumour immune microenvironment with response to anti–PD-1 therapy. Clin Cancer Res. 2014;20(19):5064–74.
61. Tumeh PC, Harview CL, Yearley JH, Shintaku IP, Taylor EJ, Robert L, Chmielowski B, Spasic M, Henry G, Ciobanu V, West AN. PD-1 blockade induces responses by inhibiting adaptive immune resistance. Nature. 2014;515(7528):568–71.
62. Herbst RS, Soria JC, Kowanetz M, Fine GD, Hamid O, Gordon MS, Sosman JA, McDermott DF, Powderly JD, Gettinger SN, Kohrt HE. Predictive correlates of response to the anti-PD-L1 antibody MPDL3280A in cancer patients. Nature. 2014;515(7528):563–7.
63. Tse BW, Collins A, Oehler MK, Zippelius A, Heinzelmann-Schwarz VA. Antibody-based immunotherapy for ovarian cancer: where are we at? Ann Oncol. 2014;25(2):322–31.
64. Le DT, Uram JN, Wang H, Bartlett BR, Kemberling H, Eyring AD, Skora AD, Luber BS, Azad NS, Laheru D, Biedrzycki B. PD-1 blockade in tumours with mismatch-repair deficiency. N Engl J Med. 2015;372(26):2509–20.
65. Llosa NJ, Cruise M, Tam A, Wicks EC, Hechenbleikner EM, Taube JM, Blosser RL, Fan H, Wang H, Luber BS, Zhang M. The vigorous immune microenvironment of microsatellite instable colon cancer is balanced by multiple counter-inhibitory checkpoints. Cancer Discov. 2015;5(1):43–51.
66. Hamanishi J, Mandai M, Ikeda T, Minami M, Kawaguchi A, Murayama T, Kanai M, Mori Y, Matsumoto S, Chikuma S, Matsumura N. Safety and antitumour activity of anti–PD-1 antibody, nivolumab, in patients with platinum-resistant ovarian cancer. J Clin Oncol. 2015;33(34):4015–22.
67. Ge J, Zhu L, Zhou J, Li G, Li Y, Li S, Wu Z, Rong J, Yuan H, Liu Y, Chi Q. Association between co-inhibitory molecule gene tagging single nucleotide polymorphisms and the risk of colorectal cancer in Chinese. J Cancer Res Clin Oncol. 2015;141(9):1533–44.
68. Jacobs J, Smits E, Lardon F, Pauwels P, Deschoolmeester V. Immune checkpoint modulation in colorectal cancer: what's new and what to expect. J Immunol Res. 2015;2015:158038.
69. Kang CW, Dutta A, Chang LY, Mahalingam J, Lin YC, Chiang JM, Hsu CY, Huang CT, Su WT, Chu YY, Lin CY. Apoptosis of tumour infiltrating effector TIM-3+ CD8+ T cells in colon cancer. Sci Rep. 2015;5(1):1–2.
70. Takamatsu M, Hirata A, Ohtaki H, Hoshi M, Ando T, Ito H, Hatano Y, Tomita H, Kuno T, Saito K, Seishima M. Inhibition of indoleamine 2, 3-dioxygenase 1 expression alters immune response in colon tumour microenvironment in mice. Cancer Sci. 2015;106(8):1008–15.
71. Tsuchiya N, Sawada Y, Endo I, Uemura Y, Nakatsura T. Potentiality of immunotherapy against hepatocellular carcinoma. World J Gastroenterol: WJG. 2015;21(36):10314.
72. Zhou E, Huang Q, Wang J, Fang C, Yang L, Zhu M, Chen J, Chen L, Dong M. Up-regulation of Tim-3 is associated with poor prognosis of patients with colon cancer. Int J Clin Exp Pathol. 2015;8(7):8018.
73. Van Cutsem E, Cervantes A, Adam R, Sobrero A, Van Krieken JH, Aderka D, Aranda Aguilar E, Bardelli A, Benson A, Bodoky G, Ciardiello F. ESMO consensus guidelines for the management of patients with metastatic colorectal cancer. Ann Oncol. 2016;27(8):1386–422.
74. Mak G, Moschetta M, Arkenau HT. Immunotherapy in colorectal cancer. In: Colorectal cancer: from pathogenesis to treatment, vol. 301. Rijeka: InTech; 2016.
75. Dudley JC, Lin MT, Le DT, Eshleman JR. Microsatellite instability as a biomarker for PD-1 blockade. Clin Cancer Res. 2016;22(4):813–20.
76. Segal NH, Kemeny NE, Cercek A, Reidy DL, Raasch PJ, Warren P, Hrabovsky AE, Campbell N, Shia J, Goodman KA, Erinjeri JP. Non-randomized phase II study to assess the efficacy of pembrolizumab (Pem) plus radiotherapy (RT) or ablation in mismatch repair proficient (pMMR) metastatic colorectal cancer (mCRC) patients. J Clin Oncol. 2016;34:3539.
77. Pandya PH, Murray ME, Pollok KE, Renbarger JL. The immune system in cancer pathogenesis: potential therapeutic approaches. J Immunol Res. 2016;2016:1.
78. Khalil DN, Smith EL, Brentjens RJ, Wolchok JD. The future of cancer treatment: immunomodulation, CARs and combination immunotherapy. Nat Rev Clin Oncol. 2016;13(5):273.

79. Overman MJ, McDermott R, Leach JL, Lonardi S, Lenz HJ, Morse MA, Desai J, Hill A, Axelson M, Moss RA, Goldberg MV. Nivolumab in patients with metastatic DNA mismatch repair-deficient or microsatellite instability-high colorectal cancer (CheckMate 142): an open-label, multicentre, phase 2 study. Lancet Oncol. 2017;18(9):1182–91.
80. Passardi A, Canale M, Valgiusti M, Ulivi P. Immune checkpoints as a target for colorectal cancer treatment. Int J Mol Sci. 2017;18(6):1324.
81. Shahda S, Noonan AM, Bekaii-Saab TS, O'Neil BH, Sehdev A, Shaib WL, Helft PR, Loehrer PJ, Tong Y, Liu Z, El-Rayes BF. A phase II study of pembrolizumab in combination with mFOLFOX6 for patients with advanced colorectal cancer. J Clin Oncol. 2017;35:3541.
82. Wang J, Yuan R, Song W, Sun J, Liu D, Li Z. PD-1, PD-L1 (B7-H1) and tumour-site immune modulation therapy: the historical perspective. J Hematol Oncol. 2017;10(1):34.
83. Overman MJ, Lonardi S, Wong KY, Lenz HJ, Gelsomino F, Aglietta M, Morse MA, Van Cutsem E, McDermott R, Hill A, Sawyer MB. Durable clinical benefit with nivolumab plus ipilimumab in DNA mismatch repair-deficient/microsatellite instability-high metastatic colorectal cancer. J Clin Oncol. 2018;36:773–9.
84. Bray F, Ferlay J, Soerjomataram I, Siegel RL, Torre LA, Jemal A. Erratum: global cancer statistics 2018: GLOBOCAN estimates of incidence and mortality worldwide for 36 cancers in 185 countries. CA Cancer J Clin. 2018;68:394–424.
85. Long L, Zhang X, Chen F, Pan Q, Phiphatwatchara P, Zeng Y, Chen H. The promising immune checkpoint LAG-3: from tumour microenvironment to cancer immunotherapy. Genes Cancer. 2018;9(5–6):176.
86. Walle T, Martinez Monge R, Cerwenka A, Ajona D, Melero I, Lecanda F. Radiation effects on antitumour immune responses: current perspectives and challenges. Ther Adv Med Oncol. 2018;10:1758834017742575.
87. Arnold M, Sierra MS, Laversanne M, Soerjomataram I, Jemal A, Bray F. Global patterns and trends in colorectal cancer incidence and mortality. Gut. 2017;66(4):683–91.
88. FDA U. FDA grants accelerated approval to pembrolizumab for first tissue/site agnostic indication. Silver Spring: US Food and Drug Administration; 2017.
89. Siegel RL, Miller KD, Fedewa SA, Ahnen DJ, Meester RG, Barzi A, Jemal A. Colorectal cancer statistics, 2017. CA Cancer J Clin. 2017;67(3):177–93.
90. Park YJ, Kuen DS, Chung Y. Future prospects of immune checkpoint blockade in cancer: from response prediction to overcoming resistance. Exp Mol Med. 2018;50(8):1–3.
91. Song W, Shen L, Wang Y, Liu Q, Goodwin TJ, Li J, Dorosheva O, Liu T, Liu R, Huang L. Synergistic and low adverse effect cancer immunotherapy by immunogenic chemotherapy and locally expressed PD-L1 trap. Nat Commun. 2018;9(1):1–1.
92. Dosset M, Vargas TR, Lagrange A, Boidot R, Végran F, Roussey A, Chalmin F, Dondaine L, Paul C, Marie-Joseph EL, Martin F. PD-1/PD-L1 pathway: an adaptive immune resistance mechanism to immunogenic chemotherapy in colorectal cancer. Onco Targets Ther. 2018;7(6):e1433981.
93. Kamatham S, Shahjehan F, Kasi PM. Immune checkpoint inhibitors in metastatic colorectal cancer: current status, recent advances, and future directions. Curr Colorectal Cancer Rep. 2019;15(4):112–21.
94. Everett KL, Kraman M, Wollerton FP, Zimarino C, Kmiecik K, Gaspar M, Pechouckova S, Allen NL, Doody JF, Tuna M. Generation of Fcabs targeting human and murine LAG-3 as building blocks for novel bispecific antibody therapeutics. Methods. 2019;154:60–9.
95. Workman CJ, Wang Y, El Kasmi KC, Pardoll DM, Murray PJ, Drake CG, Vignali DA. LAG-3 regulates plasmacytoid dendritic cell homeostasis. The Journal of Immunology. 2009;182(4):1885–91.
96. Tao W, Artama M, von Euler-Chelpin M, Hull M, Ljung R, Lynge E, Ólafsdóttir GH, Pukkala E, Romundstad P, Talbäck M, Tryggvadottir L. Colon and rectal cancer risk after bariatric surgery in a multicountry Nordic cohort study. International Journal of Cancer. 2020;147(3):728–35.
97. Nirschl CJ, Drake CG. Molecular pathways: coexpression of immune checkpoint molecules: signaling pathways and implications for cancer immunotherapy. Clinical cancer research. 2013;19(18):4917–24.

Chapter 16
Examining the Role of the MACC1 Gene in Colorectal Cancer Metastasis

Aparna S. Narayan, Jayshree Nellore, Valli C. Nachiyar, and Sujatha Peela

Abstract Positive survival outcomes for patients with colorectal cancer (CRC) are closely correlated to the metastatic dissemination of primary tumors. In fact, a staggering 90% of all deaths due to CRC are caused by its associated metastasis. At present, tumor staging and predictions as to whether the primary tumor will metastasize are done via the invasive method of histopathological staining. This chapter explores the potential of metastasis-associated in colon cancer 1 (MACC1) as a potential non-invasive biomarker in the diagnosis, staging, and prognosis of CRC. MACC1, discovered in 2009, is an evolutionarily conserved molecule which is involved in a plethora of interactions with other key biomolecules toward the development and metastasis of primary tumors in the colon. This chapter aims to provide a comprehensive overview of this molecule by deconstructing the machinations by which MACC1 upregulates and downregulates signaling pathways which influence events in the metastatic cascade of CRC. Beginning with an introduction into CRC, this chapter describes the various characteristics of the MACC1 gene and protein along with their role in activating signaling pathways such as c-MET, β-catenin/AKT, SPON2, etc. The review then explores the real-time potential of MACC1 in clinical settings as a diagnostic and prognostic marker to provide accurate information on the stage of CRC, probability of metastasis, and response to treatment. This chapter concludes with current trends and research investigating MACC1 as a potential therapeutic target for improved treatment options and interventions.

Keywords Colorectal cancer · MACC1 · Predictive biomarkers · Metastasis · Molecular therapy

---

A. S. Narayan · J. Nellore (✉) · V. C. Nachiyar
Department of Biotechnology, Sathyabama Institute of Science and Technology (Deemed to be University), Chennai, Tamil Nadu, India

S. Peela (✉)
Department of Biotechnology, Dr.B.R. Ambedkar University, Srikakulam, AP, India

G. P. Nagaraju et al. (eds.), *Colon Cancer Diagnosis and Therapy*,
https://doi.org/10.1007/978-3-030-63369-1_16

Abbreviations

5-FU	Fluorouracil
ABCG2	ATP-binding cassette sub-family G member
ACF	Aberrant crypt foci
AP-1	Activator protein 1
APC gene	Adenomatous polyposis coli 1
AS1	Antisense ribonucleic acid
ATP	Adenosine triphosphate
CAC	Colitis-associated cancer
ChIP	Chromatin immunoprecipitation
CNV	Copy number variations
CRC	Colorectal cancer
CTC	Circulating tumor cells
CTNNB1	Catenin beta-1
DD	C-terminal death domains
DNA	Deoxyribonucleic acid
EGFR	Epidermal growth factor receptor
ELISA	Enzyme-linked immunosorbent assay
EMSA	Electrophoretic mobility shift assay
EMT	Epithelial-mesenchymal transition
FAP	Familial adenomatous polyposis coli
FAS	Fas cell surface death receptor
HGF	Hepatocyte growth factor
HIF-1	Hypoxia-inducible factor 1 subunit alpha
HK2	Hexokinase 2
hTERT	Human telomerase reverse transcriptase
HTS	High-throughput screenings
LDH	Lactate dehydrogenase
lncRNA	Long non-coding ribonucleic acid
MACC1	Metastasis-associated in colon cancer 1
MET	MET proto-oncogene, receptor tyrosine kinase
miRNA/miR	Microribonucleic acid
MMR	Mismatch repair
mR-1	Major histocompatibility complex class I-related gene protein
mRNA	Messenger ribonucleic acid
PDH	Pyruvate dehydrogenase
PI3K	Phosphatidylinositol-4,5-bisphosphate 3-kinase
PTM	Post-transcriptional modifications
qRT-PCR	Real-time quantitative reverse transcription polymerase chain reaction
RNA	Ribonucleic acid
SNPs	Single nucleotide polymorphisms
Sp1	Specificity protein 1

SPON2	Spondin 2
STAT1	Signal transducer and activator of transcription 1
TAM	Tumor-associated macrophages
TCF7L2	Transcription factor 7-like 2
TGF-β	Transforming growth factor beta 1
TLR	Toll-like receptors
UTR	Untranslated region
VEGF	Vascular endothelial growth factors
VEGF-A	Vascular endothelial growth factor A
Wnt	Wingless-related integration site
μORF	Upstream open reading frames

16.1 Introduction

16.1.1 A Brief Outline of Colorectal Cancer

Colorectal cancer (CRC) is a particularly serious form of cancer which, according to a 2018 status report by GLOBOCAN, affects over 1.09 million people worldwide and causes 551,000 deaths [1]. Colorectal cancer develops in the large intestine and is synonymous with the terms "bowel cancer," "colon cancer," or "rectal cancer." 65% of all CRC cases are found to occur in developed countries [2], with a higher incidence rate among men in comparison to women [2]. Although characterized by symptoms such as blood in the stool, weight loss, lethargy, and irregular bowel movements, one in two patients with CRC does not report any symptoms in the early stages of the disease [3]. The major underlying causes which ultimately lead to the development of CRC are related to age and poor lifestyle. Obesity, sedentary lifestyles, smoking, alcohol consumption, and constant diets of red and processed meat have been found to increase an individual's risk of this disease [4]. Additionally, certain syndromes, such as Crohn's disease, ulcerative colitis, Gardner syndrome, and inflammatory bowel disease, show strong associative links to CRC [2, 5]. Estimates from a decade ago stated that more than 75% of patients with CRC show a negligible genetic propensity toward it [6, 7]. Interestingly despite these supposedly tenuous associations to underlying genetic risks, CRC's genetic mechanisms have been the subject of robust investigations with recent research shedding light on the definitive role of certain genes in the development and progression of this disease. An emphatic example for CRC's relation to inherited genetic risks is the observation that individuals with two or more first-degree relatives are two to three more times likely to develop colorectal cancers in their lifetimes. 20% of all patients with CRC have reported the presence of CRC among their first-degree kin. Most cases in this subset have Lynch syndrome which is also known as hereditary nonpolyposis colorectal cancer [7]. Another inherited genetic disorder that causes CRC is familial adenomatous polyposis [2].

Research into the molecular biology of CRC shows that acquired or inherited mutations in the Wnt signaling pathway increase the signaling activity and lead to a cascade of events that ultimately end in the uncontrollable division and proliferation of epithelial cells lining the colon or rectum [8], whereas the mutations themselves are believed to originate in the intestinal crypt stem cell [8–10]. The APC gene codes for the protein adenomatous polyposis coli which in turn controls and restricts the accumulation of β-catenin protein. Researchers have shown that APC is often a mutated gene in CRC and no longer curbs the accumulation of β-catenin which causes the latter to move into the nucleus, bind to the DNA there, and activate the transcription of proto-oncogenes [11]. Another important route that leads to CRC is that of mutations in genes which hampers the programmed cell death function. Apart from mutations in the APC gene, CRC can also occur via mutations in the CTNNB1, NKD1, TCF7L2, AXIN1, or/and AXIN2 genes [11]. TGF-β, SMAD, and DCC (deleted in colorectal cancer), which are responsible for programmed cell death, are commonly seen to be deactivated in CRC [11, 12]. TGF-β in particular has been found to have a deactivating mutation in approximately 50% of all colorectal cancers [11]. Additional genes whose mutations are linked to CRC are FAM123B, SOX9, ATM, ARID1A, ACVR2A, MSH3, SLC9A9, TGFBR2, BRAF, TCF7L2, MSH6, and MYC [13]. All these genes are involved in the Wnt and TGF-β pathways [13].

The mismatch repair (MMR) system in the cells is present to detect errors and correct them consequently maintaining the integrity of the cell's genetic material [14]. In Lynch syndrome, there is epigenetic silencing or mutations in the MMR proteins which interfere with the cells' inherent capacity to correct errors and further allow cancer mutations to progress. 15-18% of CRC tumors have been found to have aberrations in the MMR mechanism [15]. Abnormal methylation, i.e., hypomethylation or hypermethylation, of protein-coding genes and miRNA are also associated with CRCs [15, 16]. CRC shows a positive correlation with age, and several genes that show methylation with age have also been implicated in the development of CRC [15].

Mortality due to CRC is proportional to its metastasis. As discussed in this review, MACC1 is a gene that has been recorded to influence proliferation, invasion, and scattering of colon cancer cells [17]. Colorectal cancer is mostly benign in its initial stages, usually present in the form of a polyp which may become cancers as time progresses. If detected at its early stages, CRC will most likely be confined to the walls of the colon and respond positively to surgical intervention. However, when metastasis occurs, treatment becomes increasingly difficult with the patient more likely to have palliative care rather than active treatment. Many classical models tracing the progression and pathogenesis of CRC describe the polyp to cancer sequence [18]. This transformation of the polyp into a metastatic form may take several years and occur due to mutations and epigenetic and inflammatory changes [18]. The three most widely described types of polyps are adenomatous polyps (adenomas), which are pre-cancerous and may sometimes change into cancer, hyperplastic polyps and inflammatory polyps which are common but typically not pre-cancerous, and, finally, sessile serrated polyps and traditional serrated adenomas which have a considerable risk to develop into CRC [7]. Polyps are more likely to develop into CRC if they are larger than 1 cm, if there are more than three, or if they are associated with dysplasia when removed [7].

Metastasis in CRC is the leading factor that leads to patient death. Recovery rates are 90% for patients in early stages, 65% in those with initial lymph node metastases, and less than 10% in individuals with distant metastasis [19]. A staggering 50% of CRC patients develop distant metastases, and discerning the stage of CRC and predictions on whether it will metastasize are largely done using histopathological staging and describing tumor spread within surgical specimens [20]. According to a paper by Stein and Schlag in 2007 [21], colon tumors show distinct tropisms in regard to the targets of metastasis. There are a 30–70% spread into the liver, 20–40% spread in the lung, 5–10% spread in the bone, and minimal spread into the brain, ovaries, and adrenal gland [20, 21]. 25% of patients diagnosed with CRC will already have distant metastases or synchronous metastasis, while another 25% will develop distant metastases or, in this case, metachronous metastasis within 2 years of initial diagnosis and treatment. According to statistics from the National Cancer Institute, approximately 90% of all patients' deaths due to CRC are directly linked to metastatic dissemination [22]. To reduce the high mortality associated with this cancer and improve patient outcomes, it is critical to investigate and evaluate methods to identify the risk of metastasis during the early stages of the disease.

16.1.2 Metastasis-Associated in Colon Cancer 1 (MACC1)

Metastasis-associated in colon cancer 1 (MACC1) is an oncogene found to be involved in the progression and metastasis of cancer. It is located on the minus strand of the human chromosome 7 (7p21.1) at 20,146,776 to 20,223,538 (76,762 bp) [23]. Interestingly, chromosomal aneuploidy such as trisomy and tetrasomy on chromosome 7 is not only characteristic of CRC but is found in several other cancer types as well. 7p21 is associated with other cancers of the gastrointestinal tracts such as gastric, intestinal, and pancreatic cancer. The unspliced primary MACC1 transcript was found to have 7 exons and 6 introns. The longest mRNA, when spliced, had 3,188 nucleotides and all 7 exons. Further, the 5′ end of MACC1 contains several upstream open reading frames (μORFs) with the longest ORF at 2,559 nucleotides, starting at exon 4, position 310. This ORF is of particular interest and is often referred to as the MACC1 consensus coding sequence [23]. The MACC1 has several single nucleotide polymorphisms (SNPs) in weakly conserved positions with 16 present in the coding sequence. These SNPs have been found to contain premature stop codons and cause exchanges of arginine and threonine, as well as shifting reading frames.

Genome-wide searches looking to identify differentially expressed genes in CRC showed that MACC1 expression levels increase during the transition from adenoma to carcinoma. MACC1 mRNA can be detected in all stages of colon cancer and predict the possibility of metastasis to an accuracy of 74–80%, depending on the stage of the cancer. In patients with a low expression of MACC1, survival rates were placed at 80% over a course of 5 years, whereas those with high MACC1 expression levels had an 85% mortality rate [17, 20, 24]. Research shows that genes neighboring MACC1 such as TWIST and IGB8, which are involved in signal transduction, cell adhesion, and motility, may also be responsible for tumorigenesis and metastasis in CRC [25, 26].

16.1.3 MACC1 in CRC

Metastasis-associated in colon cancer 1 (MACC1) was identified by Stein and colleagues during a landmark investigation carried out in 2009 [25]. They found that this gene, located on chromosome 7, plays a definitive role in the metastatic progression of CRC. Apart from CRC, MACC1 also serves as a biomarker for the following cancer types: ovarian cancer [27], renal carcinoma [28], lung cancer [29], breast cancer [30], gallbladder cancer [31], osteosarcoma [32], hepatocellular carcinoma [33], gastric cancer [34], esophageal cancer [35], tongue squamous cancer [36], glioma [37], pancreatic cancer [38], nasopharyngeal cancer [39], salivary adenoid cystic carcinoma [40], and hilar cholangiocarcinoma [41].

MACC1 expresses itself in the critical transition of a benign polyp to its malignant phenotype. Further, according to observations by Arlt et al. [20], MACC1 protein is present in the nucleus of tumors that develop distant metastases. In non-metastasizing tumors, MACC1 was absent in the nucleus and present in the cytoplasm. This gene enables metastasis in CRC by inducing invasion and pro-tumor inflammation; sustaining proliferation; allowing the evasion of growth suppression, immune attack, and cell death; promoting tumor angiogenesis and metabolic reprogramming; and causing genetic instability along with replicative immortality [42]. Studying 103 metastatic tissues and the associated MACC1 copy numbers and mRNA expression levels showed a positive correlation between MACC1 expression and CRC metastasis [43]. Interestingly, analysis by Isella et al. in 2013 showed that MACC1 was the only independent parameter to predict the probability of recurrence in CRC [44]. A definitive advantage of MACC1 as a biomarker to predict metastasis is its non-invasive nature. Additionally, MACC1 transcripts can be detected in the plasma of patients with CRC, as shown in a study examining 312 such samples by Stein et al. [45].

16.2 Metastasis-Associated in Colon Cancer 1 (MACC1)

16.2.1 MACC1 Gene's Promoter

The MACC1 promoter, spanning from −426 to −18, is critical to its functioning as it consists of functional binding sites for various transcription factors. Some of these transcription factors include activator protein 1 (AP-1), specificity protein 1 (Sp1), and CCAAT-enhancer-binding protein (C/EBP) [46, 47]. Research has shown that these factors regulate the transcription of MACC1 by binding to its minimal essential core promoter regions. Further, observations from electrophoretic mobility shift assays (EMSA) and chromatin immunoprecipitation (ChIP) assays display that expression levels of Sp1 and c-Jun are synchronous to those of the gene itself and its propensity to influence metachronous metastases [46].

Juneja et al. [46], as mentioned above, examined the influence of transcription factors on the MACC1 promoter by observing the promoter region of MACC1 by generating truncated deletion constructs. Identification of the MACC1 promoter has come with several key advantages, one of which is the ability to utilize this knowledge to carry out high-throughput screenings (HTS) for transcriptional MACC1 inhibitors [46].

16.2.2 MACC1's Targets

MACC1 is responsible for metastasis by directly or indirectly influencing a variety of functions such as proliferation, metabolic de-regulation, apoptosis resistance, angiogenesis, and stemness. Research into the molecular mechanism by which this gene performs these functions have yielded interesting results. MACC1 starts the cascade of events leading up to and sustaining metastasis by activating its target molecules such as c-MET, NANOG, and SPON2. Among MACC1's target molecules, c-MET plays a central and critical role in the downstream signaling mechanisms of MEK/ERK, PISK/AKT/β-catenin, STAT1/3, and TWIST/VEGF. These signaling mechanisms are associated with the oncogenic cellular processes of transformation, tumor progression, and metastasis. Apart from c-MET, NANOG has been found to induce stemness, and SPON2 contributes to metastatic dissemination [42].

c-MET occurs in tandem with HGF and the HGF/MET axis. Its role, along with MACC1, in influencing the metastasis of CRC has been an area of intense research over the course of the last decade. Further, insights into this mechanism have the potential to reveal promising targets for anti-tumor and anti-metastatic intervention among CRC patients with or at risk for cancer spread [48]. MET first binds to its ligand hepatocyte growth factor (HGF) and forms a complex which in turn activates the HGF/Met signaling pathway responsible for the various stages in metastasis. It must be noted that MACC1 is a target of the MAPK signaling pathway which ensures MACC1 transcription and translation [20]. Two independent but related studies conducted by Stein et al. [17, 49] provided novel observations regarding the process by which MACC1 binds to the Met promoter fragment. They noted that certain sites within the confines of the Met promoter such as Sp1 and AP2 act as specific consensus sequences to which the MACC1 binds. This interrelationship between MACC1, Met, and HGF represents a positive feedback loop that acts as an important driving force behind metastasis in CRC. Hence, MACC1 and Met show promise as possible pacemakers to study and monitor the progression of cancer spread in patients with colorectal cancer (Fig. 16.1).

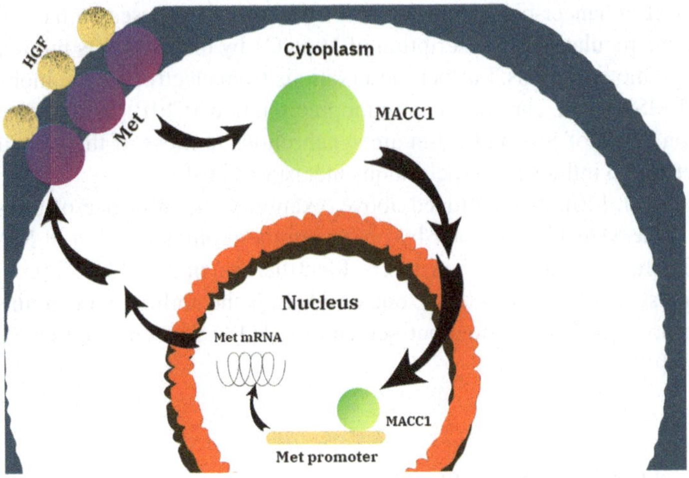

Fig. 16.1 The MACC1-Met-HGF axis. As illustrated by the figure, HGF along with Met causes the translocation of MACC1 from the cytoplasm and into the nucleus. Once in the nucleus, MACC1 binds to its target, the Met promoter, which leads to the transcription of Met mRNA and translation into more Met, hence forming a positive feedback mechanism. (Please note that the figure in the illustration above is for descriptive purposes and is not an accurate representation of the actual biomolecules)

As mentioned briefly before, MACC1 binds to several promoters of genes that may contribute to cell proliferation and motility. Schmid et al. studied the potential of SPON2 [50] and S100P [51] as targets for MACC1 and the subsequent effect after their binding. They found that both SPON2 and S100P induced cell motility in cell cultures and liver metastasis in mice. However, studies on human cell lines and details on the exact mechanism of how these transcription factors operate are still elusive.

Another interesting finding concerning MACC1 and its target molecules is the resulting resistance to chemotherapy medication cisplatin on overexpression of this gene. Although yet to be conclusively established in the case of CRC, it has been observed that the downregulation of MACC1 reduced the resistance to cisplatin in human glioblastoma U251 cells and tongue squamous cell carcinoma [36, 52]. The hypothesis that MACC1 expression may lead to cisplatin resistance is centered around the idea of the ATP-binding cassette sub-family G member 2 (ABCG2) being a transcriptional target of MACC1. It is hence theorized that the overexpression of MACC1 may cause an increase in ABCG2 and subsequent cisplatin resistance [47]. An investigation into the role of the Wnt/β-catenin pathway showed that the activation of this pathway decreased sensitization to cisplatin, whereas the inhibition of it led to a positive response to this medicine [53]. Aberrations in the Wnt pathway have been well established in CRC [8, 13]; however, the role of MACC1 in the former is yet to be explored.

An additional transcription factor demonstrated to be related to MACC1 is TWIST1/2. MACC1 works through the HGF/Met signal pathway to upregulate this

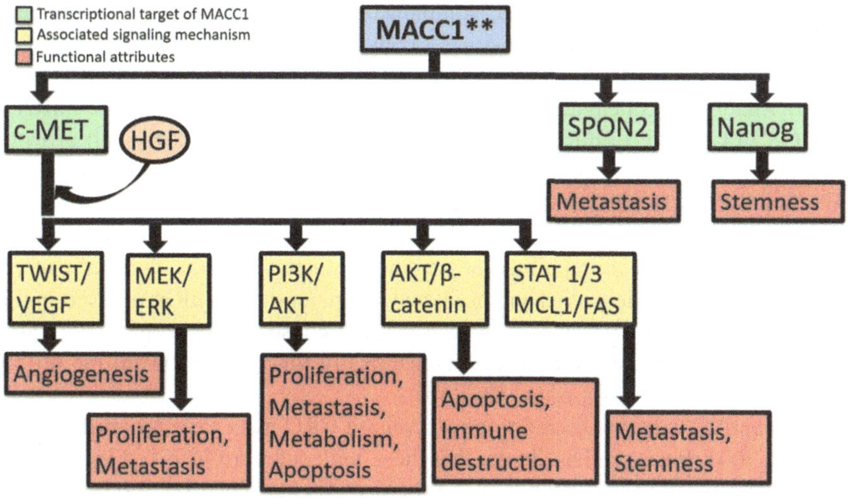

Fig. 16.2 Flowchart adapted from [42] summarizing the MACC1 targets and the resulting functional attributes. As seen in the figure, the major targets of MACC1 identified include c-MET, SPON2, and Nanog. While the associated signaling mechanism associated with c-MET has been well defined, additional investigation is still required to understand the exact pathway by which SPON2 and Nanog cause metastasis and stemness. (**Adapted from Radhakrishnan et al. [42])

transcription factor. Through this channel, MACC1 causes vasculogenic mimicry in gastric cancer tumors [54]. Although vascularization in tumors of patients with CRC is yet to be positively correlated to it, TWIST1/2 itself is an important biomarker that has been linked to epithelial-mesenchymal transition (EMT) in CRC [55, 56]. Hence, one possible route by which MACC1 has been theorized to lead to vascularization and EMT in CRC is via the HGF/MET/TWIST1/2 pathway [47] (Fig. 16.2).

16.2.3 miRNA Influence on MACC1 Expression

miRNAs are small, conserved RNA molecules with the ability to modulate the genes they target in a post-transcriptional manner. Evolutionarily directed to be conserved and endogenous, miRNA molecules have been found to play a critical role in the progression of tumors into their metastatic phenotype in CRC patients [57]. Over the last few years, the potential of miRNA to be used as a biomarker in the diagnosis and prognosis of metastasis in various cancers, including CRC, has been explored [57]. With respect to CRC in particular, the miRNA mR-1 was observed to contribute significantly to the transcriptional regulation of Met in CRC specimens, as reported by Migliore et al. in 2012 [58]. Their research yielded new and interesting insights into the delicate interplay between miR-1 and MACC1 toward causing metastasis. It was shown that miR-1 is significantly downregulated during the course of CRC progression. Ergo, simultaneous overexpression of MACC1 and downregulation of miR-1 may positively contribute toward the transformation of benign tumors into malignant ones among patients with CRC. Similar in silico analysis by Zhang and colleagues highlighted a similar downregulation of the miRNA miR-143 in CRC [59]. miR-143 plays a role in delimiting excessive cell growth, migration, and invasion by taking part in the Ras, Erk5, and Akt pathways [60]. Additionally, miRNA may also influence several signal molecules and prevent aberrations in the MAPK, PI3K/Akt, and HGF/Met pathways, serving as a novel therapeutic target for medication aimed at curbing the metastasis of colorectal cancer. Hurst et al., in 2009, described and predicted this potential of miRNAs to aid in the clinical intervention of cancer metastasis and consequently coined the term "metastamiRNA" to describe miRNAs specifically functioning toward the up- or downregulation of metastases [61].

Other miRNAs hypothesized to play a role in CRC metastasis are miR-338-3p and miR-200a. Research has shown that these molecules are involved in the transcriptional regulation and inhibition of processes such as invasion, migration, and EMT in gastric and hepatocellular carcinomas [62, 63]. miR-338-3p was found to suppress EMT in gastric cancer by taking part in cytoskeleton remodeling and motor activity and ensuring basolateral polarity formation among epithelial cells. By binding to the 3'UTR region of the MACC1 gene, this miRNA targeted the MACC1/Met/Akt pathway and prevented metastasis in gastric cancer cells [62]. However, these miRNAs' exact role in CRC is yet to be definitively identified.

Many studies studying the interplay between the HGF/Met pathway, metastasis, and HIF-1α stabilization have shown that the latter interacts with the former pathway and plays an active role in cancer progression in CRC [64]. In light of the findings of MACC1 functioning with HIF-1α stabilization, it has been suggested that the former may be stress-responsive as the latter has been established to be involved in creating hypoxic stress. Some miRNAs such as miR-511-5p and miR-483 are involved in overcoming hypoxia in CRC [65, 66]. It has also been found that methylation of miR-218 disallows the expression of MACC1; this was further proved by analyzing the expression patterns of miR-218 and the consequent inhibition of MACC1 under the influence of the methyltransferase inhibitor 5-azacytidine. Other miRNAs involved in reducing MACC1 expression were summarized in a review by Radhakrishnan et al. [42] and include miR-141, miR-433, miR-485, miR-497, miR-574-5p, miR-590-3p, miR-598, and miR-944 [67].

16.2.4 MACC1 Domain Architecture

The MACC1 protein associated with the gene is made up of 852 amino acids which form several functionally important domains and motifs. MACC1 can interact with a wide variety of biomolecules due to its uniquely arranged protein domains [23]. Characteristic oncogenic cellular mechanisms – such as proliferation, invasion, resistance to treatment, and hindrance of apoptosis – are a result of protein-protein interaction and post-translational modifications [68]. The various domains of

MACC1, i.e., ZU5; SRC Homology, 3 Domain (SH3); and two C-terminal death domains (DD), have been identified via fold recognition and homology modeling algorithms [69]. The SH3 domain and binding motif in particular have been found to play a critical role in the biological function of the protein. Observations have shown that the absence of the SH3 region disallows MACC1 from binding to its transcriptional target Met [17]. To properly gauge the exact impact of the SH3 domain in MACC1 specifically in terms of tumorigenesis and metastasis, Pichorner et al. carried out a study analyzing SW480-derived transfectants without this domain. They found that in the absence of this domain, cell motility, translocation of MACC1 into the nucleus, tumor development, and metastasis in mice were drastically reduced. Hence, the SH3 domain is crucial in MACC1 metastatic expression. The double DD architecture has been shown to trigger apoptosis and regulate innate immunity, inflammation, and directed migration [68, 70].

Additionally, the N-terminal of this protein which precedes the ZU5 region has 130 to 150 amino acids with conserved motifs including a clathrin box, two Epsin 15 Homology motifs, interacting sites, and an adaptor protein 2α binding site [23]. Motifs in the central and C-terminal region on MACC1 have been theorized to be associated with putative tyrosine phosphorylation. Phosphorylated tyrosine is central to signal transduction and receptor mediation. Residues in MACC1 with a propensity toward phosphorylation are Y379, Y598, Y695, Y768, Y789, and Y793. Loss of phosphorylation has been linked to loss of function in MACC1 [23].

16.2.5 Post-translational Modifications (PTMs) of MACC1

MACC1 regulation takes place on the transcriptional and post-transcriptional levels. As is typical of proteins, MACC1 is a target of post-translational modifications (PTMs) following its translation and folding. PTMs like phosphorylation, glycosylation, and covalent attachment mediate cellular localization, activity, interaction, stability, and binding affinity. The sites of these modifications can be predicted by algorithms. Additionally, post-transcriptional repression of MACC1 is often carried out by various miRNAs [42]. The expressions of MACC1's target genes have been hypothesized to depend on N-acetyl-glucosamine and β-catenin [23]. Therefore, therapeutic interference of MACC1 at the transcriptional and post-translational level using small molecules may serve to help improve current clinical interventions for CRC and improve patient outcomes.

16.2.6 Single Nucleotide Polymorphisms of MACC1

Lang and colleagues, in 2011, were the first to report correlations between single nucleotide polymorphisms (SNPs) of MACC1 and patient outcomes [71]. SNPs such as rs1990172 and rs975263 have been found to be linked to heightened risk toward metachronous metastasis development and shorter patient survival among cohorts above the age of 60 with stage I or II CRC tumors [42]. The MACC1 gene is associated with 16 SNPs in its weakly conserved coding region [23].

A study of 318 CRC patients examining 6 SNPs of MACC1 suggested that rs1990172, located in the intronic region of MACC1, was linked to poor patient recovery and could be used to predict overall survival rate [72]. Additionally, copy number variations (CNV) in MACC1 were shown to impact the latter's expression levels and cause large lesions, multiple metastases, and vascularization [43]. Examining the SNPs and CNVs of MACC1, individually or in combination, has the potential to be diagnostic biomarkers for CRC metastasis. Additionally, examining the status of mismatch repair may be of prognostic value and predict whether treatment via 5-FU is a viable option for patients with CRC in stage II [73].

16.3 Colon Cancer Metastasis, Routes, and Steps

16.3.1 Colon Cancer Metastasis

In 1889, Paget drew parallels to seeds in soil to explain distant metastases' characteristic organ specificity. This hypothesis laid the foundations for contemporary theories and studies regarding the various events in the "metastatic cascade" [74]. The metastatic cascade includes cell detachment from the primary tumor mass, invasion into the surrounding tissue, intravasation, extravasation, arrest at target organs, initiation of proliferation, and neo-angiogenesis [75]. The organ targets of CRC metastasis are heavily influenced by the vascular system architecture and the interaction of the tumor cells with its surrounding microenvironment [74, 76].

A characteristic feature of cancer is the presence of uncontrolled cell growth and division through unregulated cell cycles. This is done via the upregulation of growth factors and causes sustained proliferation. This ability to supersede control mechanisms allows the cells to enter a continuous growth state of rapid cell expansion and spreading. Cancer cells also show heightened resistance to apoptosis or programmed cell death and immune surveillance. Further, inflammation is often associated with metastasis and enhances the cancer's ability to spread to neighboring sites. The metastatic capability of the cancer cells is conserved through continuous genome instability caused by SNPs, CNV, and mutations. The tumor receives oxygen and metabolites and removes its waste through the development of an active vascular network formed via tumor angiogenesis and neovascularization. Oncogenes also shift the energy metabolism of the cells toward aerobic glycolysis (Warburg effect) and perpetuate unlimited replication through telomerase activity, which prevents telomere attrition [77–79].

Prognosis of cancer and patient survival rate predictions are currently based on histopathological staging which uses the parameters tumor infiltration depth (T), lymph node metastasis (N), and distant metastasis (M). While stages I and II do not show any metastasis, stage III shows lymph node metastasis, and stage IV is

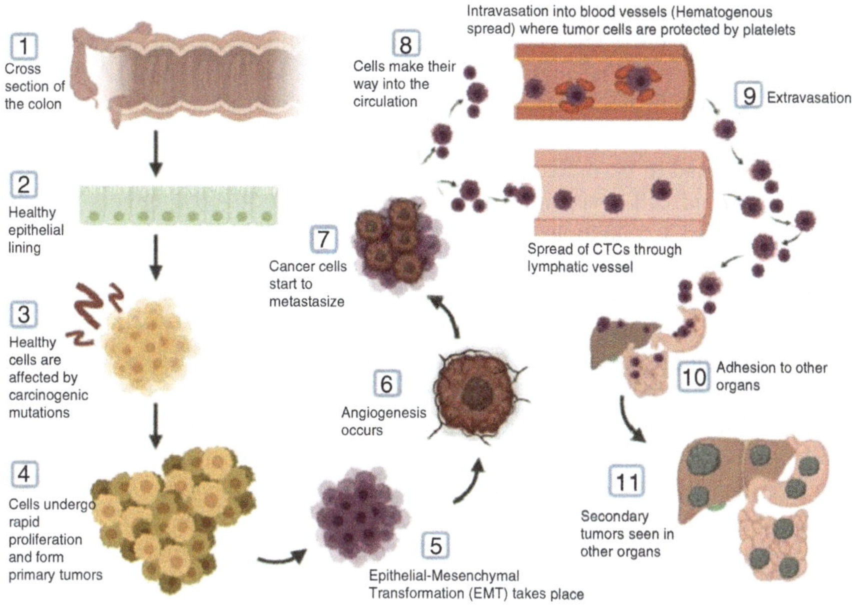

Fig. 16.3 Metastatic cascade in colorectal cancer: The epithelial cells lining the colon, under carcinogenic stress, rapidly divide and proliferate as seen in (4) in the figure above. The cells then transform into mesenchymal cells via the EMT mechanism. With angiogenesis, tumor cells receive metabolites, oxygen, and other essential requirements which allows them to continue dividing and expanding. Metastasis or the spreading of the tumor may happen either through the blood vessels and lymphatic vessels or via independent CTCs that have broken off from the primary tumor. The CRC CTCs then attach themselves to neighboring or distant organs and form secondary tumors at these sites. (Image made with BioRender and compiled using information gathered from [42] and [76])

characterized by spread to distant organs. TNM-based staging comes with several disadvantages, primary of which is its inability to predict metastasis in patients who receive treatment and recover. 30–40% of patients who have recovered from stage I or II cancer show recurrence or develop metachronous metastasis. Screening for biomolecules may solve this problem as several liquid biopsies have now been established as a non-invasive, fairly accurate method to help cyclically monitor recurrence and predict metastatic development [20, 80] (Fig. 16.3).

16.3.2 General Molecular Determinants of Tumor Progression and Metastasis

Cells undergo complex changes at the molecular level that enable them to display oncogenic characteristics such as invasiveness, motility, resistance to apoptosis, etc. Fearson and Vogelstein proposed that tumor progression which takes place from aberrant crypt foci (ACF) is the result of mutations that inactivate tumor suppressor genes and activate oncogenic ones. Important tumor suppressors that may be inactivated as a result of genetic alterations are p53, Smad 2/4, TGF-RII, and APC. APC is mutated in 85% of colon tumors and may lead to familial adenomatous polyposis coli (FAP) [81, 82]. β-Catenin, which, along with APC, plays a key role in the Wnt pathway, is found to be mutated in most CRC cells. This may cause unregulated proliferation and cell division. Signal dysregulation in 50–60% tumors may be attributed, in part, to mutations in the K-Ras oncogene. Other receptors that may be activated and cause uncontrollable proliferation are those of tyrosine kinase ErbB2 and Met [20].

Carcinogenesis is also associated with epigenetic silencing. Colon tumors work by silencing tumor suppressor genes such as p16/INK4A, hMLH1, and SFRP via promoter hypermethylation [83–85]. Other signaling pathways, such as HGF/met, TGF, and Wnt, along with their target transcription factors like Ets/AP1, Twist, and Snail have been implicated in causing EMT. These pathways suppress the expression of E-cadherin, N-cadherin, and vimentin which leads to key processes of the metastatic cascade [82]. Cancer cell proliferation may occur due to the upregulation of certain growth factors which cause the cell cycle to progress without checkpoints. This is often caused by aberrations in p53, Rb and PTEN, cyclin-dependent kinases, cyclins, CIP, KIP, and/or c-MYC [44]. Additionally, the angiogenesis process is governed by vascular endothelial growth factors (VEGFs) such as angiopoietin1, angiopoietin2, VEGFR1, VEGFR2, VEGFR3, and Tie1 [86, 87]. Wnt signaling is also activated by hTERT-β-catenin/LEF-mediated interaction by telomerase [88]. Other factors that contribute to the stemness of cancer cells are CD117, SOX2, and OCT4 [89].

16.3.3 Effect and Influence of MACC1 on the Various Stages of CRC Metastatic Progression

16.3.3.1 Activating Invasion and Metastasis

MACC1 causes CRC tumors to progress from adenomas to carcinomas by inducing cell motility [90]. During this process, the primary tumor's epithelial features give way to form an invasive front that makes its way into the underlying tissue and causing the spread of circulating tumor cells (CTCs) [91]. MACC1, which can also be detected in 55% of the tumor buds in CRC, plays a crucial role in the metastatic process by initiating and driving cell invasion [91]. This was further corroborated by findings that linked transgenic overexpression of MACC1 to the conversion of non-invasive adenomas to carcinomas in mice [92]. MACC1 brings about EMT through the MACC1/HGF/c-MET axis which relies on c-MET/AKT signaling [17]. Additionally, the TWIST1 and TWIST2 transcription factors also drive migration and invasion in CRC [93]. EMT is also caused by MACC1-regulated PI3K/AKT signaling and increased pAKT expression which results in mesenchymal differentiation [94]. Matrix remodeling, which is a characteristic of this stage in metastasis, has been shown to correlate to E-cadherin, enhanced N-cadherin, and α-smooth muscle actin [94]. Cell plasticity and motility are enhanced in CRC cells via the WNT signaling which in turn is influenced by kinase AKT, β-catenin, SNAIL½, TWIST½, and CDH1 [95]. Carcinogenesis and progression of colorectal cancer through the invasion factor MMP9 (metalloproteinase) are also associated with MACC1 [96].

16.3.3.2 Ensuring Continuous Proliferation

MACC1 is most closely associated with c-MET and the receptor tyrosine kinase promoting factor HGF. c-MET activates GAB1-SHP2-ERK/MAPK and PI3K/AKT which sustain proliferation in metastatic CRC tumor cells [97]. Before binding to c-MET, MACC1 is regulated by the ERK signaling mechanism through AP1 and SP1 [98]. Self-sustaining proliferation takes place via a positive feedback loop as illustrated in Fig. 16.2. The target genes c-MYC, cyclin D1/E, MMP2, VEGF, and MMP9 which are members of the PI3K/AKT pathway are also involved in MACC1-induced cell proliferation [99]. MMP promotes proliferation by increasing the spatial availability of growth factors, while VEGF achieves the same via angiogenesis [100, 101]. It must be noted that c-MET can also be activated without HGF. Certain point mutations in the transducer docking sites may result in oncogenic transformation [102].

16.3.3.3 Escaping Growth Suppression

Cancer cells show a distinct dysregulation in their cell division cycles which causes unrestricted cell division. MACC1 was found to cause this phenomenon by inducing uncontrolled G1/S-phase progression and silencing G0/G1 [99]. At a molecular level, MACC1 is believed to achieve this through the PI3K/AKT and β-catenin pathways which in turn cause the expression of genes such as cyclin B, D1, D2, E, c-MYC, and SPON2, all of which are involved in the regulation of certain points of the cell cycle such as initiation, G1/S-phase transition, and apoptosis [94, 99]. MACC1 may also disrupt the cell cycle through the well-documented tumor suppressor gene PTEN [42].

16.3.3.4 Evading Cell Death

MACC1 may further cause metastasis in CRC cells through its ability to evade apoptosis. MACC1 functions simultaneously with the expression of anti-apoptotic proteins BCL2 and MCL1 and the downregulation of apoptosis-inducing proteins BAX and BAD [94]. Pro-survival-based signaling is one method by which MACC1 circumvents cell death. MACC1, using the PI3K/AKT signaling, goes on to increase

BCL2, BAX, BAD, and caspase 3 expressions while downregulating MCL1 through the STAT1/3 signaling pathway [103, 104]. Resistance to apoptosis in CRC cells may also be caused as a result of the Warburg effect which upregulates glycolytic enzymes, increases ATP generation, reduces reactive oxygen species, and stabilizes mitochondrial membrane potential [96].

16.3.3.5 Immune Destruction and Inflammation

The first clue that MACC1 was simultaneously involved in metastasis and immune escape was gained by the associated downplay of FAS and upward expression of MCL1 through STAT1/3 [89]. MACC1 has also been shown to ward off immune attacks by activating TIMP1/2 and through the association with the latter, tumor-associated macrophages (TAMs) [105]. TAMs are notorious for establishing tumor-supporting microenvironments by secreting cytokines IL1, IL6, TNF-α, and TGF-β, which allow the tumors to evade T-cell-mediated tumor destruction [106]. MACC1 may also promote metastasis through the Toll-like receptor 9 (TLR9) pathway, particularly in the cell-free DNA of tumors. TRL families have previously been established to play critical roles in activating innate immunity and causing colonic inflammation [107]. Utilizing its ability to cause inflammation, MACC1 may cause conventional colitis-associated cancer (CAC) and further drive inflammatory bowel disease-associated colitis to dysplasia and consequent carcinomas [108]. The two death domains (DD) in the MACC1 C-terminus are likely to be involved in the mediation of inflammation in its targets [23].

16.3.3.6 Causing Genomic Instability

One mechanism by which cancer cells develop, transform, and continue their metastatic progression is through their correlated genome instability [100]. Markers of genome instability such as mismatch repair (MMR) have been found to be associated with MACC1 and even help predict and chart the response of CRC patients to 5-FU-based chemotherapy [73]. To date, several research endeavors have positively linked phenomenon such as copy number variations (CNVs) and SNPs to lesion size, number of metastases routes, and vascularization of CRC tumors [43]. Genomic instability may also cause allelic losses and inactivation of biomolecules such as APC, p53, Smad 2/4, and TGF-RII that function as tumor suppressors [20]. Interesting to note are the results from a study which showed that in their experimental cohort, 85% of APC in the colon tumor cells were mutated [82]. Molecules apart from APC which are central to the Wnt pathway and susceptible to mutation due to the effects of MACC1 are β-catenin, cyclin D1, S100A4, and MMP7 [83]. MACC1 has also been confirmed to have ties with KRAS G12 and KRAS G13 which undergo point mutations in their exon 2's codons 12 and 13, respectively. KRAS G12 and 13 have both been heavily implicated in metachronous metastases development [109].

16.3.3.7 Inducing Angiogenesis

The expression of VEGF-A under the influence of MACC1 upregulates TWIST and causes subsequent vasculogenesis and endothelium-dependent tumor angiogenesis [45]. Interestingly, MACC1 may also carry out vasculogenic mimicry which in turn leads to endothelium-independent angiogenesis. This "mimicry," done via the expression of VE-cadherin and TWIST, is essentially a process whereby tumor cells develop endothelial-like vasculature and use this to maintain blood supply [93]. VEGF signaling, under the direction of MACC1, also performs lymphogenesis and therefore promotes metastasis via lymphatic vessels [42].

16.3.3.8 Manipulating Cellular Energetics

The Warburg effect which has been well documented in MACC1 achieves the former through the upregulation of glycolytic enzymes such as hexokinase (HK2), pyruvate dehydrogenase (PDH) kinase, and lactate dehydrogenase (LDH) [42]. It has been found that MACC1 thrives under glucose deprivation and metabolic stress, developing phenotypes such as increased viability and apoptosis resistance as a result. MACC1 responds positively to the Warburg effect which also results in a resistance to trastuzumab. MACC1 maintains these conditions through the activation of the PI3K/AKT signaling [110]. Additionally, metabolic stress may increase the level of lncRNA MACC1-AS1 which enables metabolic plasticity and poor patient outcomes [42, 111].

16.3.3.9 Allowing Cancer Stemness and Immortality

Stem cell markers OCT4 and NANOG have been shown to work synergistically with MACC1 to promote stemness and immortality in cancer cells [92]. This is achieved through the Wnt signaling by the MACC1/PI3K/AKT/GSK3βaxis which stabilizes β-catenin that interacts with hTERT to facilitate nuclear retention and target gene expression [42, 94, 112]. In an investigation carried out by Merlos-Sua'rez and colleagues, the probability of CRC recurrence was directly linked to the expression of certain genes, one of which was MACC1 [113] (Fig. 16.4).

16.4 Prognostic and Predictive Potential of MACC1

As discussed in the previous sections, MACC1 is involved in various cellular functions that lead to the development, progression, and maintenance of CRC metastasis. Additionally, it is also found to circulate in the patient's body fluids even at the early stages of the disease and can hence be exploited as a possible non-invasive biomarker to predict the risk of metastases [19]. Apart from predictive functions,

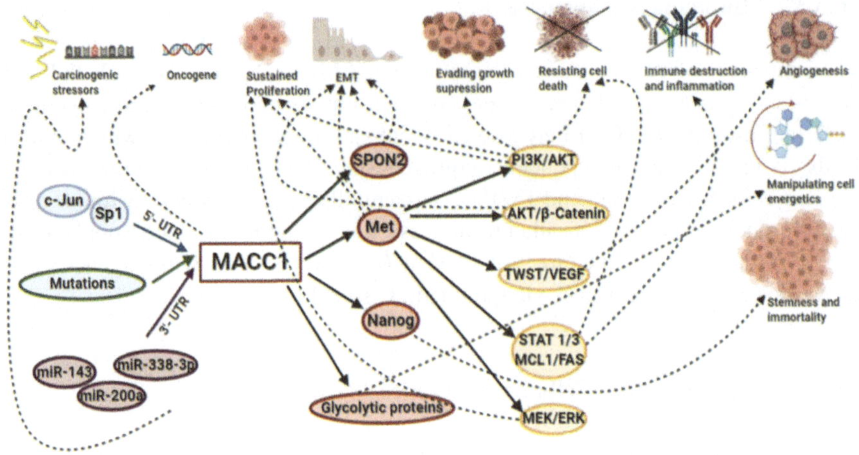

Fig. 16.4 MACC1's effect on the various stages of metastasis: MACC1, through its associated pathways, brings about metastasis in CRC through sustained proliferation, EMT, immune destruction, angiogenesis, metabolic reprogramming, stemness, etc. As illustrated in the diagram above, the PI3K/AKT pathway, in particular, takes part in several key metastatic events. Please note that the above is only an overview of the MACC1-related genetic influences on CRC metastasis. Many of these pathways may be involved in several of the cascade events. Further, there are many other signaling molecules (mentioned in the sections above) that are involved in this process but haven't been mentioned in the diagram above. (Image created using BioRender and adapted from [42] and [47])

MACC1 may also be used as a prognostic tool to discern the efficacy and response to a particular method of treatment. It can be identified in cells and tissues via qRT-PCR, immunohistochemistry, and ELISA and also be detected in cryo- and formalin-fixed paraffin-embedded samples [19]. Combining MACC1 transcripts with genes like S100A4 has been found to improve prognosis among CRC patients and indicate potential patient outcomes [45]. Detection of elevated levels of HGF in tandem with MACC1 has been reported to predict poor survival chances among patients [114].

MACC1 allows clinicians to evaluate responses to treatment in cases like rectal cancer where it is used as a prognostic marker to determine the efficacy of preoperative chemoradiotherapy [115]. Although MACC1 expression has been noted in a plethora of cancer types, it is particularly robust in indicating the risk of distant metastasis in CRC when compared to liver and lung cancers [17]. Periodic liquid biopsies to screen for high levels of MACC1 can also be used to predict postoperative recurrence [44]. As mentioned previously, MACC1 has now been found to function as an important parameter to ensure the viability and efficacy of chemotherapeutic treatment using the medication 5-fluorouracil (5-FU) in CRC patients [42, 116]. It has also been found to accurately predict when neo-adjuvant chemoradiotherapy for rectal cancer stops yielding results.

Innovative approaches using a combination of techniques to study MACC1 expression and structure along with its associated SNPs, CNVs, PTMs, and miRNAs may help drastically help in the development of panels to accurately and precisely predict the percentage risk of development and/or the stage of cancer in patients with CRC.

16.5 Impact of MACC1 on Therapy

Although MACC1 has been established by several studies to have immense potential as a therapeutic target for interventions to treat CRC, a deeper understanding of its unique morphology and cellular mechanisms may help further validate MACC1 as an important lead for drug developers to look at. While MACC1 may help diagnose CRC in its early stages and hence improve patient outcomes, it may also help personalize treatment options [19].

Currently CRC is treated via oxaliplatin, capecitabine, and irinotecan combination; however, the medial survival rate still stands at less than 2 years for stage IV patients [20]. Based on the knowledge of MACC1 pathways, drugs like cetuximab, panitumumab, and bevacizumab which target EGFR (former) and VEGF (latter) have shown promise in improving patient outcomes [20]. Additionally, molecule-based therapies using small interfering molecules (small molecule inhibitors), miRNAs, ribozymes, and antisense oligos remain largely unexplored and may provide several, targeted approaches toward treating CRC patients [67].

Targeting key signaling pathways may also prevent CRC metastasis; some approaches presently working toward this include investigating the potential of decoy-Met, Met-blocking antibodies, and small molecules like SU11274, K252a, and PHA665752, all of which may interfere with the MACC1/Met/HGF axis which is crucial for the progression of metastasis [117]. Additionally, molecules like NK4 may serve to antagonize the HGF ligand and block the associated positive feedback mechanism which perpetuates cell proliferation [117]. Recent advances in screening methods have highlighted the importance of the MACC1 promoter and its potential to serve as a foundation to identify MACC1 inhibitors. High-throughput screening and the resulting study of the MACC1 promoter and possible inhibitors have led to the development of rottlerin and lovastatin, both of which reduce MACC1 expression and consequently obstruct tumor growth, invasion, and migration in in vivo settings [118].

The current therapeutic options based around MACC1 in CRC treatment have been met with a considerable amount of success. However, to fully tap into the potential of MACC1 toward aiding CRC patients, more large-scale research studying its accuracy toward predicting metastasis need to be undertaken across different ethnicities. Further investigations into its cellular mode of operation may open up yet more doors toward understanding the exact molecular routes by which CRC cells develop and metastasize. This would then also provide more opportunities to develop treatment plans conscious of the underlying driving forces that cause this disease.

16.6 Conclusion

The development of metastasis in colorectal cancer is linked to 90% of patient mortality. Understanding the genetic mechanisms behind this disease and developing innovative therapies based on this knowledge may help significantly improve patient outcomes for this cancer type. MACC1 has emerged as a promising candidate in this endeavor. As was discussed in this chapter, MACC1 and its associated signal pathways such as Met, β-catenin, SPON2, etc. are heavily involved in processes such as cancer cell division, invasion, migration, angiogenesis, immune destruction, etc. Additionally, SNPs and miRNAs related to MACC1 have also been observed to play a critical role in the expression of this gene and the consequent development of metastasis.

The high mortality rate associated with CRC can be reduced by new, targeted molecular therapies. MACC1 can not only predict the chances of metastasis in early-stage CRC patients but can also be used to gauge the response to a particular treatment option. MACC1 has hence proven to be of immense potential both as a therapeutic target and as a lead in further studies, research, and understanding related to the cellular mechanisms of colorectal cancer.

Acknowledgments This work would not be possible without the support from the staff of the Department of Biotechnology and the School of Bio and Chemical Engineering of Sathyabama Institute of Science and Technology. Additionally, the authors take this opportunity to extend their thanks to the management of the institute and its patrons.

Funding This paper received no specific grant from any funding agency in the public, commercial, or not-for-profit sectors.

Conflict of Interests The authors declare no conflict of interest.

References

1. Bray F, Ferlay J, Soerjomataram I, Siegel R, Torre L, Jemal A. Global cancer statistics 2018: GLOBOCAN estimates of incidence and mortality worldwide for 36 cancers in 185 countries. CA Cancer J Clin. 2018;68(6):394–424.
2. Bosman FT. Chapter 5.5: Colorectal cancer. In: Stewart BW, Wild CP, editors. World cancer report. Lyon, France: The International Agency for Research on Cancer, World Health Organization; 2014. p. 392–402. ISBN 978-92-832-0443-5.
3. Juul JS, Hornung N, Andersen B, Laurberg S, Olesen F, Vedsted P. The value of using the faecal immunochemical test in general practice on patients presenting with non-alarm symptoms of colorectal cancer. Br J Cancer. 2018;119(4):471–9.
4. Theodoratou E, Timofeeva M, Li X, Meng X, Ioannidis JP. Nature, nurture, and cancer risks: genetic and nutritional contributions to cancer. Annu Rev Nutr. 2017;37:293–320.
5. Juhn E, Khachemoune A. Gardner Syndrome. Am J Clin Dermatol. 2010;11(2):117–22.
6. Watson AJ, Collins PD. Colon cancer: a civilization disorder. Dig Dis. 2011;29(2):222–8.

7. David C, Wendy A, Heinz-Josef L, Lynch HT, Minsky B r, Nordlinger B, Starling N. Colorectal cancer. Lancet. 2010;375(9719):1030–47.
8. Ionov Y, Peinado MA, Malkhosyan S, Shibata D, Perucho M. Ubiquitous somatic mutations in simple repeated sequences reveal a new mechanism for colonic carcinogenesis. Nature. 1993;363(6429):558–61.
9. Chakravarthi S, Krishnan B, Madhavan M. Apoptosis and expression of p53 in colorectal neoplasms. Indian J Med Res. 1999;86(7):95–102.
10. Khalek FJA, Gallicano GI, Mishra L. Colon cancer stem cells. Gastrointest Cancer Res: GCR. 2010;(Suppl 1):S16.
11. Markowitz SD, Bertagnolli MM. Molecular basis of colorectal cancer molecular origins of cancer. N Engl J Med. 2009;361(25):2449.
12. Mehlen P, Fearon ER. Role of the dependence receptor DCC in colorectal cancer pathogenesis. J Clin Oncol. 2004;22(16):3420–8.
13. Cancer Genome Atlas Network. Comprehensive molecular characterization of human colon and rectal cancer. Nature. 2012;487(7407):330–7.
14. Ryan E, Sheahan K, Creavin B, Mohan HM, Winter DC. The current value of determining the mismatch repair status of colorectal cancer: a rationale for routine testing. Crit Rev Oncol Hematol. 2017;116:38–57.
15. Schnekenburger M, Diederich M. Epigenetics offer new horizons for colorectal cancer prevention. Curr Color Cancer Rep. 2012;8(1):66–81.
16. Lao VV, Grady WM. Epigenetics and colorectal cancer. Nat Rev Gastroenterol Hepatol. 2011;8(12):686–700.
17. Stein U, Walther W, Arlt F, Schwabe H, Smith J, Fichtner I, et al. MACC1, a newly identified key regulator of HGF-MET signaling, predicts colon cancer metastasis. Nat Med. 2009;15(1):59–67.
18. Grady WM, Markowitz SD. The molecular pathogenesis of colorectal cancer and its potential application to colorectal cancer screening. Dig Dis Sci. 2015;60(3):762–72.
19. Stein U. MACC1–a novel target for solid cancers. Expert Opin Ther Targets. 2013;17(9):1039–52.
20. Arlt F, Stein U. Colon cancer metastasis: MACC1 and Met as metastatic pacemakers. Int J Biochem Cell Biol. 2009;41(12):2356–9.
21. Stein U, Schlag PM. Clinical, biological, and molecular aspects of metastasis in colorectal cancer. Recent Results Cancer Res. 2007;176:61–80.
22. Christofori G. New signals from the invasive front. Nature. 2006;441(7092):444–50.
23. Stein U, Dahlmann M, Walther W. MACC1—more than metastasis? Facts and predictions about a novel gene. J Mol Med. 2010;88(1):11–8.
24. Aragane H, Sakakura C, Nakanishi M, Yasuoka R, Fujita Y, Taniguchi H, et al. Chromosomal aberrations in colorectal cancers and liver metastases analyzed by comparative genomic hybridization. Int J Cancer. 2001;94(5):623–9.
25. Yang J, Mani SA, Weinberg RA. Exploring a new twist on tumor metastasis. Cancer Res. 2006;66(9):4549–52.
26. Paschos KA, Canovas D, Bird NC. The role of cell adhesion molecules in the progression of colorectal cancer and the development of liver metastasis. Cell Signal. 2009;21(5):665–74.
27. Zhang RT, Ren F, Shi HR. Expression of metastasis-associated in colon cancer-1 in different stages of epithelial ovarian cancer. Zhongguo yi xue ke xue Yuan xue bao. Acta Acad Med Sinicae. 2014;36(1):47–51.
28. Jin Z, Xu N, Guo K, Xu P, Li P, Zhang Y, et al. Increased expression of metastasis-associated in colon cancer-1 in renal cell carcinoma is associated with poor prognosis. Int J Clin Exp Pathol. 2015;8(4):3857.
29. Shimokawa H, Uramoto H, Onitsuka T, So T, Ono K, So T, et al. Macc1 amplification predicts postoperative recurrence in lung adenocarcinoma. Ann Oncol. 2010;21:24–5.
30. Huang Y, Zhang H, Cai J, Fang L, Wu J, Ye C, et al. Overexpression of MACC1 and its significance in human breast cancer progression. Cell Biosci. 2013;3(1):16.

31. Wang Y, Hong Q, Wang J, Fang Y, Hu C. Downregulated expression of metastasis associated in colon cancer 1 (MACC1) reduces gallbladder cancer cell proliferation and invasion. Tumor Biol. 2014;35(4):3771–8.
32. Zhang K, Zhang Y, Zhu H, Xue N, Liu J, Shan C, Zhu Q. High expression of MACC1 predicts poor prognosis in patients with osteosarcoma. Tumor Biol. 2014;35(2):1343–50.
33. Qiu J, Huang P, Liu Q, Hong J, Li B, Lu C, et al. Identification of MACC1 as a novel prognostic marker in hepatocellular carcinoma. J Transl Med. 2011;9(1):166.
34. Ge SH, Wu XJ, Wang XH, Xing XF, Zhang LH, Zhu YB, et al. Over-expression of metastasis-associated in colon cancer-1 (MACC1) associates with better prognosis of gastric cancer patients. Chin J Cancer Res. 2011;23(2):153–9.
35. Zhu M, Xu Y, Mao X, Gao Y, Shao L, Yan F. Overexpression of metastasis-associated in colon cancer-1 associated with poor prognosis in patients with esophageal cancer. Pathol Oncol Res. 2013;19(4):749–53.
36. Li HF, Liu YQ, Shen ZJ, Gan XF, Han JJ, Liu YY, et al. Downregulation of MACC1 inhibits invasion, migration and proliferation, attenuates cisplatin resistance and induces apoptosis in tongue squamous cell carcinoma. Oncol Rep. 2015;33(2):651–60.
37. Yang T, Kong B, Kuang YQ, Cheng L, Gu JW, Zhang JH, et al. Overexpression of MACC1 protein and its clinical implications in patients with glioma. Tumor Biol. 2014;35(1):815–9.
38. Wang G, Kang MX, Lu WJ, Chen Y, Zhang B, Wu YL. MACC1: a potential molecule associated with pancreatic cancer metastasis and chemoresistance. Oncol Lett. 2012;4(4):783–91.
39. Meng F, Li H, Shi H, Yang Q, Zhang F, Yang Y, et al. MACC1 down-regulation inhibits proliferation and tumourigenicity of nasopharyngeal carcinoma cells through Akt/β-catenin signaling pathway. PLoS One. 2013;8(4):e60821.
40. Li H, Liao X, Liu Y, Shen Z, Gan X, Li H, Huang Z. The expression of MACC 1 and its role in the proliferation and apoptosis of salivary adenoid cystic carcinoma. J Oral Pathol Med. 2015;44(10):810–7.
41. Lederer A, Herrmann P, Seehofer D, Dietel M, Pratschke J, Schlag P, Stein U. Metastasis-associated in colon cancer 1 is an independent prognostic biomarker for survival in klatskin tumor patients. Hepatology. 2015;62(3):841–50.
42. Radhakrishnan H, Walther W, Zincke F, Kobelt D, Imbastari F, Erdem M, et al. MACC1—the first decade of a key metastasis molecule from gene discovery to clinical translation. Cancer Metastasis Rev. 2018;37(4):805–20.
43. Galimi F, Torti D, Sassi F, Isella C, Corà D, Gastaldi S, et al. Genetic and expression analysis of MET, MACC1, and HGF in metastatic colorectal cancer: response to met inhibition in patient xenografts and pathologic correlations. Clin Cancer Res. 2011;17(10):3146–56.
44. Isella C, Mellano A, Galimi F, Petti C, Capussotti L, De Simone M, et al. MACC1 mRNA levels predict cancer recurrence after resection of colorectal cancer liver metastases. Ann Surg. 2013;257(6):1089–95.
45. Stein U, Burock S, Herrmann P, Wendler I, Niederstrasser M, Wernecke KD, Schlag PM. Circulating MACC1 transcripts in colorectal cancer patient plasma predict metastasis and prognosis. PLoS One. 2012;7(11):e49249.
46. Juneja M, Ilm K, Schlag PM, Stein U. Promoter identification and transcriptional regulation of the metastasis gene MACC1 in colorectal cancer. Mol Oncol. 2013;7(5):929–43.
47. Li H, Chen YX, Wen JG, Zhou HH. Metastasis-associated in colon cancer 1: a promising biomarker for the metastasis and prognosis of colorectal cancer. Oncol Lett. 2017;14(4):3899–908.
48. Raghav KPS, Eng C. Role of the MET–HGF axis in colorectal cancer: precepts and prospects. Color Cancer. 2012;1(4):329–41.
49. Stein U, Smith J, Walther W, Arlt F. MACC1 controls Met: what a difference an Sp1 site makes. Cell Cycle. 2009;8(15):2467–9.
50. Schmid F, Wang Q, Huska M, Andrade M, Fichtner I, Schlag PM, Stein U. 211 SPON2, a newly identified transcriptional target gene of MACC1, is associated with colorectal cancer metastasis. Eur J Cancer. 2012;48:63–4.

51. Schmid F, Wang Q, Huska MR, Andrade-Navarro MA, Lemm M, Fichtner I, et al. S100P, a target gene of MACC1, contributes to colorectal cancer metastasis. Cancer Res. 2013;73:416.
52. Shang C, Hong Y, Guo Y, Liu YH, Xue YX. Influence of the MACC1 gene on sensitivity to chemotherapy in human U251 glioblastoma cells. Asian Pac J Cancer Prev. 2015;16(1):195–9.
53. Gao Y, Liu Z, Zhang X, He J, Pan Y, Hao F, et al. Inhibition of cytoplasmic GSK-3β increases cisplatin resistance through activation of Wnt/β-catenin signaling in A549/DDP cells. Cancer Lett. 2013;336(1):231–9.
54. Wang L, Lin L, Chen X, Sun L, Liao Y, Huang N, Liao W. Metastasis-associated in colon cancer-1 promotes vasculogenic mimicry in gastric cancer by upregulating TWIST1/2. Oncotarget. 2015;6(13):11492.
55. Kim YH, Kim G, Kwon CI, Kim JW, Park PW, Hahm KB. TWIST1 and SNAI1 as markers of poor prognosis in human colorectal cancer are associated with the expression of ALDH1 and TGF-β1. Oncol Rep. 2014;31(3):1380–8.
56. Yu H, Jin GZ, Liu K, Dong H, Yu H, Duan JC, et al. Twist2 is a valuable prognostic biomarker for colorectal cancer. World J Gastroenterol: WJG. 2013;19(15):2404.
57. Tokarz P, Blasiak J. The role of microRNA in metastatic colorectal cancer and its significance in cancer prognosis and treatment. Acta Biochim Pol. 2012;59(4):467–74.
58. Migliore C, Martin V, Leoni VP, Restivo A, Atzori L, Petrelli A, et al. MiR-1 downregulation cooperates with MACC1 in promoting MET overexpression in human colon cancer. Clin Cancer Res. 2012;18(3):737–47.
59. Zhang Y, Wang Z, Chen M, Peng L, Wang X, Ma Q, et al. MicroRNA-143 targets MACC1 to inhibit cell invasion and migration in colorectal cancer. Mol Cancer. 2012;11(1):23.
60. Chen J, Wang MB. The roles of miRNA-143 in colon cancer and therapeutic implications. Transl Gastrointest Cancer. 2012;1(2):169–74.
61. Hurst DR, Edmonds MD, Welch DR. Metastamir: the field of metastasis-regulatory microRNA is spreading. Cancer Res. 2009;69(19):7495–8.
62. Huang N, Wu Z, Lin L, Zhou M, Wang L, Ma H, et al. MiR-338-3p inhibits epithelial-mesenchymal transition in gastric cancer cells by targeting ZEB2 and MACC1/Met/Akt signaling. Oncotarget. 2015;6(17):15222.
63. Feng J, Wang J, Chen M, Chen G, Wu Z, Ying L, et al. miR-200a suppresses cell growth and migration by targeting MACC1 and predicts prognosis in hepatocellular carcinoma. Oncol Rep. 2015;33(2):713–20.
64. Chen Z, He X, Xia W, Huang Q, Zhang Z, Ye J, et al. Prognostic value and clinicopathological differences of HIFs in colorectal cancer: evidence from meta-analysis. PLoS One. 2013;8(12):e80337.
65. Wang C, Fan HQ, Zhang YW. MiR-511-5p functions as a tumor suppressor and a predictive of prognosis in colorectal cancer by directly targeting GPR116. Eur Rev Med Pharmacol Sci. 2019;23(14):6119–30.
66. Niu ZY, Li WL, Jiang DL, Li YS, Xie XJ. Mir-483 inhibits colon cancer cell proliferation and migration by targeting TRAF1. Kaohsiung J Med Sci. 2018;34(9):479–86.
67. Ilm K, Fuchs S, Mudduluru G, Stein U. MACC1 is post-transcriptionally regulated by miR-218 in colorectal cancer. Oncotarget. 2016;7(33):53443.
68. Kokoszyńska K, Kryński J, Rychlewski L, Wyrwicz LS. Unexpected domain composition of MACC1 links MET signaling and apoptosis. Acta Biochim Pol. 2009;56(2):317–24.
69. Pichorner A, Sack U, Kobelt D, Kelch I, Arlt F, Smith J, et al. In vivo imaging of colorectal cancer growth and metastasis by targeting MACC1 with shRNA in xenografted mice. Clin Exp Metastasis. 2012;29(6):573–83.
70. Reed JC, Doctor KS, Godzik A. The domains of apoptosis: a genomics perspective. Sci Signal. 2004;2004(239):re9.
71. Lang A, Geller-Rhomberg S, Winder T, Hartmann BL, Gasser K, Kohler B, et al. Evaluation of the association between tagging polymorphisms of the MACC1 locus and overall survival in patients with colorectal cancer. J Clin Oncol. 2011;29(15_suppl):3594.

72. Schmid F, Burock S, Klockmeier K, Schlag PM, Stein U. SNPs in the coding region of the metastasis-inducing gene MACC1 and clinical outcome in colorectal cancer. Mol Cancer. 2012;11(1):49.
73. Rohr UP, Herrmann P, Ilm K, Zhang H, Lohmann S, Reiser A, et al. Prognostic value of MACC1 and proficient mismatch repair status for recurrence risk prediction in stage II colon cancer patients: the BIOGRID studies. Ann Oncol. 2017;28(8):1869–75.
74. Fidler IJ. The pathogenesis of cancer metastasis: the 'seed and soil' hypothesis revisited. Nat Rev Cancer. 2003;3(6):453–8.
75. Steeg PS. Tumor metastasis: mechanistic insights and clinical challenges. Nat Med. 2006;12(8):895–904.
76. Chambers AF, Groom AC, MacDonald IC. Dissemination and growth of cancer cells in metastatic sites. Nat Rev Cancer. 2002;2(8):563–72.
77. Weinberg RA, Hanahan D. The hallmarks of cancer. Cell. 2000;100(1):57–70.
78. Shay JW, Wright WE. Hayflick, his limit, and cellular ageing. Nat Rev Mol Cell Biol. 2000;1(1):72–6.
79. Blasco MA. Telomeres and human disease: ageing, cancer and beyond. Nat Rev Genet. 2005;6(8):611–22.
80. O'Connell JB, Maggard MA, Ko CY. Colon cancer survival rates with the new American Joint Committee on Cancer sixth edition staging. J Natl Cancer Inst. 2004;96(19):1420–5.
81. Fearon ER, Vogelstein B. A genetic model for colorectal tumorigenesis. Cell. 1990;61(5):759–67.
82. Fodde R, Smits R, Clevers H. APC, signal transduction and genetic instability in colorectal cancer. Nat Rev Cancer. 2001;1(1):55–67.
83. Blume-Jensen P, Hunter T. Oncogenic kinase signalling. Nature. 2001;411(6835):355–65.
84. Baylin SB, Ohm JE. Epigenetic gene silencing in cancer–a mechanism for early oncogenic pathway addiction? Nat Rev Cancer. 2006;6(2):107–16.
85. Suzuki H, Watkins DN, Jair KW, Schuebel KE, Markowitz SD, Chen WD, et al. Epigenetic inactivation of SFRP genes allows constitutive WNT signaling in colorectal cancer. Nat Genet. 2004;36(4):417–22.
86. Gavert N, Ben-Ze'ev A. Epithelial–mesenchymal transition and the invasive potential of tumors. Trends Mol Med. 2008;14(5):199–209.
87. Sleeman JP, Thiele W. Tumor metastasis and the lymphatic vasculature. Int J Cancer. 2009;125(12):2747–56.
88. Hannen R, Bartsch JW. Essential roles of telomerase reverse transcriptase hTERT in cancer stemness and metastasis. FEBS Lett. 2018;592(12):2023–31.
89. Zhang K, Guo Y, Wang X, Zhao H, Ji Z, Cheng C, et al. WNT/β-catenin directs self-renewal symmetric cell division of hTERT high prostate cancer stem cells. Cancer Res. 2017;77(9):2534–47.
90. Ashktorab H, Hermann P, Nouraie M, Shokrani B, Lee E, Haidary T, et al. Increased MACC1 levels in tissues and blood identify colon adenoma patients at high risk. J Transl Med. 2016;14(1):1–9.
91. Koelzer VH, Herrmann P, Zlobec I, Karamitopoulou E, Lugli A, Stein U. Heterogeneity analysis of metastasis associated in colon cancer 1 (MACC1) for survival prognosis of colorectal cancer patients: a retrospective cohort study. BMC Cancer. 2015;15(1):160.
92. Lemos C, Hardt MS, Juneja M, Voss C, Förster S, Jerchow B, et al. MACC1 induces tumor progression in transgenic mice and colorectal cancer patients via increased pluripotency markers Nanog and Oct4. Clin Cancer Res. 2016;22(11):2812–24.
93. Wang L, Zhou R, Zhao Y, Dong S, Zhang J, Luo Y, et al. MACC-1 promotes endothelium-dependent angiogenesis in gastric cancer by activating TWIST1/VEGF-A signal pathway. PLoS One. 2016;11(6):e0157137.
94. Zhen T, Dai S, Li H, Yang Y, Kang L, Shi H, et al. MACC1 promotes carcinogenesis of colorectal cancer via β-catenin signaling pathway. Oncotarget. 2014;5(11):3756.

95. Gonzalez DM, Medici D. Signaling mechanisms of the epithelial-mesenchymal transition. Sci Signal. 2014;7(344):re8.
96. Kopczyńska EK. The potential therapeutic applications and prognostic significance of metastasis-associated in colon cancer-1 (MACC1) in cancers. Contemp Oncol. 2016;20(4):273.
97. Birchmeier C, Birchmeier W, Gherardi E, Woude GFV. Met, metastasis, motility and more. Nat Rev Mol Cell Biol. 2003;4(12):915–25.
98. Zhang W, Liu HT. MAPK signal pathways in the regulation of cell proliferation in mammalian cells. Cell Res. 2002;12(1):9–18.
99. Zhang K, Tian F, Zhang Y, Zhu Q, Xue N, Zhu H, et al. MACC1 is involved in the regulation of proliferation, colony formation, invasion ability, cell cycle distribution, apoptosis and tumorigenicity by altering Akt signaling pathway in human osteosarcoma. Tumor Biol. 2014;35(3):2537–48.
100. Hanahan D, Weinberg RA. Hallmarks of cancer: the next generation. Cell. 2011;144(5):646–74.
101. Lichtenberger BM, Tan PK, Niederleithner H, Ferrara N, Petzelbauer P, Sibilia M. Autocrine VEGF signaling synergizes with EGFR in tumor cells to promote epithelial cancer development. Cell. 2010;140(2):268–79.
102. Giordano S, Corso S, Conrotto P, Artigiani S, Gilestro G, Barberis D, et al. The semaphorin 4D receptor controls invasive growth by coupling with Met. Nat Cell Biol. 2002;4(9):720–4.
103. Radhakrishnan H, Ilm K, Walther W, Shirasawa S, Sasazuki T, Daniel PT, et al. MACC1 regulates Fas mediated apoptosis through STAT1/3–Mcl-1 signaling in solid cancers. Cancer Lett. 2017;403:231–45.
104. Yao Y, Dou C, Lu Z, Zheng X, Liu Q. MACC1 suppresses cell apoptosis in hepatocellular carcinoma by targeting the HGF/c-MET/AKT pathway. Cell Physiol Biochem. 2015;35(3):983–96.
105. Erreni M, Mantovani A, Allavena P. Tumor-associated macrophages (TAM) and inflammation in colorectal cancer. Cancer Microenviron. 2011;4(2):141–54.
106. Jedinak A, Dudhgaonkar S, Sliva D. Activated macrophages induce metastatic behavior of colon cancer cells. Immunobiology. 2010;215(3):242–9.
107. Fűri I, Sipos F, Germann TM, Kalmár A, Tulassay Z, Molnár B, Műzes G. Epithelial toll-like receptor 9 signaling in colorectal inflammation and cancer: clinico-pathogenic aspects. World J Gastroenterol: WJG. 2013;19(26):4119.
108. Harpaz N, Taboada S, Mabel Ko H, Yu J, Yang Q, Xu H, Cao W. Expression of MACC1 and MET in inflammatory bowel disease-associated colonic neoplasia. Inflamm Bowel Dis. 2014;20(4):703–11.
109. Ilm K, Kemmner W, Osterland M, Burock S, Koch G, Herrmann P, et al. High MACC1 expression in combination with mutated KRAS G13 indicates poor survival of colorectal cancer patients. Mol Cancer. 2015;14(1):38.
110. Liu J, Pan C, Guo L, Wu M, Guo J, Peng S, et al. A new mechanism of trastuzumab resistance in gastric cancer: MACC1 promotes the Warburg effect via activation of the PI3K/AKT signaling pathway. J Hematol Oncol. 2016;9(1):1–15.
111. Zhao Y, Liu Y, Lin L, Huang Q, He W, Zhang S, et al. The lncRNA MACC1-AS1 promotes gastric cancer cell metabolic plasticity via AMPK/Lin28 mediated mRNA stability of MACC1. Mol Cancer. 2018;17(1):69.
112. Park JI, Venteicher AS, Hong JY, Choi J, Jun S, Shkreli M, et al. Telomerase modulates Wnt signalling by association with target gene chromatin. Nature. 2009;460(7251):66–72.
113. Merlos-Suárez A, Barriga FM, Jung P, Iglesias M, Céspedes MV, Rossell D, et al. The intestinal stem cell signature identifies colorectal cancer stem cells and predicts disease relapse. Cell Stem Cell. 2011;8(5):511–24.
114. Toiyama Y, Miki C, Inoue Y, Okugawa Y, Tanaka K, Kusunoki M. Serum hepatocyte growth factor as a prognostic marker for stage II or III colorectal cancer patients. Int J Cancer. 2009;125(7):1657–62.

115. Kawamura M, Saigusa S, Toiyama Y, Tanaka K, Okugawa Y, Hiro J, et al. Correlation of MACC1 and MET expression in rectal cancer after neoadjuvant chemoradiotherapy. Anticancer Res. 2012;32(4):1527–31.
116. Wang J, Wang W, Cai H, Du B, Zhang L, Ma W, et al. MACC1 facilitates chemoresistance and cancer stem cell-like properties of colon cancer cells through the PI3K/AKT signaling pathway. Mol Med Rep. 2017;16(6):8747–54.
117. Corso S, Comoglio PM, Giordano S. Cancer therapy: can the challenge be MET? Trends Mol Med. 2005;11(6):284–92.
118. Juneja M, Kobelt D, Walther W, Voss C, Smith J, Specker E, et al. Statin and rottlerin small-molecule inhibitors restrict colon cancer progression and metastasis via MACC1. PLoS Biol. 2017;15(6):e2000784.

Index

G. P. Nagaraju et al. (eds.), *Colon Cancer Diagnosis and Therapy*, https://doi.org/10.1007/978-3-030-63369-1

B

E

F

G

N

O

P

R

The manufacturer's authorised representative in the EU is Springer Nature Customer Service Centre GmbH, Europaplatz 3, 69115 Heidelberg, Germany. If you have any concerns regarding our products, please contact ProductSafety@springernature.com

Printed and bound by CPI Group (UK) Ltd, Croydon, CR0 4YY

30/09/2026

02225288-0009